Thrombosis and Antithrombotic Therapy

GILLES LUGASSY MD
ASSOCIATE PROFESSOR OF HEMATOLOGY
AND CHIEF, INSTITUTE OF HEMATOLOGY
THE BARZILAI MEDICAL CENTER
ASHKELON
ISRAEL

BENJAMIN BRENNER MD
ASSOCIATE PROFESSOR OF HEMATOLOGY
AND DIRECTOR
THROMBOSIS AND HEMOSTASIS UNIT
INSTITUTE OF HEMATOLOGY
RAMBAM MEDICAL CENTER
HAIFA
ISRAEL

MEYER MICHEL SAMAMA MD
PROFESSOR
SERVICE D'HÉMATOLOGIE BIOLOGIQUE
HOTEL DIEU
PARIS
FRANCE

SAM SCHULMAN MD
ASSOCIATE PROFESSOR
COAGULATION UNIT
DEPARTMENT OF MEDICINE
KAROLINSKA HOSPITAL
STOCKHOLM
SWEDEN

MARC COHEN MD
PROFESSOR OF MEDICINE AND CHIEF
DIVISION OF CARDIOLOGY
MCP HAHNEMANN UNIVERSITY
SCHOOL OF MEDICINE
ALLEGHENY UNIVERSITY OF THE HEALTH
SCIENCES
PHILADELPHIA PA
USA

MARTIN DUNITZ

© Martin Dunitz Ltd 2000

First published in the United Kingdom in 2000 by
Martin Dunitz Ltd
The Livery House
7–9 Pratt Street
London NW1 0AE

Tel: +44-(0)20-7482-2202
Fax: +44-(0)20-7267-0159
E-mail: info@mdunitz.globalnet.co.uk
Website: http://www.dunitz.co.uk

A CIP catalogue record for this book is available from the British Library

ISBN 1-85317-775-X

Distributed in the United States by:
Blackwell Science Inc.
Commerce Place, 350 Main Street
Malden MA 02148, USA
Tel: 1-800-215-1000

Distributed in Canada by:
Login Brothers Book Company
324 Salteaux Crescent
Winnipeg, Manitoba R3J 3T2
Canada
Tel: 1-204-224-4068

Distributed in Brazil by:
Ernesto Reichmann Distribuidora de Livros, Ltda
Rua Coronel Marques 335, Tatuape 03440-000
Sao Paulo,
Brazil

Composition by Wearset, Boldon, Tyne and Wear
Printed and bound in Italy by Printer Trento

Contents

Contributors

Benjamin Brenner MD
Associate Professor of Hematology and Director, Thrombosis
and Hemostasis Unit, Institute of Hematology, Rambam
Medical Center, Haifa, Israel.

Marc Cohen MD
Professor of Medicine and Chief, Division of Cardiology,
MCP Hahnemann University School of Medicine, Allegheny
University of the Health Sciences, Philadelphia PA, USA.

Pierre Desnoyers MD
Service d'Hématologie Biologique, Hotel Dieu. Paris, France.

Grigoris T Gerotziafas MD
Service d'Hématologie Biologique, Hotel Dieu, Paris, France.

Gilles Lugassy MD
Associate Professor of Hematology and Chief, Institute of
Hematology, The Barzilai Medical Center, Ashkelon, Israel.

André Planes MD
Chief, Department of Orthopedic Surgery, La Rochelle, France.

Meyer Michel Samama MD
Professor, Service d'Hématologie Biologique,
Hotel Dieu, Paris, France.

Sam Schulman MD
Associate Professor, Coagulation Unit,
Department of Medicine, Karolinska
Hospital, Stockholm, Sweden.

Preface

Venous and arterial thrombosis are major causes of morbidity and mortality in the western world. The last decade of the 20th century has witnessed impressive developments in the understanding and the management of thrombosis.

Several new syndromes, genetic or acquired, have been described and have joined the already prosperous family of thrombophilia. We now know that the majority of thromboses are in fact due to the presence of one or more thrombophilic syndromes.

Thanks to large, multicentre clinical studies, therapeutic indications for antithrombotic therapy have been established, for ischemic heart disease, deep vein thrombosis, stroke and peripheral arterial disease.

Promising new medications have, and are being developed.

It is the purpose of this book to provide comprehensive and timely coverage of the main advances in thrombosis, its pathogenesis, clinical features, prevention and therapy.

The first five chapters of the book summarize the recent knowledge on the pathogenesis and laboratory diagnosis of thrombosis and thrombophilia, Chapters 6–9 include in-depth pharmacological and clinical studies of heparins, heparinoids, direct thrombin inhibitors, with emphasis on their indications in general surgery and orthopedics.

In Chapters 10–14, the authors review the current approaches to the management of ischemic heart disease, stroke, peripheral arterial disease and venous thrombosis.

The closing chapters address the issues of thrombosis in pregnancy and in cancer patients.

The authors of the 16 chapters are acknowledged specialists in their fields, and leading contributors to large clinical trials in thrombosis and antithrombotic therapy.

We hope that this book will be of interest for general practitioners, internists, cardiologists, hematologists, neurologists, gynecologists and vascular surgeons.

Gilles Lugassy

Hemostasis and thrombosis: physiological and pathological aspects

Benjamin Brenner

Hemostasis is an intricate process that depends on the complex interactions of a number of cells and proteins within the vascular system. Blood cells involved in hemostatic processes include platelets, leukocytes and red cells. Hemostatic proteins include coagulation factors, natural anticoagulants, profibrinolytic and antifibrinolytic proteins.

Primary hemostasis

The interactions of blood cells and proteins with the vessel wall initiate procoagulant processes. The endothelial cells lining arterial and venous vessels prevent interaction between blood constituents and subendothelial and tissue components.[1] Normally, blood constituents do not interact with intact vascular endothelium. A number of mechanisms are responsible for the non-thrombogenic properties of undamaged endothelium. However, the endothelium is active in hemostatic processes through surface expression of proteins involved in platelet adhesion in procoagulants, anticoagulants and fibrinolytic mechanisms as well as in regulation of vascular tone (*Table 1.1*).[1] In the normal situation, platelets drift near the intact endothelial cell layer. Following endothelial damage,

Table 1.1
Endothelial cell protein functions in hemostasis

Protein	Function
von Willebrand factor	Adhesion, coagulation
Tissue factor	Initiation of coagulation
Tissue factor pathway inhibitor	Inhibition of coagulation
Thrombomodulin	Inhibition of coagulation
Protein C receptor	Inhibition of coagulation
Tissue plasminogen activator	Activation of fibrinolysis
Plasminogen activator inhibitor-1	Inhibition of fibrinolysis
Proteoglycans	Inhibition of coagulation
Integrins on endothelium	Adhesion

they rapidly adhere to the subendothelium. Interaction of platelets with the vessel wall is an orderly process that results in the formation of the primary hemostatic plaque, which is composed of platelet aggregates.

The interactions of red cells, leukocytes and platelets are complex and result in an increase in platelet thrombi formation. Platelets adhere to the vessel wall through interactions of platelet surface glycoproteins (GPs) with adhesion proteins (*Table 1.2*).[2] The following GP receptors and adhesion proteins (ligands) promote major platelet vessel wall interactions.

1   GPIb/V/IX with von Willebrand factor (vWF)
2   GPIa/IIa with subendothelial collagen
3   GPIc/IIa with fibronectin and laminin
4   Vitronectin receptor with vitronectin, vWF, fibronectin and thrombospondin
5   GPIIb/IIIa with fibrinogen, vWF, fibronectin, vitronectin and thrombospondin.

Table 1.2
Platelet membrane glycoproteins

Glycoprotein receptor	Ligand	Activity	Deficiency phenotype
GPIb-V-IX	vWF	Adhesion	Bleeding
GPIIb/IIIa	Fibrinogen, vWF	Aggregation	Bleeding
P-Selectin	Sialyl-Le^x	Platelet–leukocyte interactions	Infections
GPIa-IIa	Collagen	Adhesion	Bleeding

Some of the GPs are integrins such as GPIa-IIa (integrin $\alpha_1\beta_1$) or GPIIb/IIIa (integrin αIIb β_3).[3,4] Other GPs are non-integrins such as GPIV (CD36), which promotes adhesion through its ligands, thrombospondin and collagen, and P-selectin (GMP-140; CD62P), which promotes platelet–leukocyte interaction through sialyl-Lewis X.[5] GPs are essential for normal hemostasis as demonstrated by the bleeding disorders that result from inherited or acquired deficiencies of certain GPs. For example, hereditary deficiency of GPIb/IX results in Bernard–Soulier syndrome, a rare bleeding disorder manifested by spontaneous mucocutaneous and post-traumatic bleeding.[6] Similarly, inherited mutations of GPIIb/IIIa result in Glanzmann's thrombasthenia, a relatively severe mucocutaneous bleeding disorder. Acquired deficiency of the GPs may also manifest as bleeding as can be demonstrated in patients with myeloproliferative disorders.[7]

Platelet aggregation is a crucial step in the formation of the primary hemostatic plaque. This is mediated by fibrinogen, a symmetrical structural protein, which serves as the main ligand for platelet GPIIb/IIIa interactions. Normal amount (50 000 copies per platelet) and function of GPIIb/IIIa are essential for platelet aggregation as suggested by the relatively severe bleeding phenotype of Glanzmann's thrombasthenia. This is further illustrated by accumulating evidence that anti-GPIIb/IIIa antibodies are potent therapeutic agents in patients with arterial thrombosis.[8]

Platelet activation takes place through a number of other receptors. These include the platelet thrombin receptor, a seven-transmembrane G protein-coupled molecule with an amino-terminal extracellular domain. Two platelet thrombin receptors have been described: protease activated receptors 1 and 3.[9] Thrombin receptor antagonists are currently utilized in clinical settings to prevent platelet activation. Upon activation, platelets undergo shape change with pseudopodium formation and secretion of platelet granule content into the circulation. Platelet α-granules contain coagulation factors, including factor V, vWF, fibrinogen, factor XI and platelet-derived growth factor. The dense granules secrete among other constituents, ADP, serotonin and calcium. Inherited and acquired deficiencies of platelet granules result in the mild bleeding disorders — grey platelet syndrome and storage pool disease. Therapy with acetylsalicylic acid, which blocks platelet cyclo-oxygenase, results in a phenotype of acquired storage pool.[10]

von Willebrand factor is synthesized within endothelial cells and megakaryocytes. The main sources of plasma vWF are the endothelium (80%) and platelets (20%). Within the endothelium, vWF promoter is synthesized in the endoplasmic reticulum as a pre-pro-vWF dimer, the signal peptide is cleaved within the Golgi apparatus and multimerization takes place in the Weibel–Palade bodies as mature vWF.[11] Mature vWF subunit has a molecular weight of 225 kDa with multimers sized up to 20 000 kDa. vWF is secreted from endothelial cells via two pathways: constitutive secretion and stimulated secretion.[12] Stimulation can be induced by a variety of agents including thrombin, vasopressin, fibrin and histamine.

High molecular weight multimers of vWF are most potent in inducing platelet vessel wall adhesion and platelet aggregation. Mature vWF is complexed to factor VIII in plasma via a number of binding sites.[13] Factor VIII bound to vWF is reserved from cleavage by proteases such as activated protein C. In the absence of vWF, as observed for example in patients with severe von Willebrand disease (vWD) due to deletions in the vWF gene, factor VIII is degraded and a severe bleeding phenotype is manifested.[14] Similarly, mutations in vWF gene at the factor VIII binding sites, vWD-Normandy, will lead to a hemophilia A-like phenotype.[15] Heterozygous deficiency of vWF is associated with a mild bleeding phenotype.[16] Normally, the high molecular weight multimers of vWF are cleaved to smaller fragments by a 200 kDa metalloproteinase. Deficiency of this vWF proteinase results in unusually large vWF multimers, which promote adhesion of platelets to vessel walls and may result in disseminated platelet aggregation. Recently, inherited and acquired deficiency of the vWF proteinase have been reported to be the pathogenic mechanism in familial and sporadic thrombotic thrombocytopenic purpura,[17] a disorder characterized by disseminated platelet aggregation and microangiopathic hemolytic anemia.

Blood coagulation system

The blood coagulation system is a complex system of procoagulant and anticoagulant proteins (*Table 1.3*). Most coagulation factors are synthesized in the hepatocytes except for factor VIII which is synthesized in the endothelial cells of the liver.

Several of the coagulation factors undergo posttranslational modifications within the hepatocytes. The most important modification is carboxylation by γ-glutamyl carboxylase in the presence of vitamin K hydroquinone which serves as a cofactor in the carboxylation of factors II, VII, IX, X, protein C and protein S.[18] The carboxylation of these four procoagulants and two natural anticoagulants, enables the proteins to bind calcium through the γ-carboxyglutamic acid (GLA) residues thereby fostering binding of the carboxylated coagulation factors to platelet surfaces. Deficiency of vitamin K, and oral anticoagulant therapy with warfarin, which inhibits the enzyme reductase that reduces vitamin K epoxide to vitamin K hydroquinone, are the two common acquired mechanisms leading to reduced carboxylation

Table 1.3
Characteristics of coagulation factor deficiencies

Protein characteristics		Inherited deficiency state	
Pathway	**Activity**	**Prevalence**	**Bleeding phenotype**
Intrinsic			
Factor XII	Contact factor	Uncommon	None
Factor XI	Serine protease	Common (Jews)	Mild
Factor IX	Serine protease	Uncommon	Severe
Factor VIII	Cofactor	Uncommon	Severe
Extrinsic			
Tissue factor	Cofactor	Not reported	
Factor VII	Serine protease	Uncommon	Moderate to severe
Common			
Factor X	Serine protease	Rare	Moderate to severe
Factor V	Cofactor	Rare	Moderate to severe
Prothrombin	Serine protease	Rare	Moderate to severe
Fibrinogen	Structural protein	Uncommon	Moderate
Factor XIII	Fibrin network	Rare	Moderate to severe

of coagulation factors.[19] Inherited deficiency of the γ-glutamyl carboxylase resulting from a missense mutation of the enzyme has recently been reported in four siblings with severe bleeding phenotype.[20] Knockout mice models show that deficiency of the enzyme is lethal resulting in fatal in utero bleeding and bone abnormalities mimicking the teratogenic effects of the fetal warfarin syndrome.

Coagulation factors circulate in plasma as zymogens. Upon activation, the catalytic carboxy-terminal domain, which includes serine, histidine and aspartic acid, is exposed, resulting in activation of the zymogen to serine protease. The activated coagulation factor then activates another factor in the coagulation cascade. The classical interpretation of the coagulation system described an intrinsic system based on initiation of contact activation upon exposure of factors XII, XI, kallikrein and high molecular weight kininogen to collagen or negatively charged surfaces. The slow phase of contact activation results in formation of factor XIa, which then rapidly activates factor IX. The tenase complex includes factor IXa, which in the presence of cofactor VIIIa and calcium activates factor X to factor Xa on platelet surfaces. The extrinsic system begins to operate upon injury of vessel walls resulting in tissue factor and factor VII activation of factor X to factor Xa.

The prothrombinase complex then operates in the common coagulation pathway, where factor Xa in the presence of factor Va and calcium activates prothrombin to thrombin on platelet surfaces. Thrombin is an extremely potent serine protease, which rapidly degrades fibrinopeptides A and B from fibrinogen to form fibrin. Thrombin also activates the transglutaminase factor XIII, which ultimately results in cross-linking of the fibrin polymer. In addition, thrombin promotes platelet aggregation and activates factor V, factor VIII and factor XIII thereby enhancing procoagulant mechanisms.

The formation of complexes such as tenase and prothrombinase is essential for rapid coagulation activation on cell surfaces. In fact, the presence of the cofactors VIIIa and Va, calcium and phospholipids increases activation by over 200 000 fold.[21] Fibrinogen is a structural protein that is composed of two symmetric half molecules each consisting of three different polypeptide chains, Aα, Bβ and γ. Fibrinogen is synthesized in the liver, has a high plasma concentration (7 μmol/l) and a half-life of 5 days. Upon thrombin activation, fibrinopeptides A and B are released, a polymerization site is exposed, and polymerization of fibrin monomer is enhanced.

Our current understanding is that the extrinsic pathway is the main pathway for coagulation initiation. Tissue factor and factor VIIa activate factor IX and factor X to form factors IXa and Xa, which then, in the presence of factor VIII, propagate coagulation on platelet surfaces leading to thrombin formation.[22] Thrombin can also activate factor XI to factor XIa, which further activates factor IX thereby increasing thrombin formation.

More recently a cell-based model for coagulation activation has been proposed implying that coagulation initiation takes place on blood monocytes and that amplification and propagation reactions then take place on platelet surfaces.[23] Cell-based coagulation activation also operates in pathological states. For example, tumor cells may express tissue factor as well as cancer procoagulant, a direct activator of factor X, and this may explain the increased thrombotic tendency in cancer patients (see Chapter 16).[24]

Anticoagulant systems

Several major anticoagulant systems operate in order to regulate procoagulant activity (*Table 1.4*). Historically, the first to be elucidated was the antithrombin (AT) system. AT is synthesized in the liver and serves in the circulation as the major serine protease inhibitor. AT complexes to heparin sulphate that is expressed on endothelial cell surfaces and then forms complexes with the serine protease factors IIa, Xa, IXa and XIa.[25] These complexes are inactive and are removed by the liver. The second anticoagulant system includes protein C, protein S and

Table 1.4
Proteins regulating coagulation

Protein	Cofactor	Activity	Deficiency phenotype
Antithrombin	Heparin sulphate Heparin	Serine protease inhibitor	Thrombophilia
Protein C	Thrombomodulin Protein S	Degrades factors V and VIII	Thrombophilia
Tissue factor pathway inhibitor	Tissue factor	Inactivates factors VII and X	Not reported

thrombomodulin. Protein C is activated on endothelial cells by thrombin and by the endothelial cofactor thrombomodulin. Activated protein C (APC), in the presence of protein S, degrades factor V and factor VIII on platelet surfaces.[26] This system is a major anticoagulant system as suggested by inherited and acquired defects of the system components, which result in thrombotic manifestations. APC cleaves factor V at several cleavage sites. Mutations at the cleavage sites on factor V at positions 506 and 306 result in a thrombotic phenotype.[27] In contrast, mutations in factor VIII cleavage sites do not result in a thrombotic phenotype.

Tissue factor pathway inhibitor (TFPI) is the main inhibitor of the extrinsic pathway. TFPI is an endothelium-bound protein that inactivates both factors VIIa and Xa by forming quaternary complexes in the presence of phospholipid surfaces and calcium. That TFPI is essential is reflected by three lines of evidence. First, inherited deficiency of TFPI has not been detected. Second, acquired deficiency is associated with disseminated intravascular coagulation (DIC) in a model of endotoxinemia in primates.[28] Finally, knockout of TFPI in mice is not viable.[29] Following thrombin formation, endothelial cells produce prostacycline and nitric oxide, two potent vasodilators and antiaggregating agents. These are regulatory mechanisms that balance the formation of thromboxane, a potent vasoconstrictor and platelet aggregation agonist by activated platelets.[30]

Fibrinolytic system

Thrombin also induces endothelial cell secretion of tissue plasminogen activator (t-PA) and plasminogen activator inhibitor (PAI-1).[31] These plasminogen activator and inhibitor define, in part, the fibrinolytic response to thrombin formation. t-PA activates fibrin-bound plasminogen into plasmin. Both t-PA and plasminogen bind to fibrin via the first two kringle domains. Plasmin formed at the fibrin clot site degrades fibrin resulting in the formation of crosslinked fibrin degradation products characterized by the presence of D-dimer.[32]

Pathogenesis of venous and arterial thrombi

Abnormalities in blood constituents, blood flow and vessels contribute to thrombus formation. Venous thrombi differ from arterial thrombi in a number of aspects. First, venous thrombi are found in wide, high-capacity vessels compared to the relatively small elastic arterial vessels. Second, flow is slow in venous vessels and may result in stasis, which increases the likelihood of thrombosis. The venous thrombi consist mainly of red cells and fibrin (red thrombi). In contrast, arterial thrombi are formed at high shear and rapid turbulent flow conditions. vWF plays a major role in these conditions resulting in formation of platelet thrombi with fewer red cells and fibrin (white thrombi). Arterial thrombi are formed most commonly in the setting of an atheroma, often on a vulnerable atheroslerotic plaque. Finally, venous thrombi are formed usually in the distal part of the limb and slowly propagate proximally over several days or weeks. In contrast, arterial thrombi are formed

abruptly and result in ischemic symptoms within minutes to hours. An occluding arterial thrombus results in tissue ischemia and if therapy is not initiated, infarct often follows.

References

1. Born GVR, Schwartz CJ (eds). *Vascular Endothelium Physiology, Pathology and Therapeutic Opportunities.* Stuttgart, Germany: Schathauer, 1997: 1–385.

2. Ruggeri ZM. Mechanisms initiating platelet thrombus formation. *Thromb Haemost* 1997; **78**: 611–616.

3. Nurden AT. Human platelet membrane glycoprotein. In: Bloom AL, Forbes CD, Thomas DP, Tuddenham EGD (eds). *Haemostasis and Thrombosis.* Edinburgh: Churchill Livingstone, 1994: 115–165.

4. Ginsberg MH, Frelinger AL, Lam SCT. Analysis of platelet aggregation disorders based on flow cytometric analysis of membrane glycoprotein IIb IIIa with conformation specific monoclonal antibodies. *Blood* 1990; **76**: 2017–2023.

5. Wayne Smith C. Endothelial adhesion molecules and inflammation: in vitro studies on the modulating effects of interleukin-4. In: Born GVR, Schwartz CJ (eds). *Vascular Endothelium Physiology, Pathology and Therapeutic Opportunities.* Stuttgart, Germany: Schathauer, 1997: 141–155.

6. Clemetson KJ. Platelet GPIb–V–IX complex. *Thromb Haemost* 1997; **78**: 344–350.

7. Coller BS, Seligsohn U, Peretz H, Newman PJ. Glanzmann thromboasthenia: new insights from an historical perspective. *Semin Hematol* 1994; **31**: 301–311.

8. Coller BS. GPIIb/IIIa antagonists: pathophysiologic and therapeutic insights from studies of c7E3 Fab. *Thromb Haemost* 1997; **78**: 730–735.

9. Jaimieson GA. Pathophysiology of platelet thrombin receptors. *Thromb Haemost* 1997; **78**: 242–246.

10. Patrono C. Aspirin as an antiplatelet drug. *N Engl J Med* 1994; **330**: 1287–1294.

11. Sporn LA, Marder VJ, Wagner DD. Differing polarity of the constitutive regulated secretory pathways for Von Willebrand factor in endothelial cells. *J Cell Biol* 1989; **108**: 1283–1289.

12. Rand JH, Glanville RW, Wu XX et al. The significance of subendothelial Von Willebrand factor. *Thromb Haemost* 1997; **78**: 445–450.

13. Ruggeri ZM, Ware J. The structure and function of Von Willebrand factor. *Thromb Haemost* 1992; **67**: 594–599.

14. Meyer D, Fressinaud E, Gaucher C et al. Gene defects in 150 unrelated French cases with type 2 Von Willebrand disease: from the patient to the gene. *Thromb Haemost* 1997; **78**: 451–456.

15. Sadler JE. A revised classification of Von-Willebrand disease. *Thromb Haemost* 1994; **71**: 520–525.

16. Ginsburg D, Sadler JE. Von Willebrand disease — a database of point mutations, insertions and deletions. *Thromb Haemost* 1993; **69**: 177–184.

17. Furlan M, Robles R, Solenthaler M, Laemmle B. Acquired deficiency of von Willebrand factor-cleaving protease in a patient with thrombotic thrombocytopenic purpura. *Blood* 1998; **91**: 2839–2846.

18. Wu SM, Stanley TB, Mutucumarana VP, Stafford DW. Characterization of the γ-glutamyl-carboxylase. *Thromb Haemost* 1997; **78**: 599–604.

19. Furie BC, Furie B. Structure and mechanism of action of vitamin K-dependent γ-glutamyl-carboxylase. Recent advances from mutagenesis studies. *Thromb Haemost* 1997; **78**: 595–598.

20. Brenner B, Sanchez-Vega B, Wu SM et al. A missense mutation in γ-glutamyl carboxylase gene causes combined deficiency of all vitamin K-dependent blood coagulation factors. *Blood* 1998; **92**: 4554–4559.

21. Mann KG, Gafney D, Bovill EG. Molecular biology, biochemistry and lifespan of plasma coagulation factors In: Beutler E, Lichtman MA, Coller BS, Kipps TJ (eds). *Hematology.* New York: McGraw-Hill, 1995: 1206–1226.

22. Bauer KA. Activation of the factor VII-tissue factor pathway. *Thromb Haemost* 1997; **78**: 108–111.

23. Roberts HR, Monroe DM, Oliver JA et al. Newer concepts of blood coagulation. *Haemophilia* 1998; **4**: 331–334.

24. Gordon SG, Hashiba V, Poole MA et al. A cysteine proteinase procoagulant from amniochorion. *Blood* 1985; **66**: 1261–1266.

25. Lane DA, Olds RR, Thein SC. Antithrombin and its deficiency states. *Blood Coagul Fibrinolysis* 1992; **3**: 315–341.

26. Esmon CT, Ding W, Yesuhiro K et al. The protein C pathway: new insights. *Thromb Haemost* 1997; **78**: 70–74.

27. Bertina RM, Koeleman BP, Koster T et al. Mutation in blood coagulation factor V associated with resistance to activated protein C. *Nature* 1994; **369**: 64–67.

28. Sandset PM, Bendz B. Tissue factor pathway inhibitor: clinical deficiency states. *Thromb Haemost* 1997; **78**: 467–470.

29. Broze GJ. Consequences of tissue factor pathway inhibitor gene-disruption in mice. *Thromb Haemost* 1997; **78**: 699–704.

30. Patrono C, Patrignani P, Rocca B, Landolfi R. Characterization of biochemical and functional effects of antiplatelet drugs as a key to their clinical development. *Thromb Haemost* 1995; **74**: 396–400.

31. Francis CW, Markham RE, Barlow GH et al. Thrombin activity of fibrin thrombi and soluble plasmic derivatives. *J Lab Clin Med* 1983; **102**: 220–230.

32. Brenner B, Francis CW, Marder VJ. The role of soluble cross-linked fibrin in D dimer immunoreactivity of plasmic digests. *J Lab Clin Med* 1989; **113**: 682–688.

Pathogenesis of coronary arterial thrombosis

Marc Cohen

*Man lives with arteriosclerosis, and dies of the complicating
coronary thrombosis.*

J. Dedichen[1]

The acute coronary syndromes result from a sudden decrease
in blood flow through the coronary circulation. The occlusion
of the coronary artery may be complete and permanent
resulting in acute myocardial infarction or sudden cardiac
death.[2] Alternatively, the occlusion may be partially occlusive
(but severe) resulting in unstable angina. There is usually an
abrupt onset of pain, and frequently, patients experience a
cyclical, waxing and waning of pain. This is compatible with
the fundamental underlying mechanism, the rupture or
erosion of an atherosclerotic plaque within a coronary
artery.[3–20] As the plaque exposes its contents to the flowing
blood, thrombus immediately layers on top of the area of
ruptured plaque. In a small fraction of patients, thrombus
develops over an area of endothelial denudation or erosion,
without frank rupture.[21,22] The expanding thrombus can
fragment, embolize, and occlude distal intramyocardial
arteries and arterioles, precipitating ischemic necrosis.[15,16,18]

An example of an atherosclerotic coronary derived from

the pathologic archives of Professor M. Davies is seen in *Figure 2.1*.[18] Panels (a) and (b) depict the coronary artery of a person who died after coming to the hospital with unstable angina. Waxy looking plaque is taking up space within the artery, causing a narrowing in the arterial lumen. There is a precariously thin 'fibrous cap,' covering the pulp of the plaque and separating those contents from the flow of blood. As a result of some eruption that took place underneath the cap, or by some digestive process, the cap fragmented leaving a gap in the fibrous cap (panel B). The moment the plaque core is exposed to the blood, the thrombotic cascade is triggered, and fibrin and platelets are deposited as a blood clot over this 'fractured cap.' In this histological section, the thrombus

did not propagate to completely fill the lumen.

There is an evolution involving several stages and several different variables that leads to coronary thrombosis. The first element is the evolution of the atherosclerotic plaque from a simple to a complex lesion. The second element involves the cascade of events that triggers erosion or frank fracture of the overlying fibrous cap. The third element involves the induction of the overlying thrombus. The last element involves the determinants of thrombus propagation to a partially, versus completely occlusive thrombus.

The original studies conducted in these areas were published many years ago. It has taken a long time for technology (e.g.

(a)   (b)

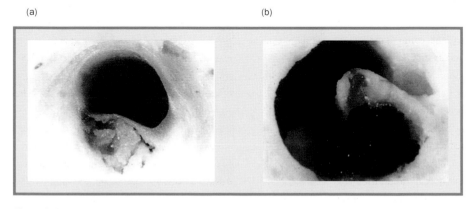

Figure 2.1
(a) Atherosclerotic plaque with a very thin but intact fibrous cap. (b) Fibrous cap is ruptured and exposed plaque overlaid by thrombus. Taken from Davies.[19]

coronary arteriography[23–25] and angioscopy[26,27]), to advance to a stage where these ideas and hypotheses can now be considered proven by virtue of these direct imaging techniques.

Substrate for thrombosis: the underlying plaque

Plaque rupture and overlying thrombus represent the very end-stage of the disease, atherosclerosis. Atherosclerosis within the vessel wall is a process with many stages. This has recently been described by an American Heart Association Task force led by Stary et al.[28] The progression of atherosclerotic plaque from a small crescent, 'a fatty streak,' to a complex, Stary class V, lesion occurs over decades but begins at a very early stage in life. In stage V, the lipid core forms an abscess. When the abscess and fibrous cap rupture, thrombosis is triggered. Unfortunately, most patients come to the attention of physicians and cardiologists at this late stage, after the 'horse is out of the barn.' Currently, the issue of how to arrest the disease in the early stages before the late stage of plaque rupture, is being addressed with vigorous risk factor reduction.

What triggers a silent plaque to rupture? Libby et al[29] and Fuster et al[30–32] have identified two groups of variables that relate to plaque rupture: (1) the intrinsic properties of plaques that may make one plaque more

vulnerable to eruption than another, plaque vulnerability, and (2) the extrinsic forces that act upon the plaque and stress or deform the plaque, external triggers.

Plaques are most vulnerable to rupture in one of two locations: on the edge of the plaque, the shoulder region, or in the middle over the soft part of the plaque. Vulnerability may be enhanced by the amount of fat within the soft region of the plaque, the number and activity of inflammatory cells underlying the fibrous cap (such as T lymphocytes, macrophages, mast cells, smooth muscle cells),[29,33] strength of the fibrous cap, and degree of luminal stenosis caused by the enlarging plaque, shear.

The area of greatest cell numbers and cellular activity is in the shoulder region at the edge of the plaque (see *Figure 2.2*). There is a balance between the smooth muscle cells that are synthesizing collagen and elastin, and the lymphocytes, macrophages, and mast cells promoting degradation of collagen and elastin.[29] The thicker fibrous cap that is a little more tenacious and not so prone to cracking or fissuring would be more protective than the thin cap.[29]

There are several external triggers that can stress an otherwise stable plaque to the point of rupture. The more common triggers are a sudden or chronic high blood pressure, constant moving, bending and flexing of the coronary artery with each beat of the heart, and a sudden change in coronary tone causing

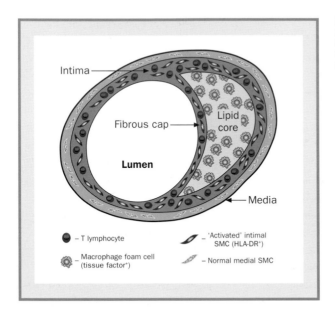

Figure 2.2
Diagram of evolving atherosclerotic plaque highlighting the multiplicity of cell types. Taken from Libby.[29]

reduction in lumen radius and changes in the velocity of blood flowing near the plaque (shear). Circadian variation in the triggering of the acute coronary syndromes has been observed and described in detail elsewhere.[34–36]

The endothelial cell is the barrier between the flowing blood and the inner aspect of the wall of the artery. It has many luminal receptors facing the blood, many synthetic functions, and also communicates with the smooth muscle cells lying in the opposite direction beneath the basement membrane. One product of endothelial cell synthesis as well as platelet synthesis is nitric oxide. This molecule has significant antithrombotic properties as well as effects on the smooth muscle cells. Cigarette smoking exerts a major toxic effect on endothelial function, and is therefore a major potential trigger for acute coronary syndromes.[22]

Clinical manifestations of plaque rupture or erosion

Not everyone who ruptures a plaque or de-endothelializes a patch of vessel wall will experience a massive myocardial infarction and sudden death.[37–39] As mentioned above, thrombus will accumulate over a ruptured or eroded plaque. The thrombus may propagate to a point that still leaves some residual lumen for blood to flow. Alternatively, the balance of forces promoting clot propagation versus clot dissolution may result in thrombus growth to a point that completely occludes the artery and stops any blood flow resulting in myocardial infarction (see *Figure 2.3*).

What determines the extent of the superimposed thrombus? (1) The extent of the exposed plaque: in one patient there may be a small erosion or fissure in the fibrous cap, while in another almost the entire fibrous cap may have sheared off leaving a large crater exposing all of the plaque gruel. (2) Local shear forces, for example in the vicinity of a branch point may be greater, which will cause more thrombus to deposit in the setting of a ruptured plaque; and (3) the thrombotic/thrombolytic equilibrium.

The balance between the thrombogenicity of the exposed plaque interior, and the thrombogenicity or prothrombolytic nature of the flowing blood[40,41] constitute the prime determinants of the individual patient's response to the ubiquitous phenomenon of endothelial denudation or erosion or even plaque rupture. For example one can imagine two patients, each with a ruptured plaque. If one patient is a smoker and has nicotine in his blood, he will have an elevated factor VII and fibrinogen level,[40] his platelets will be very 'sticky' and he may thus have an exaggerated platelet response. The other patient may be diabetic with an abnormally high level of plasminogen activator inhibitor (PAI-1). A normal patient has low levels of PAI-1 and their circulating plasminogen activators would partially dissolve the thrombus growing over their ruptured plaque. In contrast, the diabetic patient is inhibiting their plasminogen activator because of their elevated PAI-1 levels, allowing the thrombus to propagate.[42]

The interior of the plaque is intensely thrombogenic, due to a combination of the exposure of fragmented collagen to platelets, the high concentration of tissue factor produced by macrophages within the lipid core and the presence of lipid lamellae and crystals on the surface of which coagulation is very rapid. However, there is significant heterogeneity in the composition of human plaques, and accordingly, in the thrombogenicity. Experiments in which sections of plaque are exposed to platelets in vitro clearly show the lipid core to be the most thrombogenic part of the plaque.[39,43] Another plaque element affecting thrombogenicity is intraplaque tissue factor, the small glycoprotein that initiates the extrinsic coagulation cascade.[44,45] In experimental models of atherosclerosis induced by high lipid diets, the peripheral blood monocytes, even after culture and transformation to macrophages, do not express tissue factor. In contrast, there are abundant macrophages within unstable atherosclerotic plaques that express tissue factor.[46–51] The risk of further

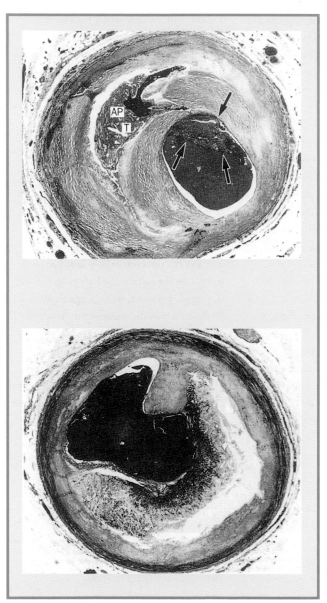

Figure 2.3
(a) Complex atherosclerotic plaque with arrows highlighting partially occlusive intraluminal thrombus. (b) Completely occlusive intraluminal thrombus at site of exposed atherosclerotic debris.

(a)

(b)

acute events relates to the proportion of monocytes expressing tissue factor.[45,50,51]

These experimental observations lay the groundwork for targeting optimal therapy in patients with plaque erosion or rupture and superimposed thrombosis.[45,52-54]

This summary suggests that minor episodes of endothelial disruption are a common event in subjects with coronary plaques and an intermittent but not infrequent stimulus to coronary thrombosis. The determinant of whether clinical symptoms of acute ischemia develop is whether intraluminal thrombus develops.

References

1. Dedichen J. Thrombosing arteriosclerosis: result of long-term anticoagulant therapy. *BMJ* 1956; ii: 1038–1039.

2. Dewood M, Spores J, Notske R et al. Prevalence of total coronary occlusion during the early hours of transmural myocardial infarction. *N Engl J Med* 1980; **303**: 897–902.

3. Duguid JB. Thrombosis as a factor in the pathogenesis of coronary atherosclerosis. *J Pathol Bacteriol* 1946; **58**: 207–212.

4. Constantinides P. Plaque fissures in human coronary thrombosis. *J Atheroscler Res* 1966; **6**: 1–17.

5. Haerem JW. Platelet aggregates in intramyocardial vessels of patients dying suddenly and unexpectedly of coronary artery disease. *Atherosclerosis* 1972; **15**: 199–213.

6. Chapman I. The cause-effect relationship between recent coronary artery occlusion and acute myocardial infarction. *Am Heart J* 1974; **87**: 267–271.

7. Duguid J. *The Dynamics of Atherosclerosis*. Aberdeen: University Press, 1976: 48.

8. Davies M, Woolf N, Robertson K. Pathology of acute myocardial infarction with particular reference to occlusive coronary thrombi. *Br Heart J* 1976; **38**: 659–664.

9. Ridolfi RL, Hutchins GM. The relationship between coronary artery lesions and myocardial infarcts: ulceration of atherosclerotic plaques precipitating coronary thrombosis. *Am Heart J* 1977; **93**: 468–486.

10. Horie T, Sekiguchi M, Hirosawa K. Coronary thrombosis in pathogenesis of acute myocardial infarction. Histopathological study of coronary arteries in 108 necropsied cases using serial section. *Br Heart J* 1978; **40**: 153–161.

11. Davies M, Fulton W, Robertson W. Relation of coronary thrombosis to ischaemic myocardial necrosis. *J Pathol* 1979; **127**: 99–110.

12. Falk E. Plaque rupture with severe pre-existing stenosis precipitation coronary thrombosis: characteristics of coronary atherosclerotic plaques underlying fatal occlusive thrombi. *Br Heart J* 1983; **50**: 127–134.

13. Davies MJ, Thomas AC. Thrombosis and acute coronary-artery lesions in sudden cardiac ischemic death. *N Engl J Med* 1984, **310**: 1137–1140.

14. Davies M, Thomas AC. Plaque fissuring — the cause of acute myocardial infarction, sudden ischaemic death and crescendo angina. *Br Heart J* 1985; **53**: 363–373.

15. Falk E. Unstable angina with fatal outcome: dynamic coronary thrombosis leading to

infarction and/or sudden death. *Circulation* 1985; **71**: 699–708.

16.   Davies M, Thomas AC, Knapman P, Hangartner R. Intramyocardial platelet aggregation in patients with unstable angina suffering sudden ischaemic cardiac death. *Circulation* 1986; **73**: 418–427.

17.   Fuster V, Badimon L, Cohen M et al. Insights into the pathogenesis of acute ischemic syndromes. *Circulation* 1988; **77**: 1213–1220.

18.   Davies MJ. A macroscopic and microscopic view of coronary thrombi. *Circulation* 1990; **82**: 1138–1146.

19.   Davies M. The contribution of thrombosis to the clinical expression of coronary atherosclerosis. *Thromb Res* 1996; **82**: 1–32.

20.   Burke AP, Farb A, Malcom GT et al. Plaque rupture and sudden death related to exertion in men with coronary artery disease. *JAMA* 1999; **281**: 921–926.

21.   Farb A, Burke AP, Tang AT et al. Coronary plaque erosion without rupture into a lipid core: a frequent cause of coronary thrombosis in sudden coronary death. *Circulation* 1996; **93**: 1354–1363.

22.   Burke AP, Farb A, Malcom GT et al. Coronary risk factors and plaque morphology in men with coronary disease who died suddenly. *N Engl J Med* 1997; **336**: 1276–1282.

23.   Levin D, Fallon J. Significance of the angiographic morphology of localized coronary stenosis: histopathologic correlations. *Circulation* 1982; **66**: 316–320.

24.   Ambrose J, Winters S, Arora R. Angiographic evolution of coronary artery morphology in unstable angina. *J Am Coll Cardiol* 1986; **7**: 472–478.

25.   Ambrose J, Tannenbaum M, Alexpooulos D

et al. Angiographic progression of coronary artery disease and the development of myocardial infarction. *J Am Coll Cardiol* 1988; **12**: 56–62.

26.   Sherman CT, Litvack F, Grundfest W et al. Coronary angioscopy in patients with unstable angina pectoris. *N Engl J Med* 1986; **315**: 913–919.

27.   Mizuno K, Miyamoto A, Satomura K et al. Angioscopic coronary macromorphology in patients with acute coronary disorders. *Lancet* 1991; **337**: 809–812.

28.   Stary HC, Chandler AB, Dinsmore RE, Fuster V. A definition of advanced types of atherosclerotic lesions and a histological classification of atherosclerosis: a report from the Committee on vascular lesions of the council on Atherosclerosis. American Heart Association. *Circulation* 1995; **92**: 1355–1374.

29.   Libby P. Molecular bases of the acute coronary syndromes. *Circulation* 1995; **91**: 2844–2850.

30.   Fuster V, Lewis A. Conner Memorial Lecture. Mechanisms leading to myocardial infarction: insights from studies of vascular biology. *Circulation* 1994; **90**: 2126–2146.

31.   Falk E, Shah PK, Fuster V. Coronary plaque disruption. *Circulation* 1995; **92**: 657–671.

32.   Fuster V, Fallon JT, Nemerson Y. Coronary thrombosis. *Lancet* 1996; **348**(Suppl I): S7–S10.

33.   Van De Wal AC, Becker AE, Van Der Loos CM, Das PK. Site of intimal rupture or erosion of thrombosed coronary atherosclerotic plaques is characterised by an inflammatory process irrespective of the dominant plaque histology. *Circulation* 1994; **89**: 36–44.

34. Muller JE, Tofler GH, Stone PH. Circadian variation and triggers of onset of acute cardiovascular disease. *Circulation* 1989; **79**: 733–743.

35. Tofler GH, Brezinski D, Schafer AI et al. Concurrent morning increase in platelet aggregability and the risk of myocardial infarction and sudden cardiac death. *N Engl J Med* 1987; **316**: 1514–1518.

36. Andreotti F, Davies GJ, Hackett DR et al. Major circadian fluctuations in fibrinolytic factors and possible relevance to time of onset of myocardial infarction, sudden cardiac death and stroke. *Am J Cardiol* 1988; **62**: 635–637.

37. Davies MJ, Bland JM, Hangartner JRW et al. Factors influencing the presence or absence of acute coronary artery thrombi in sudden ischaemic death. *Eur Heart J* 1989; **10**: 203–208.

38. Davies MJ, Richardson PD, Woolf N et al. Risk of thrombosis in human atherosclerotic plaques: role of extracellular lipid, macrophage, and smooth muscle cell content. *Br Heart J* 1993; **69**: 377–381.

39. Badimon L, Badimon JJ, Cohen M et al. Vessel wall-related risk factors in acute vascular events. *Drugs* 1991; **42**(Suppl 5): 1–9.

40. Meade T, Brozovic M, Chakrabarti P. Haemostatic function and ischaemic heart disease: principal results of the Northwick Park Study. *Lancet* 1986; **ii**: 533–537.

41. Thompson SG, Kienast J, Pyke SDM et al for the European Conserted Action on Thrombosis and Disabilities Angina Pectoris Study Group. Hemostatic factors and the risk of myocardial infarction or sudden death in patients with angina pectoris. *N Engl J Med* 1995; **332**: 635–641.

42. Hamsten A, De Faire U, Walldius G et al. Plasminogen activator inhibitor in plasma: risk factor for recurrent myocardial infarction. *Lancet* 1987; **ii**: 3–9.

43. Fernandez-Ortiz A, Badimon J, Falk E et al. Characterization of the relative thrombogenicity of atherosclerotic plaque components: implications for consequences of plaque rupture. *J Am Coll Cardiol* 1994; **23**: 1562–1569.

44. Wilcox J, Smith S, Schwartz S, Gordon D. Localization of tissue factor in the normal vessel wall and atherosclerotic plaque. *Proc Natl Acad Sci USA* 1989; **86**: 2839–2843.

45. Badimon JJ, Lettino M, Toschi V et al. Local inhibition of tissue factor reduces the thrombogenicity of disrupted human atherosclerotic plaques: effects of tissue factor pathway inhibitor on plaque thrombogenicity under flow conditions. *Circulation* 1999; **99**: 1780–1787.

46. Escaned J, Van Suylen RJ, Macleod DC et al. Histologic characteristics of tissue excised during directional coronary atherectomy in stable and unstable angina pectoris. *Am J Cardiol* 1993; **71**: 1442–1447.

47. Moreno P, Falk E, Palacios I et al. Macrophage infiltration in acute coronary syndromes: implication for plaque rupture. *Circulation* 1994; **90**: 775–778.

48. Leatham EW, Bath PM, Tooze J, Camm AJ. Increased monocyte tissue factor expression in coronary disease. *Br Heart J* 1995; **73**: 10–13.

49. Annex BH, Denning SM, Channon KM et al. Differential expression of tissue factor protein in directional atherectomy specimens from patients with stable and unstable coronary syndromes. *Circulation* 1995; **91**: 619–622.

50. Barstad RM, Hamers MJ, Kierulf P et al. Procoagulant human monocytes mediate tissue factor/factor VIIa-dependent platelet-

thrombus formation when exposed to flowing nonanticoagulated human blood. *Arterioscler Thromb Vasc Biol* 1995; **15**: 11–16.

51. Muhlfelder TW, Teodorescu V, Rand J, Rosman A. Human atheromatous plaque extracts induce tissue factor activity (TFa) in monocytes and also express constitutive TFa. *Thromb Haemost* 1999; **81**: 146–150.

52. Meyer BJ, Badimon JJ, Mailhac A et al. Inhibition of growth of thrombus on fresh mural thrombus: targeting optimal therapy. *Circulation* 1994; **90**: 2432–2438.

53. Zesheng W, Hebert D, Kaplan AV et al. Local delivery of tissue factor pathway inhibitor (TFPI) decreases mural thrombus formation induced by balloon angioplasty. *J Am Coll Cardiol* 1996; **27**(Suppl A): 334A.

54. The Medical Research Council's General Practice Research Framework. Thrombosis prevention trial: randomized trial of low-intensity oral anticoagulation with warfarin and low-dose aspirin in the primary prevention of ischemic heart disease in men at increased risk. *Lancet* 1998; **351**: 233–241.

Inherited thrombophilia

Sam Schulman

3

A tendency to thrombosis, thrombophilia, may be due to acquired abnormalities, for example cancer, systemic lupus erythematosus, cardiolipin antibodies, or to inherited predisposing defects. The latter conditions will be reviewed in this chapter. The genetic defects are shown in *Table 3.1*. The term thrombophilia was initially reserved for cases with severe or unusual thromboembolic manifestations at an early age, and it was further defined as familial or inherited if there was a family history of similar events. With recent advances in molecular biology the term inherited thrombophilia is based on biochemical and molecular genetic evidence and the importance of the clinical manifestations has decreased somewhat.

Deep vein thrombosis has an annual incidence of approximately 1/1000 inhabitants and pulmonary embolism of 0.5–1/1000. The prevalence of inherited thrombogenic abnormalities has hardly ever been investigated in a representative subset of this population, since patients above a certain age or those who were too ill for participation or with fatal pulmonary embolism at first presentation were usually excluded. In a study of 2132 consecutive patients with venous thromboembolism, performed before 1993, that is prior to

Table 3.1
Causes of inherited thrombophilia

Deficiency of antithrombin, protein C or protein S
APC resistance due to factor V Leiden mutation (G1691A)
Hyperprothrombinemia due to G20210A polymorphism
Hyperhomocysteinemia due to deficiency of cystathionine-β-synthase,
methylenetetrahydrofolate reductase or thermolabile methylenetetrahydrofolate reductase

Other possible candidates
Elevated factor VIII
Dysfibrinogenemia
Dys- or hypoplasminogenemia
Deficiency of heparin cofactor II
Deficiency of histidine-rich glycoprotein
Abnormal thrombomodulin

---

the era of recently described mutations in factor V or prothrombin, 12.85% had a thrombogenic protein deficiency (*Figure 3.1*).[1]

Clinical picture

Although the cardinal manifestations of inherited thrombophilia are deep vein thrombosis and pulmonary embolism, the symptomatology differs slightly between some of these conditions. In general arterial thrombosis, including myocardial infarction, ischaemic stroke etc. is not part of the picture. The exception to this rule is hyperhomocysteinemia. In addition, activated protein C (APC) resistance has been reported to increase the risk of juvenile transitory ischaemic attacks.[2] Superficial thrombophlebitis appears to be more common in deficiency of protein C or protein S and in APC-resistance than in the other conditions. A diagnosis of inherited thrombophilia is often reached after biochemical investigation of patients with mesenteric vein thrombosis or cerebral vein thrombosis. Almost 50% of the venous thromboembolic events are preceded by an identifiable risk situation, mainly surgery, puerperium and pregnancy (*Figure 3.2*).[3]

In the homozygous form deficiency of antithrombin, type I (activity and immunological antithrombin equally affected), is incompatible with life[4] and deficiency of protein C or protein S causes purpura fulminans at an early age, whereas APC-resistance may remain asymptomatic until late in life and thermolabile methylenetetrahydrofolate reductase only becomes a risk factor for venous thromboembolism in this form.

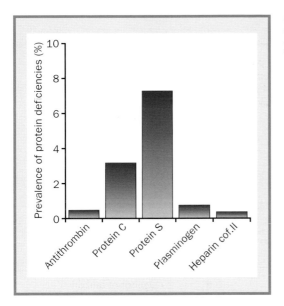

Figure 3.1
Prevalence of protein deficiencies in 2132 patients with venous thromboembolism. (Data adapted from Mateo et al.[1])

The median age for the first clinical presentation is about 25 in deficiency of antithrombin, 40 in deficiency of protein C, and in APC-resistance only 25% of affected individuals have had a venous thromboembolic episode by age 50. The risk of thromboembolic complications during pregnancy is 40–50% in deficiency of antithrombin, compared to 10–20% in deficiency of protein C or protein S.[3,5]

Other clinical manifestations, which lately have been recognized, are non-thrombotic complications during pregnancy. In a cohort study, accounting for 2543 pregnancies, stillbirth was almost four times more frequent and miscarriage also more common in those with thrombophilia compared to controls.[6] In another study 71 of 110 consecutive women with pre-eclampsia, abruptio placentae, fetal growth retardation or stillbirth had the G1691A mutation, G20210A mutation, C677T mutation, deficiency of protein C, protein S or of antithrombin or cardiolipin antibodies.[7]

Combinations of defects yield a high risk of venous thromboembolism[8] and an odds ratio of 14.3 for stillbirth.[6]

Antithrombin deficiency

This was the first kind of inherited thrombophilia to be described in 1965.[9]

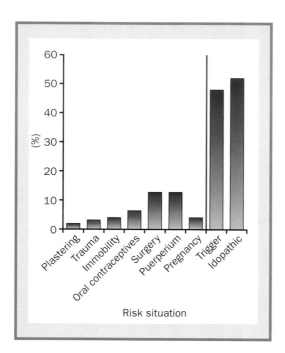

Figure 3.2
Relative impact of various clinical risk factors for the development of venous thromboembolism in patients with inherited thrombophilia. (Data adapted from de Stefano et al.[3])

Antithrombin is a serine protease inhibitor (serpin), which inhibits thrombin, kallikrein and the activated forms of factors IX, X, XI and XII. This reaction occurs when the serine protease tries to cleave antithrombin at the reactive centre and forms a stoichiometric 1:1 complex. The reaction is slow but is speeded up 1000 times by heparin or proteoglycans bound to the endothelium.

Antithrombin deficiency is classified as type I when both antigen and activity levels are reduced and as type II when activity is reduced but the antigen level is normal.

Depending on which of the functions of antithrombin is affected, type II is subclassified as type II RS with a defect in the reactive site, type II HBS with a defect in the heparin binding site, and type II PE with multiple functional defects (pleiotropic effect). In the database of antithrombin gene mutations 80 distinct mutations and 12 deletions of more than 30 bp corresponding to type I defects have been registered. Furthermore, 12 distinct mutations causing type II RS, 12 mutations causing type II HBS and 11 mutations causing type II PE or altogether 127 different mutations have been registered.[10] The prevalence of antithrombin deficiency in the population is about 1:5000, in consecutive patients with the first episode of deep vein thrombosis 1:100 and among patients with thrombophilia 4–7%.[11] A functional assay that quantitates the heparin cofactor activity of antithrombin should be used in the screening for this defect, and an international standard is available. Antithrombin is synthesized in the liver and acquired deficiency occurs in liver failure and also protein-losing nephropathy and enteropathy and these conditions have to be excluded before a diagnosis of congenital deficiency of antithrombin is made. The plasma level is also reduced during pregnancy and during medication with heparin (binding) and asparaginase. The decrease of antithrombin can be used as a prognostic marker in disseminated intravascular coagulation.

Fatal cases of thromboembolism have been described in some families with antithrombin deficiency, but in two large retrospective studies no indication of increased mortality among individuals with this defect could be found.[12,13]

Protein C deficiency

Deficiency of protein C was originally described in 1981.[14] Protein C is a vitamin K-dependent glycoprotein, synthesized in the liver. Protein C is activated by thrombin and 20 000 times faster by the endothelial-bound thrombin–thrombomodulin complex to APC, a serine protease. APC cleaves selectively, and thereby inactivates, factors Va and VIIIa.

Protein C deficiency is, in analogy with antithrombin deficiency, classified into type I and type II deficiency (see above). The functional defects may be a defective activation by thrombin–thrombomodulin, a decreased binding to phospholipids or poor interaction with cofactors or substrates. A functional assay should be used in the screening for deficiency mutations, but none of the assays will identify all type II defects. An international standard is available. Congenital deficiency should be differentiated from acquired deficiency due to vitamin K deficiency or liver disease. During treatment with vitamin K antagonists determinations of the protein C level are difficult to interpret. Of 160 different mutations identified in the protein C gene, 107 are missense mutations, and a vast majority of the mutations are responsible for type I deficiency.[15]

The prevalence of protein C deficiency in the population is 0.2–0.4%, in patients with first episode of deep-vein thrombosis 3% and in most studies of patients with thrombophilia 6–9%.[11] In a retrospective study there was no evidence of an excess mortality in this population.[16] The prevalence of homozygous protein C deficiency was estimated to be in the range 1:160 000–1:360 000.[17] Depending on the protein C level being undetectable or a few percent, the condition will manifest itself with purpura fulminans neonatally or within the first years of life. When the protein C levels in the homozygotes are at least 5% the manifestations will be similar to those in the heterozygotes. Purpura fulminans is caused by thrombosis in small vessels, resulting in cutaneous and subcutaneous ischaemic necrosis.[18]

The reason for an increased incidence of superficial thrombophlebitis in protein C deficiency — as opposed to antithrombin deficiency — is probably related to the antiinflammatory activity of protein C.

Protein S deficiency

In 1984 two groups reported on patients with thrombophilia and protein S deficiency.[19,20] This is also a vitamin K-dependent glycoprotein, but in addition to synthesis in the liver it is also produced by the endothelium, megakaryocytes and Leydig cells in the testis. In its free form (40%) protein S serves as a cofactor for APC, whereas 60% is bound in a 1:1 stoichiometric complex to the β-chain of C4b-binding protein. The cofactor effect is non-enzymatic and expressed by an increment of the APC-affinity for the negatively charged phospholipid surfaces of endothelium or platelets, enhancing localized complex formation with factors Va and VIIIa. Protein S may also have an APC-independent

inhibiting effect on the tenase complex (FIXa-FVIIIa) and the prothrombinase complex (FXa-FVa).

The subclassification of protein S deficiency has been less straightforward than for the other deficiencies due to the existence of a free and a bound form. The combination of low total and free antigen and low activity is type I. A reduction of protein S activity alone is type II or IIb and when this is accompanied by a reduction of free protein S antigen the subclass is type III or IIa, depending on the system chosen. Functional assays for protein S have not been widely adopted due to an interference in cases with APC-resistance. An assay for the free protein S antigen is most suitable as a screening test. Acquired deficiency is seen due to vitamin K deficiency or liver disease, during treatment with vitamin K antagonists and pregnancy. Investigations of mutations causing protein S deficiency have been complicated by the existence of two protein S genes, one active and one pseudogene, in close proximity to each other on chromosome 3. In the database of mutations 126 mutations, which are detrimental, and 19 sequence variations, which probably are polymorphisms, have been reported.[21]

The prevalence of protein S deficiency in the general population has not been determined in a sufficiently large study but is probably close to that of protein C deficiency. Among patients with a first episode of deep vein thrombosis 1–2% are diagnosed with protein S deficiency, whereas among thrombophilic cases the prevalence can amount to 6–13%.[11]

The clinical manifestations in heterozygotes as well as homozygotes are virtually identical to those seen in the corresponding forms of protein C deficiency (described above).

APC-resistance (factor V Leiden mutation)

The most frequent cause of inherited thrombophilia, so far, was detected in 1993, when it was reported that the plasma in some of these patients was resistant to the anticoagulant effect of APC.[22] The condition turned out to be associated with a point mutation (G1691A — the factor V Leiden mutation) leading to replacement of 506Arg by Gln in the factor V molecule,[23] which slows down the inactivation of factor Va by APC. Factor Va is also cleaved by APC at Arg306 and Arg679. Mutations A1090G and G1091C result in Gly306 and Thr306 (factor V Hong Kong and factor V Cambridge), respectively, with an associated tendency to venous thromboembolism.[24,25] Since the factor V Leiden mutation is common in the Caucasian population, with a prevalence of 3–7%,[11] and virtually absent in other races, it was suspected that the mutation has a single origin. The finding of a single FV:R506Q

haplotype in homozygotes[26] supports the hypothesis of a common ancestor, estimated to have lived 30 000 years ago.

An explanation for the exceptionally high prevalence of this thrombophilic condition has been connected to the finding of a significantly lower risk of intrapartum bleeding complications in women with this phenotype.[27] The prevalence of APC-resistance in patients presenting with the first episode of deep vein thrombosis is about 20% and in patients with thrombophilia approximately 50%.[11] The risk of venous thromboembolism in patients with APC-resistance is five times higher than in a control population. However, thrombi forming in these patients seem less likely to cause symptomatic or fatal pulmonary embolism[28,29] and there is no excess mortality in this group either.[30] Superficial thrombophlebitis is not an uncommon feature in APC-resistance and accordingly it is not surprising to find a trend to a higher incidence of early saphenous vein graft occlusion after coronary artery bypass grafting in carriers of the mutation.[31] Patients with the homozygous form of factor V Leiden mutation have a higher incidence of, but not different or more severe, thromboembolic complications than the heterozygotes. The prevalence of homozygous carriers is 0.06–0.25%.

Hyperprothrombinemia (G20210A polymorphism)

In 1996 another relatively common biochemical risk factor for venous thromboembolism was discovered.[32] A dimorphism with a G to A transition in the 3′ untranslated region of the prothrombin gene was associated with elevated plasma levels of prothrombin and with a relative risk of venous thromboembolism of about 4. The mechanism whereby the prothrombin level is increased is not known.

The prevalence of the condition in the normal population varies between 0.7 and 6.5% among Caucasians with predominance in Southern Europe.[33,34] The clinical manifestations are similar to those of the other inherited thrombophilias. Very few homozygotes have been described, and in analogy with the homozygous factor V Leiden mutation, this condition does not appear to cause different symptoms but only with a higher incidence.

Hyperhomocysteinemia

Hyperhomocysteinemia is a risk factor for deep vein thrombosis, as demonstrated in consecutive patients younger than 70 years of age with a first episode thereof.[35] There are several inherited as well as acquired conditions that can cause hyperhomocysteinemia, and among the latter are low levels of folate,

cobalamin or pyridoxine due to dietary deficiency or interaction with methotrexate, anticonvulsants, theophylline or cigarette smoking, pernicious anaemia, old age, chronic renal insufficiency, hypothyroidism and several types of cancer.[36] Among the severe inherited defects in homocysteine metabolism, cystathionine β-synthase deficiency is the most common, with a prevalence of homozygotes of 1:200 000. These individuals have congenital homocysteinuria and suffer from severe mental retardation, skeletal deformities, ectopia lentis, severe atherosclerosis and venous thromboembolism. Heterozygotes with this defect have moderately elevated levels of plasma homocysteine and the prevalence in the general population is 0.3–1.4%. About 5–10% of the severe cases have a homozygous deficiency of N^5,N^{10}-methylene-tetrahydrofolate reductase (MTHFR), manifesting itself with neurological defects, psychomotor retardation, seizures, premature vascular disease and thromboembolism. A thermolabile mutant of this enzyme results in a reduction by 50% of the normal enzyme activity, associated with an increased risk of coronary artery disease.[37] The thermolabile MTHFR was shown in 1995 to be caused by a C to T substitution at nucleotide 677 with an alanine to valine substitution in the protein.[38] The prevalence of this condition in the homozygous form is 5–15%.[36]

It has been convincingly shown that

hyperhomocysteinemia is a risk factor for venous thromboembolism with an odds ratio of 2–3[35] as well as for recurrence.[39] The importance of the thermolabile MTHFR in this respect is, however, controversial.[40–41]

Elevated FVIII

Factor VIII levels above 1.5 IU/ml had a prevalence of 25% in a population with deep-vein thrombosis and was a risk factor independent of blood group and von Willebrand factor.[42] It has also been demonstrated that elevated factor levels are rarely due to inflammatory reactions, they are persistent and often familial, although the genetic abnormality has not yet been identified.[43]

Management of inherited thrombophilia

Primary prophylaxis

Primary prophylaxis against venous thromboembolism on a long-term basis is not considered indicated in any of the inherited thrombophilias. The reason is the absence of evidence of excess mortality in deficiency of antithrombin[12,13] or protein C[16] or in APC-resistance[30] together with the incidence of major or fatal haemorrhages of 0.6–0.7% per month on full dose anticoagulation with vitamin K antagonists (international normalized ratio, INR = 2–3).[44,45] Conversely, short-term prophylaxis in high-risk situations is highly cost-effective, since

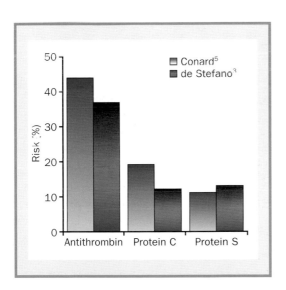

Figure 3.3
The risk of developing thromboembolic complications during pregnancy in patients with the three major coagulation inhibitor deficiencies. (Data adapted from Conard et al.[5] and de Stefano et al.[3])

half of the thromboembolic episodes in patients with inherited thrombophilia are preceded by such events (*Figure 3.2*).[3] Such a policy will improve the clinical outcome, especially in patients under 40 years of age.[3] In previously asymptomatic women with inherited thrombophilia the risk of venous thromboembolism during pregnancy seems to be increased eight-fold compared to nondeficient women.[46] The risk is most pronounced, reaching 50–70%, in women with antithrombin deficiency (*Figure 3.3*), and an active approach for this subset with prophylaxis during the entire pregnancy is advocated by many centres. Standard prophylaxis with heparin 5000 units three times per day, which does not prolong the activated partial thromboplastin time (APTT),

fails to protect 25% of the antithrombin deficient pregnant women.[47] Several optional regimens are used for these patients during pregnancy (*Table 3.2*).

For asymptomatic patients with any of the other inherited thrombophilias prophylaxis during pregnancy should be considered if family members have had thromboembolic complications in this risk situation. Screening for the common factor V Leiden mutation in pregnant women with the intention to provide prophylaxis for the carriers is not cost-effective.[48] At the time of delivery high doses of heparin may cause haemorrhage at the same time as the risk of thromboembolism is pronounced. The dose should at this point not exceed 10 000–15 000 units per 24 hours and for patients with antithrombin deficiency

Table 3.2
Alternatives for prophylaxis during pregnancy in antithrombin deficiency

Agent	Target
1. Heparin	Adjusted to prolong APTT 1.3–1.5 × normal at trough or: anti-factor Xa 0.1–0.2 IU/ml at trough
2. Low molecular mass heparin	Adjusted to reach anti-factor Xa 0.1–0.2 IU/ml at trough
3. 1 or 2 in trimester 1 and 3 and vitamin K antagonist in trimester 2	As above INR 2–3
4. Antithrombin concentrate* + any of 1–3	Antithrombin levels around 1.0 IU/ml

*Indicated for patients who have failed on anticoagulant therapy or for obstetric complications.

one or two doses of antithrombin concentrate is given to keep the plasma level above 0.8 IU/ml.[49] Protamin sulphate may be required to neutralize high doses of heparin if delivery starts abruptly.

During the puerperium the risk of thromboembolic complications is at its peak,[3] and all patients with inherited thrombophilia deserve prophylaxis during this period. Oral anticoagulation with warfarin is allowed, since it is not detectable in the plasma of the infant.[50]

Surgery is another risk factor of the same magnitude as puerperium,[3] and prophylaxis against venous thromboembolism is mandatory, but routine doses of heparin or low molecular mass heparin are sufficient. The only exception may be antithrombin deficiency, since heparin causes a decrease of the plasma level of antithrombin and substitution with antithrombin concentrate may be indicated.[3,51] The experience of substitution with protein C concentrate or fresh frozen plasma in patients with deficiency of protein C or S, respectively, is very limited.[3]

Other short-term risk situations which indicate prophylaxis are immobilization in bed or treatment with plaster cast.

Treatment

The treatment of established venous thromboembolism does not differ from the routine in nonthrombophilic individuals. This is also true for the vast majority of patients with antithrombin deficiency,[52] but a close watch should be kept at the APTT, with prompt increment of the dose of heparin to reach the desired prolongation. In patients with deficiency of protein C or protein S the vitamin K antagonists must be introduced very gradually to minimize the risk of skin necrosis.[53]

Purpura fulminans in neonates with homozygous protein C or protein S deficiency is treated with protein C concentrate or fresh frozen plasma, respectively. When the lesions have healed vitamin K antagonists can be started very gradually, and when this treatment becomes effective the parenteral substitution is discontinued.

Secondary prophylaxis

The intensity of secondary prophylaxis with vitamin K antagonists should follow the routine for all patients. The duration of the prophylaxis should be adjusted according to general risk factors for recurrence (extension of deep vein thrombosis, presence of symptomatic pulmonary embolism, unknown triggering factor). The heterozygous forms of the factor V Leiden mutation and the G20210A polymorphism do not appear to cause an increased risk of recurrence.[54] For patients with a deficiency of antithrombin, protein C or protein S the annual incidence of a first recurrence was about 10% during the first years after the initial event in a retrospective family cohort study.[55] This is higher than in a regular cohort of patients with venous thromboembolism.[54] A reassessment should therefore be performed after 6 months of anticoagulant therapy and then yearly in these patients. The benefit of continued prophylaxis should be weighed against the risks of haemorrhage, poor compliance and the inconvenience perceived by the patient.[56] After life-threatening thromboembolic events, such as massive pulmonary embolism, cerebral vein or visceral vein thrombosis lifelong secondary prophylaxis is advisable in all cases with inherited thrombophilia.

Avoidance of risk

The risk induced by oral contraceptives is well known and it has been estimated that women with the factor V Leiden mutation, receiving these agents have a 30-fold increase of the risk of venous thromboembolism.[57] Still, screening for this mutation in young women, who are for the first time prescribed oral contraceptives, is probably not cost-effective.[58] On the other hand, whenever a case with inherited thrombophilia has been diagnosed family investigations should be carried out. This kind of selective screening, where each of the first degree relatives has a 50% chance of carrying the defect, yields a high degree of

benefit. The asymptomatic carriers should then receive qualified information about all risk factors and how these should be managed.

References

1. Mateo J, Oliver A, Borrell M et al. Laboratory evaluation and clinical characteristics of 2132 consecutive unselected patients with venous thomboembolism — results of the Spanish multicentric study on thrombophilia (EMET-study). *Thromb Haemost* 1997; 77; 444–451.

2. De Lucia D, Cerbone AM, Belli A et al. Resistance to activated protein C in adults with a history of juvenile transient ischemic attacks. *Thromb Haemost* 1996; **76**: 627–631.

3. De Stefano V, Leone G, Mastrangelo S et al. Clinical manifestations and management of inherited thrombophilia: retrospective analysis and follow-up after diagnosis of 238 patients with congenital deficiency of antithrombin III, protein C, protein S. *Thromb Haemost* 1994; **72**: 352–358.

4. Hakten M, Deniz U, Ozbay G, Ulutin ON. Two cases of homozygous antithrombin III deficiency in a family with congenital deficiency of AT. In: Senzinger H, Vinazzer H (eds). *Thrombosis and Haemorrhagic Disorders.* Wurzburg, Germany: Schmitt and Meyer, 1989: 177.

5. Conard J, Horellou MH, Van Dreden P et al. Thrombosis and pregnancy in congenital deficiencies in AT III, protein C or protein S: study of 78 women. *Thromb Haemost* 1990; **63**: 319–320.

6. Preston FE, Rosendaal FR, Walker ID et al. Increased fetal loss in women with heritable thrombophilia. *Lancet* 1996; **348**: 913–916.

7. Kupferminc MJ, Eldor A, Steinman N et al. Increased frequency of genetic thrombophilia in women with complications of pregnancy. *N Engl J Med* 1999; **340**: 9–13.

8. Koeleman BP, Reitsma PH, Allaart CF, Bertina RM. Activated protein C resistance as an additional risk factor for thrombosis in protein C-deficient families. *Blood* 1994; **84**: 1031–1035.

9. Egeberg O. Inherited antithrombin deficiency causing thrombophilia. *Thromb Diath Haemorrh* 1965; **13**: 516–529.

10. Lane DA, Bayston T, Olds RJ et al. Antithrombin mutation database: 2nd (1997) update. *Thromb Haemost* 1997; 77: 197–211.

11. Lane DA, Mannucci PM, Bauer KA et al. Inherited thrombophilia: Part 1. *Thromb Haemost* 1996; 76: 651–652.

12. Rosendaal FR, Heijboer H, Briët E et al. Mortality in inherited antithrombin III deficiency 1830 to 1989. *Lancet* 1991; 337: 260–262.

13. van Boven HH, Vandenbroucke JP, Westendorp RGJ, Rosendaal FR. Mortality and causes of death in inherited antithrombin deficiency. *Thromb Haemost* 1997; 77: 452–455.

14. Griffin J, Evatt B, Zimmerman T et al. *J Clin Invest* 1981; **68**: 1370–1373.

15. Reitsma PH, Bernardi F, Doig RG et al. Protein C deficiency: a database of mutations, 1995 update. *Thromb Haemost* 1995; **73**: 876–889.

16. Allaart CF, Rosendaal FR, Noteboom WMP, Briët E. Survival in families with hereditary protein C deficiency, 1820 to 1993. *BMJ* 1995; **311**: 910–913.

17. Tuddenham EGD, Cooper DN. Protein C and protein C inhibitor. In: Tuddenham EGD, Cooper DN (eds). *The Molecular Genetics of Haemostasis and its Inherited Disorders*. New York: Oxford University Press, 1994: 149.

18. Tripodi A, Franchi F, Krachmalnikoff A, Mannucci PM. Asymptomatic homozygous protein C deficiency. *Acta Haematol* 1990; **83**: 152–155.

19. Comp P, Esmon C. Recurrent venous thromboembolism in patients with a partial deficiency of protein S. *N Engl J Med* 1984; **311**: 1525–1528.

20. Schwarz HP, Fischer M, Hopmeier P et al. Plasma protein S deficiency in familial thrombotic disease. *Blood* 1984; **64**: 1297–1300.

21. Gandrille S, Borgel D, Ireland H et al. Protein S deficiency: a database of mutations. *Thromb Haemost* 1997; 77: 1201–1214.

22. Dahlbäck B, Carlsson M, Svensson PJ. Familial thrombophilia due to a previously unrecognized mechanism characterized by poor anticoagulant response to activated protein C: prediction of a cofactor to activated protein C. *Proc Natl Acad Sci USA* 1993; **90**: 1004–1008.

23. Bertina RM, Koeleman BP, Koster T et al. Mutation in the blood coagulation factor V associated with the resistance to activated protein C. *Nature* 1994; **369**: 64–67.

24. Chan WP, Lee CK, Kwong YL et al. A novel mutation of Arg306 of factor V gene in Hong Kong Chinese. *Blood* 1998; **91**: 1135–1139.

25. Williamson D, Brown K, Luddington R et al. Factor V Cambridge: A new mutation (Arg[306]→Thr) associated with resistance to activated protein C. *Blood* 1998; **91**: 1140–1144.

26. Zöller B, Hillarp A, Dahlbäck B. Activated protein C resistance caused by a common

factor V mutation has a single origin. *Thromb Res* 1997; **85**: 237–243.

27. Lindqvist PG, Svensson PJ, Dahlbäck B, Marsál K. Factor V Q^{506} mutation (activated protein C resistance) associated with reduced intrapartum blood loss — a possible evolutionary selection mechanism. *Thromb Haemost* 1998; **79**: 69–73.

28. Martinelli I, Cattaneo M, Panzeri D, Mannucci PM. Low prevalence of factor V:Q506 in 41 patients with isolated pulmonary embolism. *Thromb Haemost* 1997; **77**: 440–443.

29. Vandenbroucke JP, Bertina RM, Holmes ZR et al. Factor V Leiden and fatal pulmonary embolism. *Thromb Haemost* 1998; **79**: 511–516.

30. Heijmans BT, Westendorp RGJ, Knook DL et al. The risk of mortality and the factor V Leiden mutation in a population based cohort. *Thromb Haemost* 1998; **80**: 607–609.

31. Moor E, Silveira A, van't Hooft F et al. Coagulation factor V (Arg506→Gln) mutation and early saphenous vein graft occlusion after coronary artery bypass grafting. *Thromb Haemost* 1998; **80**: 220–224.

32. Poort SR, Rosendaal FR, Reitsma PH, Bertina RM. A common genetic variation in the 3′-untranslated region of the prothrombin gene is associated with elevated plasma prothrombin levels and an increase in venous thrombosis. *Blood* 1996; **88**: 3698–3703.

33. Rosendaal FR, Doggen CJM, Zivelin A et al. Geographic distribution of the 20210 G to A prothrombin variant. *Thromb Haemost* 1998; **79**: 706–708.

34. Souto JC, Coll I, Llobet D et al. The prothrombin 20210 A allele is the most prevalent genetic risk factor for venous thromboembolism in the Spanish population. *Thromb Haemost* 1998; **80**: 366–369.

35. den Heijer M, Koster T, Blom HJ et al. Hyperhomocysteinemia as a risk factor for deep-vein thrombosis. *N Engl J Med* 1996; **334**: 759–762.

36. Welch GN, Loscalzo J. Homocysteine and atherothrombosis. *N Engl J Med* 1998; **338**: 1042–1050.

37. Kang S-S, Wong PWK, Susmano A et al. Thermolabile methylene tetrahydrofolate reductase: an inherited risk factor for coronary artery disease. *Am J Hum Genet* 1991; **48**: 536–545.

38. Frosst P, Blom HJ, Milos R et al. A candidate genetic risk factor for vascular disease: a common mutation in methylenetetrahydrofolate reductase. *Nature Genetics* 1995; **10**: 111–113.

39. den Heijer M, Blom HJ, Gerrits WB et al. Is hyperhomocysteinemia a risk factor for recurrent venous thrombosis? *Lancet* 1995; **345**: 882–885.

40. Margaglione M, D'Andrea G, d'Addedda M et al. The methylenetetrahydrofolate reductase TT677 genotype is associated with venous thrombosis independently of the coexistence of the FV Leiden and the prothrombin A^{20210} mutation. *Thromb Haemost* 1998; **79**: 907–911.

41. Kluijtmans LAJ, den Heijer M, Reitsma PH et al. Thermolabile methylenetetrahydrofolate reductase and factor V Leiden in the risk of deep-vein thrombosis. *Thromb Haemost* 1998; **79**: 254–258.

42. Koster T, Blann AD, Briët E et al. Role of clotting factor VIII in effect on von Willebrand factor on occurrence of deep-vein thrombosis. *Lancet* 1995; **345**: 152–155.

43. Kraaijenhagen RA, in't Anker PS, Koopman MMW et al. High plasma concentration of factor VIIIc is a major risk factor for venous thromboembolism. *Thromb Haemost* 2000; **83**: 5–9.

44. Research Committee of the British Thoracic Society. Optimum duration of anticoagulation for deep-vein thrombosis and pulmonary embolism. *Lancet* 1992; **340**: 873–876.

45. Hull RD, Raskob GE, Rosenbloom D et al. Heparin for 5 days as compared with 10 days in the initial treatment of proximal venous thrombosis. *N Engl J Med* 1990, **322**: 1260–1264.

46. Friedrich PW, Sanson B-J, Simioni P et al. Frequency of pregnancy-related venous thromboembolism in anticoagulant factor-deficient women: Implications for prophylaxis. *Ann Intern Med* 1996; **125**: 955–960.

47. De Stefano V, Finazzi G, Mannucci PM. Inherited thrombophilia: pathogenesis, clinical syndromes, and management. *Blood* 1996; **87**: 3531–3544.

48. McColl MD, Ramsay JE, Tait RC et al. Risk factor for pregnancy associated venous thromboembolism. *Thromb Haemost* 1997; **78**: 1183–1188.

49. Hellgren M, Tengborn L, Abildgaard U. Pregnancy in women with congenital antithrombin III deficiency. Experience of treatment with heparin and antithrombin. *Gynecol Obstet Invest* 1982; **14**: 127–141.

50. Orme MLE, Lewis PJ, de Swiet M et al. May mothers given warfarin breast-feed their children? *BMJ* 1977; **1**: 1564–1565.

51. Menache D. Replacement therapy in patients with hereditary antithrombin III deficiency. *Semin Hematol* 1991; **28**: 31–38.

52. Schulman S, Tengborn L. Treatment of venous thromboembolism in patients with congenital deficiency of antithrombin III. *Thromb Haemost* 1992; **68**: 634–636.

53. Sallah S, Thomas DP, Roberts HR. Warfarin and heparin-induced skin necrosis and the purple toe syndrome: infrequent complications of anticoagulant treatment. *Thromb Haemost* 1997; **78**: 785–790.

54. Lindmarker P, Schulman S, Sten-Linder M et al. The risk of recurrent venous thromboembolism in carriers and non-carriers of the G1691A allele in the coagulation factor V gene and the G20210A allele in the prothrombin gene. *Thromb Haemost* 1999; **81**: 684–689.

55. van den Belt AGM, Sanson B-J, Simioni P et al. Recurrence of venous thromboembolism in patients with familial thrombophilia. *Arch Intern Med* 1997; **157**: 2227–2232.

56. Lane DA, Mannucci PM, Bauer KA et al. Inherited thrombophilia: Part 2. *Thromb Haemost* 1996; **76**: 824–834.

57. Vandenbroucke JP, Koster T, Briet E et al. Increased risk of venous thrombosis in oral-contraceptive users who are carriers of factor V Leiden mutation. *Lancet* 1994; **344**: 1453–1457.

58. Schambeck CM, Schwender S, Haubitz I et al. Selective screening for the factor V Leiden mutation: Is it advisable before the prescription of oral contraceptives? *Thromb Haemost* 1997; **78**: 1480–1483.

Acquired hypercoagulable states

Sam Schulman

4

The aetiology of venous thromboembolism is still connected with the triad described by Rudolf Virchow in 1856,[1] namely slowing of the blood stream, changes in the vessel wall and changes in the blood itself. All the risk factors identified so far can be related to one, two or all three elements in Virchow's triad. Venous thromboembolism without any identified risk factor occurs in only 4%,[2] and often more than one risk factor is present.

In many cases the acquired hypercoagulable conditions will act in synergy with an inherited defect to cause clinical thrombosis. In fact, half of the venous thromboembolic events in patients with inherited thrombophilia are triggered by an acquired, temporary hypercoagulable state (see Chapter 3).[3] The acquired conditions can be classified as (a) iatrogenic, (b) conditions secondary to another disease or (c) physiological (*Table 4.1*).

Iatrogenic risk factors

Surgery

Surgery may induce venous thromboembolism via all the components of Virchow's triad. General anaesthesia and

Table 4.1
Acquired conditions with an increased risk of venous thromboembolism

---

Iatrogenic
Major surgery, estrogen treatment, protease inhibitors, L-asparaginase, heparin-induced thrombocytopenia, indwelling intravenous catheters

Secondary to another disease
Cancer, myeloproliferative disorders with thrombocytosis, paroxysmal nocturnal haemoglobinuria, trauma, fracture, stroke, congestive heart failure, myocardial infarction, obesity, immobility due to infection, cardiolipin antibodies or lupus anticoagulant ± systemic lupus erythematosus, Cushing's syndrome, nephrotic syndrome, inflammatory bowel disease, hyperhomocysteinemia, hypofibrinolysis, varicose veins (?)

Physiological
Age ≥40, puerperium, pregnancy, seasonal variation, long travels (?)

---

immobility per- and postoperatively slow down the blood flow. During surgery, vessel walls may be traumatized, as for example the twisting of the femoral vein during total hip replacement.[4] Finally changes in the haemostatic parameters are known to occur, such as significant reductions of the levels of antithrombin and protein C immediately after total hip replacement,[5] acute phase reactions with increased fibrinogen, thrombocytosis and platelet activation with increased aggregability, increased levels of factors II, VII, VIII and XIII and fibrinolytic shutdown after an initial activation of the fibrinolytic system.[6]

Surgery lasting for less than 30 minutes is not considered to cause any significant increase in the risk of thrombosis. The use of local or regional anaesthesia also reduces the risk. Thrombi in the deep veins of the legs have been documented with radiolabeled fibrinogen and with venography in 20–30% of patients after general surgery and in 50–80% of patients after various orthopaedic operations (*Table 4.2*). The highest incidence is observed after total knee replacement (*Figure 4.1*). In most cases the thrombosis will not result in clinical manifestations, and after the patient has been mobilized, recanalization will occur. This may, however, leave permanent damage on the venous valves, and evidence of chronic venous insufficiency is seen in 17% at 3–5 years after a postoperative calf vein thrombosis, verified by fibrinogen scanning.[7] Occasionally the thrombus will be dislodged and cause pulmonary embolism, which may be silent, clinical or fatal.

The risk of postoperative thrombosis is not

Table 4.2
Risks (in %) of venous thromboembolism after general versus orthopedic surgery without prophylaxis

	General surgery	**Orthopedic surgery**
Deep-vein thrombosis	25	50
Clinically manifested	9	23
Proximal	7	20
Pulmonary embolism	1.6	5–10
Fatal	0.8	2–5

limited to the first week or the duration of hospitalization. This is explained by a further increase in the activation of coagulation at the end of the first week at the same time as the venous flow remains reduced for a few weeks.

The incidence of venographically verified deep-vein thrombosis until day 35 in patients who received postoperative prophylaxis with low molecular mass heparin (dalteparin) for only a week after hip replacement is over 30%

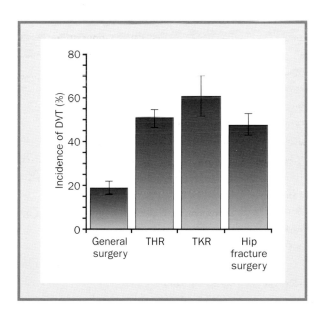

Figure 4.1
Incidence of venographically verified deep-vein thrombosis (DVT) after different kinds of surgery (mean and 95% confidence interval). THR and TKR are total hip or knee replacement, respectively. (Data adapted from Clagett et al.[58])

and that of symptomatic pulmonary embolism 3%.[8] An overview analysis indicated that the vast majority of patients with late postoperative venous thromboembolism already has an asymptomatic thrombosis at the time of discharge.[9] In spite of efforts to improve surgical techniques, anaesthesia, postoperative mobilization and prophylactic regimens, the incidence of fatal pulmonary embolism has not decreased over the years, and this continues to be the major cause of death after hip replacement.[10]

Kidney and liver transplantations are pronounced risk factors for development of thrombosis in the renal and liver veins, respectively. The incidence in prospective paediatric series with these procedures was 10–12%[11] and 7%,[12] respectively.

Oestrogen treatment

The first generation of oral contraceptives, which contained 50–100 mg of oestrogen per tablet, produced a significant risk of venous thromboembolism.[13] Subsequently the contents of the oestrogen component have been progressively reduced with a concomitant favourable effect on the risk of thromboembolism. During the last decade the gestagen component was modified, and unexpectedly there was an increase in the risk of venous thromboembolism.[14]

For the small amounts of oestrogen used in hormone replacement therapy after menopause there is a three-fold increase in the risk of deep-vein thrombosis[15] and two-fold in pulmonary embolism[16] (*Figure 4.2*). When oestrogens in rather high doses are given for prostate cancer there is a substantial risk of venous thromboembolism.[17]

Protease inhibitors

The highly active antiretroviral therapy for patients infected with human immunodeficiency virus consists of a combination of reverse transcriptase inhibitors and a protease inhibitor and has demonstrated remarkable effects on the infection. Unfortunately, some patients develop intolerable side-effects. Among these is a metabolic syndrome with hyperlipidaemia, decreased glucose tolerance and elevated levels of plasminogen activator inhibitor (PAI-1). It is possible that the recently reported increase in occurrence of venous thromboembolism on treatment with protease inhibitors[18] can be related to that syndrome.

L-Asparaginase

In the treatment of acute lymphatic leukaemia L-asparaginase is often used as one of the chemotherapeutic agents. It induces a reduction of the antithrombin level, possibly via decreased synthesis in the liver, and several reports of thromboembolic complications have been published.[19]

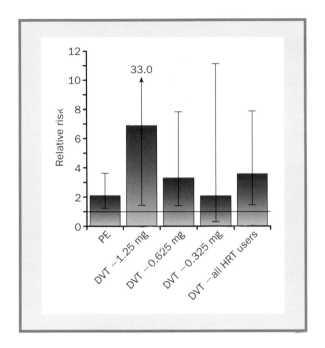

Figure 4.2
Relative risk of idiopathic deep-vein thrombosis (DVT) or pulmonary embolism (PE) in postmenopausal women receiving hormonal replacement therapy. Bar is 95% confidence interval, mg denotes oestrogen dose. (Data adapted from Jick et al[15] and Grodstein et al.[16])

Heparin-induced thrombocytopenia

Patients with heparin-induced thrombocytopenia are at a very high risk of venous and arterial thrombotic complications. In a study of patients receiving thromboprophylaxis with heparin after hip surgery the relative risks of proximal deep-vein thrombosis and of pulmonary embolism were 27 and 93, respectively, in patients with heparin-induced thrombocytopenia compared to those who did not have evidence of this syndrome.[20] An injured blood vessel is the *locus resistentia minoris* for developing thrombosis.

Indwelling intravenous catheters

The most common predisposing factor for deep-vein thrombosis and pulmonary embolism in children is indwelling catheters, being responsible for 21% of the events.[21] In many of these cases additional risk factors for thrombosis are present, such as cancer, septicaemia and sickle cell anaemia. Large vessel thrombosis or pulmonary embolism was found on autopsy in 24% of children who had received critical care support and had not always been clinically diagnosed.[22]

Secondary venous thromboembolism to another disease

Cancer

The classical association between venous thromboembolism and cancer was described in 1865 by Trousseau.[23] It is typically mucin-producing adenocarcinomas that have the highest propensity to cause deep-vein thrombosis. The detection rate of cancer during 2 years after a first episode of venous thrombosis was 7.6% if the thrombotic event was considered idiopathic but significantly lower (1.9%) if it was secondary to an identified triggering factor.[24] The risk of detecting cancer after a venous thromboembolic event is pronounced during the initial 6 months, whereas it is only minimally increased thereafter (see Chapter 16).[25]

Myeloproliferative disorders

In these patients thrombocytosis as well as polycytaemia vera with high blood viscosity are risk factors for venous thromboembolism.

Paroxysmal nocturnal haemoglobinuria

In this haematopoietic disorder with intravascular haemolysis, venous thromboembolism occurs in about 40% of the patients, often repeatedly and with life-threatening episodes.[26] Long-term anticoagulant therapy is therefore recommended for patients with this disorder.

Trauma and fractures

The incidence of venographically verified deep-vein thrombosis in patients with major trauma reaches 58% with proximal-vein thrombosis in 18%,[27] and pulmonary embolism is one of the three main causes of death after the first 24 hours. Additional risk factors in these patients are old age, surgery, blood transfusion, fracture of femur or tibia and spinal cord injury.[28] In patients with leg fractures, treated with plaster cast immobilization, the incidence of symptomatic deep-vein thrombosis, verified with venography, is 4% in patients without any prophylaxis.[28]

Stroke

One of the major causes of death after acute stroke is pulmonary embolism, which was responsible for 13% of the fatalities in one study.[29] Fibrinogen scanning reveals deep-vein thrombosis in 60% of the paralysed limbs and in 7% of the unaffected limbs in patients with stroke.[30] The incidence of symptomatic deep-vein thrombosis was, however, only 1% during the first 10 days in the placebo group of a randomized trial.[31]

Myocardial infarction and congestive heart failure

The increased incidence of venous thromboembolism seen during the short-term recovery after myocardial infarction is related to a combination of risk factors, including immobilization, old age and congestive heart failure. The myocardial infarction is not in itself an independent risk factor, and in the era of rapid administration of acetylsalicylic acid to these patients, treatment with heparin adds a negligible benefit. Congestive heart failure impairs the cardiopulmonary capacity and thereby reduces the likelihood of tolerating pulmonary emboli.

Obesity

The reports regarding obesity as a risk factor for thrombosis are conflicting, which partly can be due to the lack of a uniform definition of this condition. Obesity does not appear to be an independent risk factor for thrombosis and in order to increase the risk of postoperative thrombosis the obesity has to be pronounced, which probably is confounded by a delayed mobilization.

Immobility due to infection

An important risk factor for fatal pulmonary embolism is associated with immobility, which in most cases is unrelated to surgery.[32]

Among patients admitted to the department of infectious disease, there was a fatality rate in pulmonary embolism of 0.4% in those of at least 55 years of age.[33] This is a high incidence, even when compared with surgical studies.

Cardiolipin antibodies/lupus anticoagulant

Patients with systemic lupus erythematosus (SLE) have a high prevalence of venous thromboembolism, often but not always in combination with phospholipid (cardiolipin) antibodies and/or lupus anticoagulant.[34] When phospholipid antibodies are detected in patients with venous and/or arterial thrombosis but the criteria for SLE are not fulfilled, the condition is called primary antiphospholipid syndrome. Thrombocytopenia and habitual, spontaneous abortions are also typical features of this syndrome.[35] The lupus anticoagulants interfere with the prothrombin–phospholipid complex and the cardiolipin antibodies are actually directed against a β2-glycoprotein I-phospholipid complex.[36] The mechanism whereby this causes thrombosis is unclear, but increased expression of procoagulant lipid surfaces with activated platelets, interference with the protein C pathway or with fibrinolysis have been implicated. The prevalence of the syndrome depends partly on the sensitivity of the tests performed, but in a study of 1124 patients with venous thromboembolism, 15% had cardiolipin antibodies.[37] The risk of recurrent venous thromboembolism was doubled and the mortality almost tripled among the patients with antibodies during a 4-year period of observation, including 6 months of anti-vitamin K therapy after the initial event (*Figure 4.3*).[36] Regular intensity of anticoagulation, aiming at an international normalised ratio (INR) of 2–3, appears sufficient for these patients but not for those with SLE and the phospholipid antibody syndrome, in whom INR of at least 3 is advisable.[38]

Behçet's disease

Arterial and venous thrombosis, as well as superficial thrombophlebitis are seen in about one third of the patients. The pathogenesis has not been elucidated and autoantibodies have not been associated with the phenomena.

Cushing's syndrome

The severity of the hormonal changes in Cushing's syndrome is positively correlated with the elevation of factor VIII levels in plasma, and venous thromboembolic complications are common, especially in connection with adrenalectomy.[39]

Nephrotic syndrome

Thromboembolic complications are common in patients with nephrotic syndrome, with an incidence of 33% during 2 years in a prospective study.[40] These patients demonstrate several haemostatic abnormalities, including reduced levels of antithrombin and protein S and increased levels of fibrinogen and factor VIII. The thrombotic events have a predilection for the renal vein, possibly due to the pronounced reduction of antithrombin there after losses due to leakage via the glomeruli to the urine. Pulmonary embolism is also a common feature, demonstrated in seven of 26 children with nephrotic syndrome.[41]

Inflammatory bowel disease

There is a moderate increase in the risk of thromboembolic complications in inflammatory bowel disease, and some of the patients have elevated levels of PAI-1, of fibrinogen or of cardiolipin antibodies, whereas others have a reduced level of antithrombin.[42]

Hyperhomocysteinemia

Inherited enzyme defects may cause mild or severe forms of hyperhomocysteinemia (see Chapter 3). A multitude of acquired risk factors also influences the metabolism of

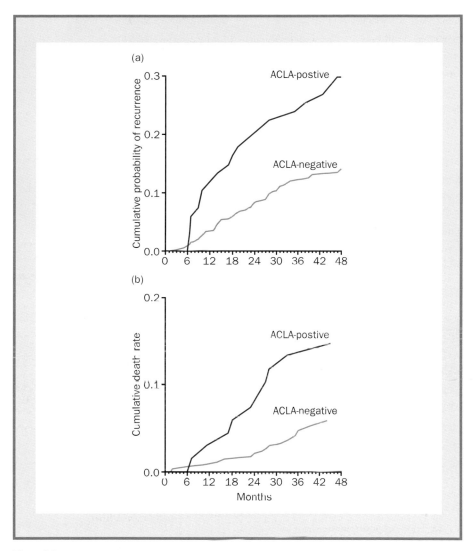

Figure 4.3
Probability of recurrent venous thromboembolism and death rate during 4 years after the first event and 6 months of secondary prophylaxis in patients with and without cardiolipin antibodies. The differences are statistically significant with P = 0.0013 and P = 0.01, respectively, at 48 months. (Reprinted from Am J Med, *vol 104, Schulman et al,[37] copyright 1998, with permission from Excerpta Medica Inc.)*

homocysteine.[43] Moderately increased levels are seen in chronic renal failure and pernicious anaemia. Cancer of the breast, ovary or pancreas, as well as acute lymphoblastic leukaemia can also result in marked elevations. Mildly increased levels have been observed in association with treatment with methotrexate, phenytoin or theophylline and also in smokers. Hypothyroidism and, finally, old age also result in higher homocysteine levels. Hyperhomocysteinemia leads to an increased risk of arterial and venous thromboembolism[43,44] and increases the risk of recurrence of the latter.[45]

Hypofibrinolysis

A reduced fibrinolytic capacity, with typically elevated levels of PAI-1, is usually an acquired condition. It is often seen in patients with metabolic disorders, such as hyperlipidaemia and diabetes, and a normalization can be achieved after improvement of the life style.[46] Laboratory evidence of hypofibrinolysis has been reported in 7–37% of patients with venous thromboembolism in descriptive studies.[47] Conversely, in a prospective cohort study with age- and smoking-matched control subjects, PAI-1 antigen and tissue-type plasminogen activator (t-PA) antigen without venous occlusion did not predict future venous thromboembolism in healthy persons.[48] In a prospective study of patients with venous thromboembolism, randomized

regarding the duration of secondary prophylaxis, increased levels of functional PAI-1 and t-PA antigen correlated with development of a recurrent episode within the next 3–6 years.[49] However, the effect of PAI-1 was weak and the influence of t-PA antigen was dependent on the age of the patient. Thus, although the presence of hypofibrinolysis is of epidemiological interest, the tests are not useful as predictors in the individual case.

Varicose veins

Varicose veins may be a sign of chronic venous disease of the extremity and thus a sequel after deep vein thrombosis. Still, this risk factor is very weak, since among 30 000 patients with varicose veins, treated with surgery, only one succumbed to pulmonary embolism.[50]

Physiological factors
Age

There is a logarithmic increase in the risk of venous thromboembolism with age.[51] Thus, the disease is very rare in children and from age 20 to age 80 there is a 200-fold increase in the incidence. This is associated with increasing levels of fibrinogen, von Willebrand factor, t-PA antigen and homocysteine.

Pregnancy and puerperium

The risk of venous thromboembolism is increased six-fold during pregnancy, rendering this complication the most common cause of maternal death.[52] Fatal pulmonary embolism has been reported at an incidence of 1–3 per 100 000 deliveries.[53] The aetiology is mainly a decreased venous flow, due to obstruction of the iliac veins by the expanding uterus and procoagulant changes in the coagulation and fibrinolytic system. The levels of fibrinogen, factor VIII, von Willebrand factor and the vitamin K-dependent factors II, VII, IX and X as well as of the plasminogen activator inhibitors, PAI-1 and PAI-2 increase. At the same time the protein S level decreases, to some extent also antithrombin and a state of resistance to activated protein C is acquired. See also Chapter 13.

During the puerperium the risk of venous thromboembolism is even higher, with for example three times as many events than during pregnancy in patients with inherited thrombophilia.[3]

Seasonal variation

In some epidemiological studies an increase in the incidence of venous thromboembolism was observed during the winter season.[34] This may be at least partly explained by an observed seasonal variation in fibrinogen, which was 0.34 g/l higher during the winter in a cohort of 7983 persons.[55] One can also assume, that the cluster of hip fractures during the winter contributes in some countries.

Long travels

There are numerous anecdotal reports of venous thromboembolism after long travels, especially by aeroplane, nicknamed 'the economy class syndrome.'[56] However, in a study of elderly volunteers, travelling 8–16 hours by bus, there was no abnormality in parameters of activation of coagulation or of fibrinolysis at the end of the journey.[57] Only the thrombin–antithrombin complex increased, but still remained within the normal range.

Conclusion

A large number of conditions can thus contribute to an increased risk of thromboembolism. The strongest of these risk factors should be considered as important also for asymptomatic individuals. For patients with a previous event of venous thromboembolism all these factors may be crucial when the secondary prophylaxis has been discontinued. By increasing the awareness among medical staff and by educating the patient of such risk factors, it should be possible to reduce the risk of a recurrence.

References

1. Virchow R. *Abhandlungen zur Wissenschafligen Medizin*. Von Medinger Sohn & Co, 1856.

2. Anderson FA Jr, Wheeler HB. Physician practices in the management of venous thromboembolism: a community-wide survey. *J Vasc Surg* 1992; **15**: 707–714.

3. De Stefano V, Leone G, Mastrangelo S et al. Clinical manifestations and management of inherited thrombophilia: retrospective analysis and follow-up after diagnosis of 238 patients with congenital deficiency of antithrombin III, protein C, protein S. *Thromb Haemost* 1994; **72**: 352–358.

4. Stamatakis JD, Kakkar VV, Sagar S et al. Femoral vein thrombosis and total hip replacement. *BMJ* 1977; **66**: 194–201.

5. Flordal PA, Ljungström K-G, Svensson J et al. Effects on coagulation and fibrinolysis of desmopressin in patients undergoing total hip replacement. *Thromb Haemost* 1991; **66**: 652–656.

6. Bergqvist D. *Postoperative Thromboembolism. Frequency, Etiology, Prophylaxis.* Berlin: Springer Verlag, 1983.

7. Lindhagen A, Bergqvist D, Hallböök T. Deep venous insufficiency after postoperative thrombosis diagnosed with ^{125}I-labelled fibrinogen uptake test. *Br J Surg* 1984; **71**: 511–515.

8. Dahl OE, Müller C, Mathiesen P et al. Prolonged prophylaxis following hip replacement surgery — results of a double-blind, prospective, randomised, placebo-controlled study with dalteparin (Fragmin). *Thromb Haemost* 1997; **77**: 26–31.

9. Ricotta S, Iorio A, Parise P et al. Post discharge clinically overt venous thromboembolism in orthopaedic surgery patients with negative venography — an overview analysis. *Thromb Haemost* 1996; **76**: 887–892.

10. Campling EA, Devlin HB, Hoile RW, Lunn JN. The report of the National Confidential Enquiry into Peri-Operative Deaths (NCEPOD), London, UK: Pub, 1993.

11. van Lieburg AF, de Jong MCJW, Hoitsma AJ et al. Renal transplant thrombosis in children. *J Pediatr Surg* 1995; **30**: 615–619.

12. Lallier M, St-Vil D, Dubois J et al. Vascular complications after pediatric liver transplantation. *J Pediatr Surg* 1995; **30**: 1122–1126.

13. Vessey MP, Doll R. Investigation of relation between use of oral contraceptives and thromboembolic disease. *BMJ* 1968; **2**: 199–205.

14. Spitzer WO, Lewis MA, Heinemann LAJ et al. Third generation oral contraceptives and risk of venous thromboembolic disorders: an international case-control study. *Lancet* 1996; **312**: 83–88.

15. Jick H, Derby LE, Myers MW et al. Risk of hospital admission for idiopathic venous thromboembolism among users of postmenopausal oestrogens. *Lancet* 1996; **348**: 981–983.

16. Grodstein F, Stampfer MJ, Goldhaber SZ et al. Prospective study of exogenous hormones and risk of pulmonary embolism in women. *Lancet* 1996; **348**: 983–987.

17. Lundgren R, Sundin T, Colleen S et al. Cardiovascular complications of estrogen therapy for nondisseminated prostatic carcinoma. A preliminary report from a randomized multicenter study. *Scand J Urol Nephrol* 1986; **20**: 101–105.

18. Carr A, Brown D, Cooper DA. Portal vein thrombosis in patients receiving indinavir, a

protease inhibitor. *AIDS* 1997; **11:** 1657–1658.

19. Conard J, Cazenave B, Maury J et al. L-asparaginase, antithrombin III and thrombosis. *Lancet* 1980; **i:** 1091.

20. Warkentin TE, Levine MN, Hirsh J et al. Heparin-induced thrombocytopenia in patients treated with low-molecular-weight heparin or unfractionated heparin. *N Engl J Med* 1995; **332:** 1330–1335.

21. David M, Andrew M. Venous thromboembolic complications in children. *J Pediatr* 1993; **123:** 337–346.

22. Derish MT, Smith DW, Frankel LR. Venous catheter thrombus formation and pulmonary embolism in children. *Pediatr Pulmonol* 1995; **20:** 349–354.

23. Trousseau A. Phlegmasia alba dolens. In: *Clinique Médicale de l-Hôtel Dieu de Paris*, 5th edn. Paris: JB Baillière et Fils, 1865; 639–654.

24. Prandoni P, Lensing AWA, Büller H et al. Deep-vein thrombosis and the incidence of subsequent cancer. *N Engl J Med* 1992; **327:** 1128–1133.

25. Sørensen HT, Mellemkjær L, Steffensen FH et al. The risk of a diagnosis of cancer after primary deep venous thrombosis or pulmonary embolism. *N Engl J Med* 1998; **338:** 1169–1173.

26. Hillmen P, Lewis SM, Bessler M et al. Natural history of paroxysmal nocturnal hemoglobinuria. *N Engl J Med* 1995; **333:** 1253–1258.

27. Geerts WH, Code KI, Jay RM et al. A prospective study of venous thromboembolism after major trauma. *N Engl J Med* 1994; **331:** 1601–1606.

28. Kock H-J, Schmidt-Neuerburg KP, Hanke J et al. Thromboprophylaxis with low-molecular-weight heparin in outpatients with plaster-cast immobilisation of the leg. *Lancet* 1995; **346:** 459–461.

29. Bounds JV, Wiebers DO, Whisnant JP, Okazaki H. Mechanisms and timing of deaths from cerebral infarction. *Stroke* 1981; **12:** 474–477.

30. Warlow C, Ogston D, Douglas AS. Venous thrombosis following strokes. *Lancet* 1972; **i:** 1305–1306.

31. Kay R, Wong KS, Yu YL et al. Low-molecular-weight heparin for the treatment of acute ischemic stroke. *N Engl J Med* 1995; **333:** 1588–1593.

32. Saeger W, Genzkow M. Venous thromboses and pulmonary embolisms in post-mortem series: probable causes by correlation of clinical data and basic diseases. *Pathol Res Pract* 1994; **190:** 394–399.

33. Gårdlund B. Fatal pulmonary embolism in hospitalized non-surgical patients. *Acta Med Scand* 1985; **218:** 417–421.

34. Long AA, Ginsberg JS, Brill-Edwards P et al. The relationship of antiphospholipid antibodies to thromboembolic disease in systemic lupus erythematosus. *Thromb Haemost* 1991; **66:** 520–524.

35. Asherson RA, Khamashta MA, Ordi-Ros J et al. The 'primary' antiphospholipid syndrome: major clinical and serological features. *Medicine (Baltimore)* 1989; **68:** 366–374.

36. McNeil HP, Simpson RJ, Chesterman CN, Krillis SA. Antiphospholipid antibodies are directed against a complex antigen that includes a lipid-binding inhibitor of coagulation: β2-glycoprotein I (apolipoprotein H). *Proc Natl Acad Sci USA* 1990; **87:** 4120–4124.

37. Schulman S, Svenungsson E, Granqvist S and the Duration of Anticoagulation Trial Study Group. The predictive value of anticardiolipin antibodies in patients with venous thromboembolism. *Am J Med* 1998; **104:** 332–338.

38. Khamashta MA, Cuadrado MJ, Mujic F et al. The management of thrombosis in the antiphospholipid-antibody syndrome. *N Engl J Med* 1995; **332:** 993–997.

39. Sjöberg HE, Blombäck M, Granberg PO. Thromboembolic complications, heparin treatment and increase in coagulation factors in Cushing's syndrome. *Acta Med Scand* 1976; **199:** 95–98.

40. Llach F, Arieff AI, Massry SG. Renal vein thrombosis and nephrotic syndrome. A prospective study of 36 adult patients. *Ann Intern Med* 1975; **83:** 8–14.

41. Hoyer PF, Gonda S, Barthels M et al. Thromboembolic complications in children with nephrotic syndrome. Risk and incidence. *Acta Paediatr Scand* 1986; **75:** 804–810.

42. Vecchi M, Cattaneo M, de Franchis R, Mannucci PM. Risk of thromboembolic complications in patients with inflammatory bowel disease. Study of hemostasis measurements. *Int J Clin Lab Res* 1991; **21:** 165–170.

43. Welch GN, Loscalzo J. Homocysteine and atherothrombosis. *N Engl J Med* 1998; **338:** 1042–1050.

44. den Heijer M, Koster T, Blom HJ et al. Hyperhomocysteinemia as a risk factor for deep-vein thrombosis. *N Engl J Med* 1996; **334:** 759–762.

45. Eichinger S, Stümpflen A, Hirschl M et al. Hyperhomocysteinemia is a risk factor of recurrent venous thromboembolism. *Thromb Haemost* 1998; **80:** 566–569.

46. Schulman S, Lindmarker P, Johnsson H. Influence of changes in life style on fibrinolytic parameters and recurrency rate in patients with venous thromboembolism. *Blood Coag Fibrinol* 1995; **6:** 311–316.

47. Prins MH, Hirsh J. A critical review of the evidence supporting a relationship between impaired fibrinolytic activity and venous thromboembolism. *Arch Intern Med* 1991; **151:** 1721–1731.

48. Ridker PM, Vaughan DE, Stampfer MJ et al. Baseline fibrinolytic state and the risk of future venous thrombosis. A prospective study of endogenous tissue-type plasminogen activator and plasminogen activator inhibitor. *Circulation* 1992; **85:** 1822–1827.

49. Schulman S, Wiman B and the Duration of Anticoagulation (DURAC) Trial Study Group. The significance of hypofibrinolysis for the risk of recurrence of venous thromboembolism. *Thromb Haemost* 1996; **75:** 607–611.

50. May R. Varicose veins. In: May R (ed). *Surgery of the Veins of the Leg and Pelvis.* Stuttgart: Thieme, 1979.

51. Anderson FA, Wheeler HB, Goldberg RJ et al. A population-based perspective of the hospital incidence and case-fatality rates of deep vein thrombosis and pulmonary embolism. *Arch Intern Med* 1991; **151:** 933–938.

52. Turnball A, Tindall VR, Beard RW. Report on confidential enquiries into maternal death in England and Wales 1982–1984. London: HMSO, 1989; 28–36.

53. Tooke JE, McNicol GP. Thrombotic disorders associated with pregnancy and the pill. *Clin Haematol* 1981; **10:** 613–630.

54. Gallerani M, Manfredini R, Ricci L et al. Sudden death from pulmonary

thromboembolism: chronobiological aspects. *Eur Heart J* 1992; **13**: 661–665.

55. van der Bom JG, de Maat MPM, Bots ML et al. Seasonal variation in fibrinogen in the Rotterdam Study. *Thromb Haemost* 1997; **78**: 1059–1062.

56. Cruickshank JM, Goprlin R, Jennett B. Air travel and thrombotic episodes: the economy class syndrome. *Lancet* 1988; **i**: 497–498.

57. Tardy B, Tardy-Poncet B, Bara L et al. Effects of long travels in sitting position in elderly volunteers on biological markers of coagulation activation and fibrinolysis. *Thromb Res* 1996; **83**: 153–160.

58. Clagett GP, Anderson FA, Geerts WH et al. Prevention of venous thromboembolism. *Chest* 1998; **114** (**Suppl**): 531S–560S.

Laboratory evaluation of prothrombotic risk

Benjamin Brenner

5

Hemostasis and thrombosis are complex and dynamic phenomena involving numerous proteins and a number of cells that participate in an orderly and intricate fashion in these processes. Thrombosis may occur when prothrombotic processes overrun the natural antithrombotic mechanisms.

By clinical definition, the hemostatic system can present three phenotypes related to thrombosis. First, the clinically normal phenotype can be characterized by either balanced hemostasis or a subclinical prothrombotic state. The second phenotype shows local thrombosis in venous or arterial vessels manifesting as deep-vein thrombosis, cerebral arterial thrombosis, coronary thrombosis, etc. The third phenotype shows systemic thrombosis potentially involving the entire vascular system manifested as disseminated intravascular coagulation (DIC).

Ideally, measurement of the prothrombotic risk should define the potential for thrombosis thereby enabling optimization of therapeutic modalities in an individual at a certain clinical situation. This chapter focuses on current laboratory evaluation of inherited and acquired prothrombotic risk factors.

Screening tests

Screening tests are widely used for evaluation of hemorrhagic disorders and bleeding tendency. Thus, one can predict bleeding following a surgical procedure by measuring the prothrombin time (PT), activated partial thromboplastin time (APTT), platelet count and the bleeding time. Furthermore, abnormalities in one or more of these screening assays may allow focused laboratory work-up directed toward identification of an inherited or an acquired bleeding disorder.

In contrast, these screening tests of hemostasis are not useful for evaluation of thrombotic tendency. In fact, abnormalities in PT, APTT, platelet counts and bleeding time are largely confined to the extreme situation of DIC, a systemic thrombotic disorder with an excessive consumption of platelets and coagulation factors.[1] However, in patients with local venous or arterial thrombosis these screening tests are usually normal. This is not really surprising, as it is hard to imagine how a local thrombus can influence the systemic circulation. In fact, it is easier to imagine that a systemic prothrombotic state, which can potentially be evaluated in the systemic circulation, may, upon local conditions, lead to expression of thrombosis at a specific vessel.

However, in certain situations a large local thrombus can be detected in the systemic circulation. For example, presence of deep-vein thrombosis in the leg, which can measure up to 80 ml in volume, may lead to an increase in fibrin degradation products like D-dimer in the systemic circulation.[2] In contrast, a small clot in a coronary artery measuring 0.1 ml would not result in an increase of D-dimer in the peripheral blood.[3] A predictive role of APTT and PT assays as a prothrombotic marker has not been established. The APTT may be shortened in pregnant women presenting with vascular complications of pregnancy like pre-eclampsia due to an increase in plasma coagulation factors levels.[4] A shortened APTT can be found in some patients with activated protein C (APC) resistance.[5] Similarly, a shortened PT can be found in some patients with APC-resistance due to factor V Leiden as well as in certain patients with factor II G20210A mutation, which is characterized by a 20–50% increase in prothrombin plasma levels.[6] However, the PT and APTT cannot detect most patients with these clinical presentations or those with other thrombophilic mutations. Thus, these assays cannot be used to screen for the prothrombotic risk.

Why the PT and APTT are useful for screening for bleeding disorders, characterized by prolongation of these tests, and not useful for detection of prothrombotic risk characterized by shortened PT and APTT is not entirely clear. However, one potential clue is related to the tests themselves. If the normal PT is 10–12 seconds, it is easier to detect prolongation than to detect significant shortening of this already relatively short time. If this assumption is correct, coagulation assays with longer normal coagulation time can potentially improve screening for thrombotic disorders. This is highly warranted as thrombotic disorders are much more common than bleeding disorders and as current evaluation involves work-up for a large number of inherited and acquired prothrombotic risk factors that is both time consuming and costly.

Evaluation of thrombophilia (Tables 5.1 and 5.2)

Currently, the three most common inherited thrombophilic states are factor V Leiden, which results in APC-resistance, methylenetetrahydrofolate reductase (MTHFR) C677T, which may lead to hyperhomocysteinemia; and factor II

G20210A mutation. Altogether these three mutations account for 50–60% of all venous thrombotic events.[7,8] In addition, about 5–10% of venous thromboses can be related to other less common inherited thrombophilias including protein C, protein S and antithrombin deficiencies.[9,10] Fewer than 1% of patients with inherited thrombophilias are found to have dysfibrinogenemia.[10] More recently, mutations in the thrombomodulin gene have been reported to be associated with thrombophilia.[11]

The presence of antiphospholipid antibodies is searched for as a part of the evaluation for acquired thrombophilia. These antibodies are involved in 5–15% of all cases of thrombosis while thrombosis is manifested in 30% of patients with antiphospholipid antibodies.[12] Thus altogether, testing for all of the above mentioned abnormalities will result

Table 5.1
Evaluation of thrombophilia

Plasma-based assays	Assay type
Antithrombin activity	Coagulation, amidolytic
Antithrombin antigen	EIA, ELISA
Protein C activity	Coagulation, amidolytic
Protein C antigen	ELISA
Protein S activity	Coagulation
Protein S antigen	ELISA
Activated protein C resistance	Coagulation
Thrombin time	Coagulation

Table 5.2
PCR-based assays for common thrombophilias

Mutation	Biochemical alteration	Prevalence (%)	Ethnic predisposition	Thrombotic risk (OR)
Factor V Leiden	APC-resistance	1–15	Caucasians	6–8
Prothrombin G20210A	Prothrombin elevation	1–5	Caucasians	3
MTHFR C677T	Hyperhomocysteinemia	10–15	No	1–2

in identification of abnormalities in about 65–75% of all evaluated patients.

Of the three common thrombophilic states, factor V Leiden is the most important regarding the thrombotic risk involved, which is estimated to be 6–8-fold in heterozygotes and 50–100-fold in homozygotes.[13,14] In addition, the relatively high prevalence in the Caucasian population[15] implies that screening for factor V Leiden in Caucasians with thrombosis is highly warranted.

It is still debatable whether homozygosity for the MTHFR C677T mutation by itself is a risk factor for venous and arterial thrombosis.[16,17] However, hyperhomocysteinemia is a common risk factor for venous and arterial thrombosis as well as for recurrence of venous thrombosis.[18–20]

In view of the limitations of a screening test for evaluation of thrombophilia, recent innovative efforts have resulted in the description of novel global protein C-pathway screening tests. These tests are designed to screen for all potential inherited and acquired abnormalities in the protein C system including those involving protein C, protein S, thrombomodulin, APC-resistance and factor V Leiden.[21,22]

Acquired APC-resistance not related to factor V Leiden mutation is probably an important and relatively common prothrombotic risk factor. It is being increasingly reported in young women on oral contraceptives, and in women who receive hormone replacement therapy.[23,24] In addition, acquired APC-resistance has been reported during normal pregnancy and more often in women with vascular complications of pregnancy such as pre-eclampsia and pregnancy loss.[25,26] APC-resistance can be found in 30–50% of patients with antiphospholipid syndrome[27] and in fact, may be one of the mechanisms for thrombosis in patients with antiphospholipid syndrome.[28] Other conditions associated with abnormalities of the protein C system include cancer in which decreases in protein C and protein S plasma levels[29] and acquired APC-resistance have all been reported.

Infectious diseases of various types including bacterial, viral and ricketsial disease can lead to consumption of protein C and protein S occasionally in association with devastating purpura fulminans.[30] Inflammatory disorders in general and autoimmune diseases in particular are associated with changes in free protein S and C_4 bound-protein S plasma levels.[31] Preliminary results of studies evaluating the protein C global assay suggest that the assay is highly sensitive in detecting patients with factor V Leiden mutation (100%) and protein C deficiency (97%).[22] The test can identify individuals with factor V Leiden who are on anticoagulant therapy. However, the assay has a lower sensitivity for detection of protein S deficiency (77%) and is less useful for detection of changes in women on oral contraceptives or to detect the effect of lupus anticoagulant.[22]

Thrombophilic polymorphism analysis by PCR-based assays (Table 5.2)

Currently, the three most commonly performed polymerase chain reaction (PCR) based assays are those involving factor V Leiden, MTHFR C677T and factor II G20210A. The methodology for performing these assays includes PCR amplifications and restriction enzyme analysis.

To start, 5 ml 3.8% citrated blood is collected by venepuncture. Genomic DNA is extracted from blood leukocytes by standard techniques.

- **Factor V G1691A**: a 208-bp genomic DNA fragment of factor V around nucleotide 1691 is amplified by PCR and then digested with *Mnl*-I as previously described.[14,32]
- **Factor II G20210A**: a 253-bp DNA fragment of the 3'-untranslated region of the prothrombin gene that includes the nucleotide 20210 is amplified with the primer 5'-CAACCGCTGGTATCAAA-TGG-3' and a mutagenic primer as described by Poort et al.[6] The amplified fragment is then digested with *Hind* III.
- **TT-MTHFR C677T**: the MTHFR 677C→T substitution is analysed by an amplification of a 198-bp DNA fragment followed by *Hinf*1 digestion, as described by De Franchis et al.[33]

Digested fragments are electrophoresed on 10% polyacrylamide gels and visualized by ethidium bromide staining.

APC-resistance assays

Following the original observation by Dahlback et al[34] that clotting assays of plasma from certain patients with venous thrombosis are not increased sufficiently in the presence of activated protein C, a growing number of APC-resistant tests have been developed.

The standard APC-resistance assay measures APTT of plasma in the presence or absence of a standardized amount of APC. Results are calculated as a ratio where APC-sensitivity ratio (APC-SR) is defined as APTT in the presence of APC divided by APTT without APC. Normal individuals have an APC-SR greater than 2.0 while patients heterozygous for factor V Leiden mutation usually have an APC-SR of 1.5–2.0 and homozygotes usually demonstrate an APC-SR of 1.1–1.4. Some overlap does occur and occasionally a patient with factor V Leiden may be found to have an APC-SR of 2.0–2.3. Some of these tests were designed to overcome the effect of oral anticoagulant therapy — a common clinical reality in patients with thrombosis.[35] These assays applied sample plasma prediluted with factor V-depleted plasma and have been reported to overcome diagnostic problems related to presence of heparin and lupus anticoagulant as well.[36]

These modified tests, which now include a number of assays based on the degree of APC-induced prolongation of Russel viper venom factor X activation, bring the sensitivity and specificity of factor V Leiden detection close to 100%. However, use of these tests solely will not detect cases of acquired APC-resistance, which can be detected by the original nonmodified APC-resistance assays. Thus, as the role of acquired APC-resistance is increasingly recognized in a variety of clinical settings, one should apply the original nonmodified APC-resistance test along with a PCR-based test to detect factor V Leiden mutation.

Protein C

Protein C is a vitamin K-dependent protein, which is synthesized in hepatocytes and then carboxylated by γ-glutamyl carboxylase in the liver cells. Protein C activity is determined by a functional assay based on activation of protein C to APC in test plasma, by thrombin, by the complex of thrombin–thrombomodulin or by Protac, a snake venom. This is followed by detection of amidolytic activity or anticoagulant activity of APC determined by prolongation of APTT in a clot-based assay.

The advantage of Protac is that it is a selective activator of protein C. Impaired amidolytic activity is detected when the active site of protein C cannot be activated. The clot-based assay provides further information on potential functional defects involving the interaction of APC with phospholipids, factor V and factor VIII.

The normal range for protein C plasma levels is 70–130 U/dl. Heterozygotes for protein C deficiency usually have activity levels of 40–60 U/dl with similar levels obtained by immunological methods measuring protein C antigen.[37] By definition, 2% of the population will have borderline-low protein C levels. These individuals rarely have clinical manifestations of thrombosis and therefore have only low laboratory values, which do not have direct clinical implications.[38] Protein C levels are reduced in patients on oral anticoagulant treatment and in this case protein C levels should be compared to plasma levels of other vitamin K-dependent factors. Likewise, in patients with vitamin K deficiency and in patients harboring the rare mutation in the γ glutamyl-carboxylase gene[39] plasma levels of protein C and all other vitamin K-dependent factors are decreased. Over 160 mutations in the protein C gene have been reported. Mutation analysis is performed at a specialized laboratory.[40]

A rare but potentially devastating manifestation in protein C-deficient patients is skin necrosis or purpura fulminans. This severe thrombotic phenomenon results from thrombosis of vessels at the dermis and has been reported in three clinical settings. First, neonatal purpura fulminans is a life-threatening presentation of neonates with homozygous protein C deficiency.[41] Second, infants and young children may present with severe acquired decrease in protein C level during infections. Finally, patients on oral anticoagulant therapy may present with warfarin skin necrosis.[42]

About 10–15% of patients with protein C deficiency may harbor another thrombophilic defect, most commonly factor V Leiden which increases the risk for thrombosis implying the clinical and practical necessity for comprehensive evaluation of thrombophilia.[43,44]

Protein S

Protein S, a vitamin K-dependent protein synthesized in the liver cells is a cofactor for protein C in the degradation reaction of factor V and factor VIII. Deficiency of protein S has been reported to result in thrombosis in heterozygotes and in purpura fulminans in homozygote neonates. Detection of protein S deficiency is based upon determination of a decrease in protein S plasma activity and antigen levels. As protein S circulates in two forms, free and C_4-protein bound, the concentrations of protein S and C_4-binding protein determine the free protein S plasma level.

Three types of hereditary heterozygous protein S deficiency have been recognized.[45] Type I is dominated by reduced total and free protein S antigen levels and reduced free protein S activity. Type II deficiency is characterized by abnormal protein S molecules, therefore antigen level is normal but activity is low. Type III deficiency is defined by reduced free protein S antigen and activity but normal total protein S levels.

Protein S activity is measured by the degree of prolongation of APTT following incubation of test plasma diluted with protein S-depleted plasma, with either Protac, which activates protein C, or with a fixed amount of APC. Total and free protein S antigen levels are measured by immunological methods. These have included in the past electroimmunoassay and more recently enzyme-linked immunosorbent assays (ELISA). A variety of different ELISAs has been employed but the interpretation of these assays may still occasionally remain a diagnostic problem.

One potential caveat resulting from these assays is related to misdiagnosis of protein S deficiency in patients with APC-resistance. Although the modified APC-resistance tests and several recently developed assays for protein S, have reduced the diagnostic problem of determination of protein S deficiency in the presence of APC-resistance,[46] the problem has not yet been entirely solved.

It has been reported that about 5–15% of patients with protein S deficiency may have combined thrombophilia most likely with factor V Leiden mutation.[47] Protein S plasma levels are reduced in patients with liver disease, pregnancy, certain infectious diseases and in subjects on oral anticoagulant therapy. Patients with autoimmune disorders like the antiphospholipid syndrome or systemic lupus erythematosus often present with low free protein S levels resulting from an increase in binding of protein S by the C_4-binding protein.

Thrombomodulin

Thrombomodulin is expressed on endothelial cells following coagulation activation and serves as a cofactor for the activation of protein C to APC by thrombin. While acquired defects resulting from antibodies directed toward thrombomodulin have been previously searched for,[48] inherited defects in the thrombomodulin gene have only recently been described.[11] It is still unclear whether these mutations, reported to be uncommon in the general population, are indeed associated with a thrombotic phenotype. Analysis of these mutations is currently restricted to specialized research laboratories.

Antithrombin

Antithrombin inhibits thrombin and other serine proteases including factors IXa, Xa, XIa and XIIa. This inhibition is increased 2000-fold in the presence of heparin or heparin sulfate molecules on endothelial cells.

Inherited deficiency of antithrombin was the first reported inherited thrombophilic state. Antithrombin deficiency is an autosomal dominant inherited thrombophilia.[49] This deficiency results in a thrombotic phenotype that mainly involves the venous system. Antithrombin plasma levels decrease in liver disease, massive thrombosis, nephrotic syndrome, inflammatory bowel disease, disseminated intravascular coagulation and during heparin therapy.

Antithrombin has two functional domains, the reactive center $Arg^{393}Ser^{394}$ and the heparin-binding site located at the N-terminus of the molecule. Thrombin cleaves the reactive site and forms the inactive thrombin–antithrombin complex. Mutations near the active site of antithrombin have been reported.[49] Likewise, other point mutations were reported near the heparin-binding site. Laboratory evaluation of antithrombin deficiency includes functional and immunological assays. Antithrombin antigen level is detected by immunological assays including electroimmunoassay and ELISA.

The four types of antithrombin deficiency include the quantitative type I deficiency where both activity and antigenicity levels are reduced. In addition, three type II functional type antithrombin deficiencies are now recognized.[49] These include reactive site defects, heparin-binding site defects and pleomorphic type defects. Crossed-immunoelectrophoresis is often useful to document an abnormal migration of a defective antithrombin molecule.

Dysfibrinogenemia

Inherited abnormalities in fibrinogen structure and function may result in different clinical phenotypes including bleeding, thrombosis or no overt clinical symptoms. Inherited dysfibrinogenemia can be detected by relatively simple screening assays. While the PT and APTT are usually normal, the thrombin time is prolonged and performing the assay by using different concentrations of thrombin can help in this regard. Fibrinogen level is usually normal. Further analysis of a particular dysfibrinogenemia requires biochemical evaluation of fibrin formation[50] and imaging procedures such as scanning electron-microscopy or atomic force microscopy.[50]

Antiphospholipid antibodies (Table 5.3)

These autoantibodies are directed to complexes of proteins and negatively charged phospholipids. The clinically relevant antibodies are mostly of the IgG type, although other types like IgM and IgA have been reported. These antibodies can be detected in a variety of disease states including autoimmune disorders, infectious diseases, malignancies or in relation to drugs as well as in normal individuals.[51]

The clinical implications of these autoantibodies are related to the degree of

Table 5.3
Evaluation of antiphospholipid antibodies

Detection of lupus anticoagulant
(1) Prolongation of coagulation assays by dRVVT, TTI, KCT
(2) Failure to normalize prolongation by mixing studies
(3) Normalization by high concentrations of phospholipids

Detection of anticardiolipin antibodies
IgG, IgM, IgA, ELISA
anti-β_2 GPI antibodies

Other antibodies
Antiendothelial cell antibodies
Antiprothrombin antibodies
Antiannexin V antibodies

involvement of tissues or organs. Multiple autoantibodies directed toward several tissues can be detected in an individual patient. Most commonly, these antibodies have been reported in patients with the antiphospholipid syndrome manifested by thrombosis in arterial and venous vessels, pregnancy loss and thrombocytopenia.

Screening assays for antiphospholipid antibodies include ELISA for anticardiolipin and tests for lupus anticoagulant. The latter is detected and confirmed by the following triad[52]:

1. Prolongation of a coagulation assay such as a lupus anticoagulant sensitive APTT, thromboplastin titration index (TTI), diluted Russel viper venom test (dRVVT) or kaolin clotting time (KCT).

The APTT and KCT are based on contact activation of the intrinsic pathway, the TTI on activation of the extrinsic pathway and the dRVVT on direct activation of factor X.

2. Demonstration that the prolonged coagulation assay is not corrected by mixing studies with normal plasma.

3. Normalization of the prolonged coagulation time by high concentration of phospholipids such as those used in the platelet neutralization test.

It is now well established that other autoantibodies may be involved in the thrombotic tendency observed in patients with antiphospholipid antibodies. These include antiendothelial cell antibodies, antiprothrombin and antiannexin V antibodies[51,53] as well as antibodies directed to specific phospholipids such as phosphatidyl serine, phosphatidyl choline, phosphatidyl inositol and phosphatidyl ethanolamine. Patients with the antiphospholipid syndrome phenotype may have one or more of these autoantibodies even without harboring the classical lupus anticoagulant or anticardiolipin antibodies.

Plasma homocysteine (Table 5.4)

Homocysteine is a nonessential amino acid which is rapidly remethylated to methionine or transulfurated to cystathionine. These are established by a number of enzymes and by several cofactors including vitamin B12, folic acid, vitamin B6 and betaine. Enzymatic deficiencies or polymorphisms and nutritional deficiencies may result in hyperhomocysteinemia.[54] For detection of homocysteine levels, blood is obtained with 3.8% sodium citrate. Samples should be taken on the morning after fasting due to circadian changes in homocysteine levels. Normal plasma levels are in the range 5–15 μmol/l. These levels are determined by HPLC. Mild to moderate elevations of 15–50 μmol/l are detected mostly in patients with nutritional deficiencies as well as with those harboring the common thermolabile methylene-tetrahydrofolate reductase C677T polymorphism. Marked elevations over

Table 5.4
Causes of hyperhomocysteinemia

		Prevalence	HC level (μmol/l)
(a)	**Genetic**		
	Homozygous enzyme defects	1/250 000	>100
	TL-MTHFR C677T	1/10	5–25
b)	**Metabolic**		
	Renal failure	1/1000	>50
	Antiphospholipid syndrome	1/500	15–25
(c)	**Nutritional**		
	Folic acid deficiency	1/20	15–25
	Vitamin B12 deficiency	1/50	15–25
(d)	**Drugs**		
	Methotrexate	1/1000	15–50

100 μmol/l can be detected in patients with homozygous hyperhomocysteinemia or homocysteinuria, a rare disorder characterized by severe thrombotic tendency in childhood.[32]

Heparin-induced thrombocytopenia

Laboratory diagnosis of heparin-induced thrombocytopenia has important clinical implications regarding discontinuation of heparin therapy and institution of danaparoid or hirudin in the appropriate clinical setting. Diagnosis is supported by two types of assays: functional tests and immunoassays. The most sensitive functional assay (>90%) involves ^{14}C serotonin release. However, for practical reasons the most convenient and widely used assay is aggregation of platelets obtained from normal donors, in the presence of patient serum, with heparin.[55] This assay can be performed in a routine hemostasis laboratory. However, the sensitivity of this test is low (~50%).

Immunoassays for diagnosis of heparin-induced thrombocytopenia include several ELISAs which measure IgG, IgM or IgA that bind to platelet factor 4–heparin complexes on microtiter plates.[56] The sensitivity of these ELISAs is high (80–90%). For practical reasons, diagnosis of heparin-induced thrombocytopenia requires performance of a rapid functional assay and ELISA.

Table 5.5
Prothrombotic markers

		Clinical correlation
(a)	**Coagulation factors**	
	Fibrinogen	MI, CVA
	Factor VII	MI, CVA
	Factor VIII	VTE
(b)	**Activation peptides**	
	Fibrinopeptide A	AT, VTE, Anticoagulant therapy
	Prothrombin fragment 1 + 2	AT, VTE
(c)	Thrombin–antithrombin complexes	AT, VTE, DIC
(d)	Fibrin degradation products (D-dimer)	VTE, AT, DIC

MI, myocardial infarction; CVA, cerebral vascular accident; VTE, venous thromboembolism; AT, arterial thrombosis; DIC, disseminated intravascular coagulation.

Coagulation factors and activation markers (Table 5.5)

An increase in coagulation factor plasma levels has been reported to be associated with arterial and venous thrombosis. For example, an increase in factor VII and fibrinogen levels were associated with myocardial infarction (MI) and increased factor VIII levels were recently reported in patients with venous thrombosis.[8]

Activation markers of coagulation are peptides, which can be detected in plasma following activation of certain coagulation factors. The most frequently used are prothrombin fragment 1 + 2 formed in the process of activation of prothrombin to thrombin and fibrinopeptide A formed following cleavage of fibrinogen by thrombin. Another marker of coagulation activation is the thrombin–antithrombin (TAT) complexes.

These markers of coagulation activation have been used to detect the prothrombotic potential in patients with inherited or acquired thrombophilia as well as to analyse the safety of coagulation concentrates manufactured for treatment of patients with bleeding disorders. Activation markers are reported to be increased in women receiving hormone replacement therapy, explaining in part their increased thrombotic tendency.

Owing to its long half-life (150 minutes), factor VIIa can be detected in plasma following activation of factor VII. Other coagulation enzymes cannot be easily detected in blood due to their extremely short half-lives. In contrast, activation peptides and coagulation enzyme-inhibitor complexes have longer half-lives, which facilitate their detection.

Fibrinopeptide A was the first reported marker of coagulation activation. The short half-life (3–5 minutes) implies that radioimmunoassay or immunoenzymatic assay of fibrinopeptide A detects only very recent coagulation activation.[57] Prothrombin fragment 1 + 2 has a longer half-life (90 minutes). The application of this ELISA is for detection of prothrombotic events relating to activation of prothrombin.[58] TAT complex is also detected by ELISA. The half-life of the TAT complex is short (15 minutes).

The above-mentioned assays are often used to detect coagulation activation in research projects as well as in certain clinical situations. These include venous and arterial thromboembolism, in patients with inherited thrombophilias, or in acquired thrombophilic states like acute promyelocytic leukemia or endotoxinemia. It has been reported that anticoagulant therapy leads to a decrease and even normalization of elevated activation markers in patients with thrombosis, suggesting that these markers may be useful for monitoring the efficacy of anticoagulant therapy.[59]

Endogenous thrombin potential

As thrombin is the most potent procoagulant, estimation of the potential for thrombin generation is warranted as a measure of the prothrombotic state. It has been suggested that determination of endogenous thrombin potential is useful for detection of the prothrombotic state.[60]

Future perspectives

The number of characterized thrombophilias is growing rapidly, and it is anticipated that the majority of inherited thrombophilic states will be characterized in the coming years. Efforts should be directed toward better screening tests for the prothrombotic state. Progress in these directions will improve cost-effective detection of individuals with increased thrombotic risk, and potentially will enable prevention of thrombosis in large populations at risk.

References

1. Bick RL. Disseminated intravascular coagulation: objective clinical and laboratory diagnosis, treatment and assessment of therapeutic response. *Semin Thromb Hemostas* 1996; **22**: 69–88.

2. Brenner B, Francis CW, Totterman S et al. Non-invasive quantitation of clot lysis in patients with deep vein thrombosis using a modified D-dimer assay. *Circulation* 1990; **81**: 1818–1825.

3. Brenner B, Francis CW, Fitzpatrick PG et al. Relation of pre- and post-thrombolytic treatment plasma D-dimer concentrations to coronary artery reperfusion in patients with acute myocardial infarction. *Am J Cardiol* 1989; **63**: 1179–1184.

4. Brenner B, Zwang E, Bronstein M, Seligsohn U. von Willebrand factor multimer patterns in pregnancy induced hypertension. *Thromb Haemost* 1989; **62**: 715–717.

5. Griffin JH, Heeb MJ, Kojima Y et al. Activated protein C resistance: molecular mechanisms. *Thromb Haemost* 1995; **74**: 444–448.

6. Poort SW, Rosendaal FR, Reitsma PH, Bertina RM. A common genetic variation in the 3'-untranslated region of the prothrombin gene is associated with elevated plasma prothrombin levels and an increase in venous thrombosis. *Blood* 1996; **88**: 3698–3703.

7. Solomon O, Steinberg DM, Zivelin A et al. Single and combined prothrombotic factors in patients with idiopathic venous thromboembolism. *Arterioscl Thromb Vasc Biol* 1999; **19**: 511–518.

8. Rosendaal FR. Thrombosis in the young: epidemiology and risk factors. A focus on venous thrombosis. *Thromb Haemost* 1997; **78**: 1–6.

9. Taberno MD, Tomas JF, Alberca I et al. Incidence and clinical characteristics of hereditary disorders associated with venous thrombosis. *Am J Hematol* 1991; **36**: 249–254.

10. Cote HCF, Lord ST, Pratt KP. γ-chain dysfibrinogenemias: molecular structure function relationship of naturally occurring

mutations in the γ chain of human fibrinogen. *Blood* 1998; **92**: 2195–2212.

11. Öhlin AK, Norlund L, Marlar RA. Thrombomodulin gene variations and thromboembolic disease. *Thromb Haemost* 1997; **78**: 396–400.

12. Galli M, Finazzi G, Barbui T. Antiphospholipid antibodies. Predictive value of laboratory tests. *Thromb Haemost* 1997; **78**: 75–78.

13. Svensson PJ, Dahlback B. Resistance to activated protein C as the basis for venous thrombosis. *N Engl J Med* 1994; **330**: 517–522.

14. Bertina RM, Koeleman BPC, Koster T et al. Mutation in blood coagulation factor V associated with resistance to activated protein C. *Nature* 1994; **369**: 64–67.

15. Zivelin A, Griffin JH, Xu X et al. A single genetic origin for a common Caucasian risk factor for venous thrombosis. *Blood* 1997; **89**: 397–402.

16. Frosst P, Blom HJ, Milos R et al. A candidate genetic risk factor for vascular disease: a common mutation in methylenetetrahydrofolate reductase. *Nat Genet* 1995; **10**: 111–113.

17. Stampfer MJ, Malinow MR, Willett WC et al. A prospective study of plasma homocyst(e)ine and risk of myocardial infarction in US physicians. *JAMA* 1992; **268**: 877–881.

18. Falcon CR, Cattaneo M, Panzeri D et al. High prevalence of hyperhomocyst(e)inemia in patients with juvenile venous thrombosis. *Arterioscler Thromb* 1994; **14**: 1080–1083.

19. den Heijer M, Blom HJ, Gerrits WB et al. Is hyperhomocysteinaemia a risk factor for recurrent venous thrombosis? *Lancet* 1995; **345**: 882–885.

20. Fermo I, Vigano, DS, Paroni R et al. Prevalence of moderate hyperhomocystinemia in patients with early-onset venous and arterial occlusive disease. *Ann Intern Med* 1995; **123**: 747–753.

21. Kraus M. The anticoagulant potential of the protein C system in hereditary and acquired thrombophilia: pathological mechanisms and new tools for assessing its clinical relevance. *Semin Thromb Hemost* 1998; **24**: 337–354.

22. Haas FJML, van Sterkenburg-Kamp BM, Scheepers HMM. A protein C pathway (PCP) screening test for the detection of APC resistance and protein C or S deficiencies. *Semin Thromb Hemost* 1998; **24**: 355–362.

23. Henkerns CMA, Bom VJJ, Seinen AJ, van der Meer J. Sensitivity of activated protein C: influence of oral contraceptives and sex. *Thromb Haemost* 1995; **73**: 402–404.

24. Rosing J, Tans G, Nicolaes GA et al. Oral contraceptives and venous thrombosis: different sensitivities to activated protein C in women using second- and third-generation oral contraceptives. *Br J Haematol* 1997; **97**: 233–238.

25. Rai R, Regan L, Hadely E et al. Second-trimester pregnancy loss is associated with activated protein C resistance. *Br J Haematol* 1996; **92**: 489–490.

26. Brenner B, Mandel H, Lanir N et al. Activated protein C resistance can be associated with recurrent fetal loss. *Br J Haematol* 1997; **97**: 551–554.

27. Zangvill E, Jabareen A, Lanir N, Brenner B. Resistance to activated protein C antiendothelial antibodies and other markers of thrombophilia in patients with

antiphospholipid antibodies syndrome. *Br J Haematol* 1996; **93**(Suppl 2): 315 (1190).

28. Bokarewa MI, Blomback M, Bremme K. Phospholipid antibodies and resistance to activated protein C in women with thrombophilia. *Blood Coagul Fibrinolysis* 1995; **6**: 417–422.

29. Hesselvik JF, Malm J, Dahlback B, Blomback M. Protein C, protein S and C4b-binding protein in severe infection and septic shock. *Thromb Haemost* 1991; **65**: 126–129.

30. Powars D, Larsen R, Johnson J et al. Epidemic meningococcemia and purpura fulminans with induced protein C deficiency. *Clin Infect Dis* 1993; **3**: 247–249.

31. Hessing M. The interaction between complement component C4b-binding protein and the vitamin K-dependent protein S forms a link between blood coagulation and the complement system. *Biochem J* 1991; **277**: 581–592.

32. Mandel H, Brenner B, Berant M et al. Coexistence of hyperhomocysteinemia and factor V Leiden mutation: Impact on expression of thrombosis. *N Engl J Med* 1996; **334**: 763–768.

33. De Franchis R, Mancini FP, D'Angelo A et al. Elevated total plasma homocysteine and C→T mutation of 5,10 methylenetetra-hydrofolate reductase gene in thrombotic vascular disease. *Am J Hum Genet* 1996; **59**: 262–264.

34. Dahlback B, Carlsson M, Svensson PJ. Familial thrombophilia due to previously unrecognized mechanism characterized by poor anticoagulant response to activated protein C: prediction of a cofactor to activated protein C. *Proc Natl Acad Sci USA* 1993; **90**: 1004–1008.

35. Tripodi A, Negri B, Bertina RM, Mannucci PM. Screening for the FV: Q^{506} mutation. Evaluation of thirteen plasma-based methods for their diagnostic efficacy in comparison with DNA analysis. *Thromb Haemost* 1997; 77: 436–439.

36. Aboud MR, Ma DDF. A comparison between two activated protein C resistance methods as routine diagnostic tests for factor V Leiden mutation. *Br J Haematol* 1997; **97**: 798–803.

37. Mannucci PM, Boyer C, Tripodi A et al. Multicenter comparison of five functional and two immunological assays for protein C. *Thromb Haemost* 1987; **57**: 44–48.

38. Miletich JP, Sherman I, Broze G. Absence of thrombosis in subjects with heterozygous protein C deficiency. *N Engl J Med* 1987; **317**: 991–996.

39. Brenner B, Sanchez-Vega B, Wu SM et al. A missense mutation in γ-glutamyl carboxylase gene causes combined deficiency of vitamin K dependent blood coagulation factors. *Blood* 1998; **92**: 4554–4559.

40. Reitsma PH. Protein C deficiency: from gene defects to disease. *Thromb Haemost* 1997; **78**: 344–350.

41. Seligsohn U, Berger A, Abend M et al. Homozygous protein C deficiency manifested by massive venous thrombosis in the newborn. *N Engl J Med* 1984; **310**: 559–562.

42. Griffin JH. Anticoagulants and skin necrosis. *Adverse Drug React Toxicol Rev* 1994; **13**: 157–167.

43. Koeleman BPC, Reitsma PH, Allaart CF, Bertina RM. Activated protein C resistance as an additional risk factor for thrombosis in protein-C deficient families. *Blood* 1994; **84**: 1031–1035.

44. Brenner B, Zivelin A, Lanir N et al. Venous thromboembolism associated with double

heterozygosity for R506Q mutation of factor V and for T298M mutation of protein C in a large family of a previously described homozygous protein C deficient newborn with massive thrombosis. *Blood* 1996; **88:** 877–880.

45. Zoller B, Garcia de Frutos P, Dahlback B. Evaluation of the relationship between protein S and C4b-binding protein isoforms in hereditary protein S deficiency demonstrating type I and type III deficiencies to be phenotypic variants of the same genetic disease. *Blood* 1995; **85:** 3524–3531.

46. Faioni EM, Franchi F, Asti D et al. Resistance to activated protein C in nine thrombophilic families: interference in a protein S functional assay. *Thromb Haemost* 1993; **70:** 683–690.

47. Zoller B, Bernsdotter A, Garcia de Frutos P, Dahlback B. Resistance to activated protein C as an additional genetic risk factor in hereditary deficiency of protein S. *Blood* 1995; **85:** 3518–3523.

48. Gibson J, Nelson M, Brown R et al. Autoantibodies to thrombomodulin: development of an enzyme immunoassay and a survey of their frequency in patients with the lupus anticoagulant. *Thromb Haemost* 1992; **67:** 507–509.

49. Bayston TA, Lane DA. Antithrombin: molecular basis of deficiency. *Thromb Haemost* 1997; **78:** 339–343.

50. Henschen AH. Human fibrinogen — structural variants and functional sites. *Thromb Haemost* 1993; **70:** 42.

51. Triplett DA. Protean clinical presentations of antiphospholipid antibodies. *Thromb Haemost* 1995; **74:** 329–337.

52. Exner T. Diagnostic methodologies for circulating anticoagulants. *Thromb Haemost* 1995; **74:** 338–344.

53. Rand JH, Wu X-X, Andree HAM et al. Pregnancy loss in the antiphospholipid-antibody syndrome — a possible thrombogenic mechanism. *N Engl J Med* 1997; **337:** 154–160.

54. Selhub J, D'Angelo A. Hyperhomocysteinemia and thrombosis: acquired conditions. *Thromb Haemost* 1997; **78:** 527–531.

55. Amiral J, Bridey F, Dreyfus M et al. Platelet factor 4 complexed to heparin is the target for antibodies generated in heparin-induced thrombocytopenia. *Thromb Haemost* 1992; **68:** 95–96.

56. Amiral J. Diagnostic tests in heparin-induced thrombocytopenia. *Platelets* 1997; **8:** 68–72.

57. Nossel HL, Yudelman I, Canfield RE. Measurement of fibrinopeptide A in human blood. *J Clin Invest* 1974; **54:** 43–54.

58. Pelzer H, Schwarz A, Stuber W. Determination of human prothrombin activation fragment 1 + 2 in plasma with an antibody against a synthetic peptide. *Thromb Haemost* 1991; **65:** 153–159.

59. Millenson MM, Bauer KA, Kistler JP et al. Monitoring "mini-intensity" anticoagulation with warfarin: comparison of a prothrombin time using a sensitive thromboplastin with prothrombin fragment 1 + 2 levels. *Blood* 1992; **79:** 2034–2038.

60. Hemker HC, Beguin S. Thrombin generation in plasma: its assessment via the endogenous thrombin potential. *Thromb Haemost* 1995; **74:** 134–138.

Low molecular weight heparins: a comparative review of pharmacodynamic, clinical pharmacology

Meyer Michel Samama, Pierre Desnoyers and Grigoris T Gerotziafas

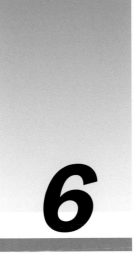

Introduction

Low molecular weight heparins (LMWHs) are actually the medication of choice in the prophylaxis of deep vein thrombosis (DVT) and pulmonary embolism (PE) in either medical or postsurgical patients. Recently, LMWHs have been recommended for the treatment of DVT and PE. They also have indications in cardiovascular disease, stroke and hemodialysis.[1,2] They are obtained from different preparations of standard heparin according to various procedures. Thus, they are different in their biochemical and pharmacological properties.[3,4] These differences may influence the clinical profile of LMWHs. The anti-IIa and anti-Xa specific activities of standard heparin are practically identical, whereas in the case of a specific LMWH the anti-IIa and anti-Xa specific activities are different and moreover, the differences are variable from one LMWH to another. Although the ex vivo anticoagulant effect of LMWHs is observed at doses averred to as antithrombotic, these heparins may have a significant antithrombotic effect in vivo, with no detectable anticoagulant effect in vitro. The mechanism of their antithrombotic activity is still obscure.[5] About 12 years ago it was discovered that after intravenous or subcutaneous administration, LMWHs induce the release of tissue factor pathway inhibitor (TFPI) from its vascular pool.[6] This effect contributes to their antithrombotic effect. Finally the hemorrhagic risk associated with LMWHs may vary from one preparation of LMWH to another.

In this chapter we compare the mode of preparation of the various commercial LMWHs, their physical constants and their biological activities. We also compare the pharmacokinetic constants, subcutaneous absorption, distribution and clearance rate as well as the dose adjustment of the various LMWHs in the case of renal insufficiency and elderly patients.

Pharmacodynamic properties

Mode of preparation of the various LMWHs

Low molecular weight heparins are generally obtained using five different procedures from standard heparin that is extracted from porcine intestinal mucosa (*Table 6.1*): depolymerization by nitrous acid; depolymerization by isoamylic nitrate; digestion by a heparinase; cleavage of standard bovine heparin induced by peroxidation and alkaline hydrolysis following benzylation.

The question that arises is do these different procedures for the production of LMWHs result in similar products? Several studies compared the antithrombotic efficacy of different fragments of heparin, isolated and prepared using the different procedures, on animal experimental models (particularly rabbits).[7,8]

Cade et al[9] studied the influence of the production method on the physiological properties of LMWHs. LMWHs were prepared by different methods: they had different mean molecular weights, different distributions of their molecular weights and they had different antithrombotic activity (in experimental models of thrombosis and/or in humans). By contrast, three preparations of LMWHs with identical mean molecular weights and distribution of molecular weight, obtained using three different procedures (enzymatic depolymerization using the flavobacterium *Heparinum*, chemical degradation by nitrous acid and fractionated dissolution) had a similar thromboprophylactic effect. The antithrombotic effect expressed as inhibition of the formation of hemostatic clot in a rabbit mesenteric arteriolar segment or as inhibition of clot formation in the jugular vein of rabbit after endothelial lesion combined with a reduction of the blood flux, was dose-dependent.[10]

Biochemical and pharmacological studies have shown that LMWHs produced by each of the procedures previously described, show chemical, biochemical and pharmacological differences. Chemical modifications of the

Table 6.1
Currently available LMWHs

LMWH	Commercial name	Pharmaceutical manufacturer	Production method
Dalteparin	Fragmin	Pharmacia Upjohn (Sweden)	Depolymerization by nitrous acid
Enoxaparin	Lovenox Clexane	Avantis (France)	Benzylation and alkaline hydrolysis
Nadroparin	Fraxiparin Seteparin	Sanofi-Synthelabo (France)	Depolymerization by nitrous acid
Certoparin	Sandoparin	Sandoz (Switzerland-Germany)	Depolymerization by isoamylic nitrate
Ardeparin	Normiflo	Wyeth-Ayerst (USA)	Cleavage by peroxidation
Parnaparin	Fluxum	Opocrin-Alpe Warrem (Italy)	Peroxidation
Tinzaparin	Innohep Logiparin	Novo-Dupont (Denmark)	Digestion by heparinase
Reviparin	Clivarin	Knoll (Germany)	Depolymerization by nitrous acid
RO 11	Boxol	Rovi (Spain)	Depolymerization by nitrous acid

final domains and the internal structure of the molecule as well as the degree of the desulfation during the manufacturing process modify the biological behavior of each LMWH. For example, depolymerization induces a modification of the antithrombin binding sites and consequently reduces the antithrombotic activity of LMWH. The interaction with heparin cofactor II and the platelet factor (PF4), the neutralization by protamine sulfate and the cellular interactions may also vary from one LMWH to another.[11] Interestingly, it has been shown that the mode of preparation of LMWHs affects not only the chemical structure but also their pharmacokinetic and biological properties.[12]

This subject has been recently reviewed.[13] Moreover, the manufacturing process for one LMWH may change over time. Nadroparin calcium is such an example, since it was first obtained by a fractionation method and now is prepared by depolymerization of unfractionated heparin (UFH) using nitrous acid. Similarly, enoxaparin sodium was prepared by depolymerization using alkaline hydrolysis after benzylation; a procedure that required the addition of large amounts of sodium bisulfite in order to prevent the oxidation of the terminal domains. A modern procedure eliminated the use of sodium bisulfite. However the product of this procedure possesses similar pharmacological properties to the product obtained by the procedure using the sodium bisulfite. Thus, the important question of whether the available LMWH preparations are the same is disputed.[14]

Physical properties

Molecular weight

The mean molecular weight (MW) varies from 3500 to about 6000 daltons. The observed differences of mean molecular weights may induce variations of the ratio (R) of proportionality of the areas under the curve obtained after injection of 30 U/kg of two different LMWHs. However, no clear correlation was seen between the mean molecular weights of enoxaparin (3500–5500 D), nadroparin (4200–4800 D),

dalteparin (5000 D), tinzaparin (4900 D), ardeparin (5500–6500 D) and the pharmacokinetics of these different LMWHs (*Table 6.2*).[4,15]

Distribution of heparin fragments

The distribution of heparin fragments was studied with two different methods: spectral analysis (HNMR) and the analysis of size distribution with quasi-clastic light scattering (QCLS) using an argon laser at 488 nm.[16] Five LMWHs (dalteparin, enoxaparin, tinzaparin, certoparin and ardeparin) were compared (*Table 6.2*).

1. For dalteparin the distribution peak was situated at 100 nm with a small number of macromolecules with larger size distributed up to 700 nm.

2. The distribution peak for tinzaparin was more concentrated around 100 nm and a small number of macromolecules was distributed up to 1000 nm.

3. In enoxaparin the majority of the particles were distributed at 100 nm with a small number of macromolecules over 1000 nm.

4. In certoparin most molecules were located at 200 nm with some large molecules at up to 1400 nm.

5. The distribution of histogram for ardeparin was different from that of the other LMWHs. The peak was situated

Table 6.2
Biological constants

LMWH	Molecular weight (daltons)	Molecular weight distribution	
		<3000 D	>8000 D
First international standard*	5000–6000		
Dalteparin sodium (Fragmin)	5000–5950	9.1 (3–15)	19.5 (14–26)
Enoxaparin sodium (Lovenox, Clexane)	4200 (3500–5500)	40.1	9.2
Nadroparin calcium (Fraxiparine)	4500 (4200–4800)	28.9	8.2
Ardeparin (Normiflo)	5500–6500	2000–15 000	
Parnaparin sodium (Fluxum)	4000–5000	19.7	22.2
Tinzaparin sodium (Logiparin-Innohep)	5800–6750*	31.9	14.0
Reviparin sodium (Clivarin)	3550–4650	—	—
Bemiparin sodium RO 11	3000–4200	40	<15

* A reference preparation of dalteparin.

at 500 nm, with a large number of fragments distributed up to 1500 nm and another large group of macromolecules with a size of about 5000 nm. These characteristics indicated that the distribution of ardeparin's fragments was not very different from that of standard unfractionated heparin.

The distribution of the fragments comprising the LMWHs, characterizes the various preparations of LMWHs. It is most likely that the distribution of molecular weight is more important than the mean molecular weight. This criterion allows a more confident distinction between a LMWH and unfractionated heparin. Comparable results were presented by Komatsu et al[17] who studied LMWHs with calibrated molecular weights using high performance chromatography with gel permeability (HPCGP).

Finally dalteparin, in contrast to tinzaparin and enoxaparin, possesses no negatively charged sulfated amino groups at the reduced extremity of its molecule. This structure probably reduces the cellular interactions and protects the larger fragments from elimination. Thus these molecules remain in the circulation and contribute to the expression of the anti-Xa activity via the binding to TFPI.[6]

Binding to platelets

The binding of heparin to the platelet membrane is specific, saturable and reversible. It is independent of the presence of calcium ions and platelet glycoproteins (GpIIb-IIIa, GpIb, GpV, GpIX).[18] Activated platelets expose on their surface binding sites of high and low affinity for heparin. When platelets are activated by thrombin or ADP they bind more heparin than inactivated platelets.[18–20] The pentasaccharide domain is not necessary for the binding of heparin to platelet membranes. Moreover, heparin fragments with low affinity or high affinity for AT bind to platelet membranes with similar affinity. The mean molecular weight, the degree of sulfation and the electronegative charge of heparin fragments are the determining

parameters for the affinity of heparin for the platelet membrane. The affinity increases when these parameters increase.[20,21]

LMWHs bind less than unfractionated heparin to platelet surfaces because the smaller sized fragments of LMWHs have low affinity for the heparin binding sites. They do not induce platelet activation and consequently the number of heparin binding sites exposed on platelet membranes is reduced.

Heparin binds by covalent bonds to several proteins secreted from activated platelets, such as platelet factor 4 (PF4), von Willebrand factor, β-thromboglobulin, thrombospondin, fibronectin, vitronectin and histidine-rich glycoprotein.[22,23] These proteins are present on platelet membranes as well as in plasma. The affinity of heparin fragments for these proteins is reduced by reduction of the mean molecular weight, the degree of sulfation and the electronegative charge.[24] The affinity of LMWHs for these proteins is lower than the affinity of unfractionated heparin.

Fragments without the pentasaccharide domain have low affinity for AT (and no anticoagulant effect). These fragments have higher affinity for the above-mentioned platelet proteins than the fragments that possess the pentasaccharide. Fragments with low affinity for AT remove the fragments with high affinity for AT that are bound on platelet and plasma proteins. It has been proposed that the presence of fragments with low affinity for AT in a preparation of LMWH could improve the anticoagulant effect of LMWH.[25,26]

The biological constants

All LMWHs are salts of sodium except nadroparin, which is a calcium salt. Bender and Aronson[27] demonstrated that after subcutaneous administration of LMWH the sodium and calcium salts are bioequivalent. However, anti-Xa activity of unfractionated heparin is reduced in the absence of calcium. This phenomenon is not observed in the case of LMWH.[28] The absorption of LMWH after subcutaneous injection depends on the nature of the salt and its concentration in the injected solution. Absorption is slower with a calcium salt compared with a sodium salt.

Antithrombotic profile

The anti-Xa and anti-IIa specific activities of LMWHs have been extensively studied in order to define their antithrombotic and anticoagulant properties. However, regardless of the necessity for standardization of LMWHs[29] and the introduction of the first international standard of LMWH in 1988,[30] an international consensus for in vitro comparison between LMWHs and UFH has never been established.

Specific anti-Xa and anti-IIa activities of the various LMWHs

There are variations in the titration of the specific activities of LMWH for the same LMWH using different methods. The titration of the anti-Xa and anti-IIa specific activity of the same LMWH preparation varies from one study to another depending on the method used. Thus, the anti-Xa and anti-IIa activities of dalteparin sodium vary according to different authors from 30 to 60 IU/mg for the anti-IIa activity (50% variation) and from 122.5 to 165 IU/mg for anti-Xa activity (26% variation) (*Table 6.3*).

Variation of the titration of the specific activities of different LMWHs using the same method and the same reagents was studied in five different laboratories.[31] Between the lower and the higher values the percentage of variation is 5.7% for nadroparin, 11.8% for enoxaparin and 9.3% for dalteparin.

Comparison of different LMWHs after intravenous administration

A single daily intravenous injection of dalteparin, nadroparin or enoxaparin was administered to 12 healthy volunteers. The kinetics of the anti-Xa of the three LMWHs shows monoexpotential function. The half-life of the three LMWHs was not statistically different, and the terminal half-life of the

Table 6.3
Biological constants

LMWH	Anti-IIa activity (versus the 1st International standard for LMWHs) (IU/mg)	Anti-Xa activity (versus the 1st International standard for LMWHs) (IU/mg)	Ratio anti-Xa/anti-IIa activity
First international standard*	68	168	2.47[29]
Dalteparin sodium	30	122.5	4
(Fragmin)	40	165	4
	60	148	2.47
		160	
Enoxaparin sodium (Lovenox-Clexane)	28	100	3.57[31]
Nadroparin calcium (Fraxiparine)	30	97	3.23
		88	
Ardeparin (Normiflo)	60	120	2
Parnaparin sodium (Fluxum)	35	85	2.43
Tinzaparin sodium (Logiparin-Innohep)	50	75	1.5
		90	1.8
Reviparin sodium (clivarin)	40	130	3.25
Bemiparin sodium RO 11	10–15	80–90	6–9

* A reference preparation of dalteparin.

anti-IIa activity in plasma was not different. Only the clearance of the anti-IIa activity (lh^{-1}) shows significant differences for enoxaparin versus dalteparin or nadroparin.[32]

The administration of nadroparin and enoxaparin is associated with similar prolongations of activated partial thromboplastin time (APTT), whereas dalteparin induces a much longer duration APTT.

Comparison of different LMWHs after subcutaneous administration

For most of the LMWHs the maximum concentration peak of anti-Xa activity in plasma is achieved 4–6 hours after the subcutaneous injection. However, the concentrations of LMWH obtained in plasma are different for each LMWH (*Table 6.4*). The anti-Xa plasma activity peak and the area under the curve (AUC) are in general higher for enoxaparin and dalteparin and lower for tinzaparin. Enoxaparin and dalteparin can be considered bioequivalent products with respect to their anti-Xa activity. Considering anti-IIa activity, however, no equivalence could be demonstrated. Dalteparin is different with an almost double C_{max} and AUC compared with exoxaparin and tinzaparin.[33]

In prophylactic doses the concentrations of the anti-Xa plasma activity 4–6 hours after subcutaneous injection of 3075 anti-Xa IU of nadroparin calcium or 3200 anti-Xa IU of parnaparin sodium are very similar: 0.31 anti-Xa IU/ml versus 0.30 anti-Xa IU/ml, respectively. On the contrary after subcutaneous injection of 2500 anti-Xa IU of tinzaparin the anti-Xa plasma activity is 0.12 anti-Xa IU/ml. The concentration of the anti-IIa plasma activity measured 4–6 hours after injection of 3075 anti-Xa IU of nadroparin and 2500 anti-Xa IU of tinzaparin are 0.05 IU/ml and 0.03 anti-IIa IU/ml respectively.

In therapeutic doses the differences among the LMWHs are more remarkable when the injected doses are greater than those given prophylactically. The mean peak concentration of the anti-Xa activity in plasma 4–6 hours after subcutaneous administration of 10 000 anti-Xa IU of tinzaparin is 0.46 anti-Xa IU/ml. It is about 0.80 anti-Xa IU/ml after subcutaneous injection of 12 550 anti-Xa IU. The concentration of the anti-Xa activity in plasma 4–6 hours after subcutaneous administration of 185 anti-Xa IU/kg of nadroparin calcium (about 11 100 anti-Xa IU for an individual of 60 kg) is 1.55 anti-Xa IU/ml in plasma. The concentration of the anti-Xa plasma activity after subcutaneous injection of 12 800 anti-Xa IU of parnaparin is 0.8 to 0.9 anti-Xa IU/ml.[34–36] Thus, at equivalent anti-Xa IU administered therapeutic doses a significant difference of the peak anti-Xa activity in plasma is observed.

Comparison of the effect of dalteparin, enoxaparin and certoparin on hemostasis

A study compared three markers of activation of coagulation and platelets: thrombin–antithrombin complex (TAT), the prothrombin fragments 1 and 2 (F 1 + 2) and β-thromboglobulin (β-TG) in the blood obtained after skin incision in healthy volunteers. The three LMWHs studied induced a slight diminution of the F 1 + 2

Table 6.4
Pharmacokinetic parameters of LMWHs after subcutaneous injection

	Cmax (anti-Xa IU/ml)	Tmax	AUC Anti-Xa IU/hour/ml	AUC Anti-IIa IU/hour/ml
Dalteparin				
2500 anti-Xa IU/sc	0.22 ± 0.07	2.82 ± 0.92*	1.26 ± 0.4*	
5000 anti-Xa IU/sc	0.48 ± 0.30	3.0 ± 0.06**	3.17 ± 0.82	0.57 ± 0.15**
Enoxaparin sodium				
2000 anti-Xa IU/sc	0.28 ± 0.06	2.35 ± 0.56*	1.96 ± 0.55*	0.25 ± 0.07**
(20 mg)				
4000 anti-Xa IU/sc	0.42 ± 0.11**	4.28 ± 0.58**	3.47 ± 0.6**	
(40 mg)	0.45 ± 0.05**	3.1 ± 0.4***	3.0 ± 0.69***	0.66 ± 0.25
	0.57 ± 0.14**	2.91 ± 0.5*	4.57 ± 1.04*	
Nadroparin calcium				
3075 anti-Xa IU/sc	0.32 ± 0.09	3.62 ± 0.73*	2.35 ± 0.63*	
Reviparin sodium				
3300 anti-Xa IU/sc	0.42 ± 0.06	3.10 ± 0.5	2.44 ± 0.59	—
Tinzaparin sodium				
sc mg of 4500 anti-Xa IU	0.18 ± 0.04	3.08 ± 0.79	1.35 ± 0.90	0.30 ± 0.1

* Reference 33; ** Reference 66; *** Reference 72; SC: subcutaneously.

formation in venous blood. Dalteparin and enoxaparin but not certoparin also inhibited the formation of TAT. None of the LMWHs significantly affected the concentration of β-TG.[37]

Hemorrhagic profile: neutralization

The ex vivo effect of LMWH on platelets was studied in rabbits treated with LMWH. Inhibition of collagen induced platelet aggregation was significantly reduced after administration of an LMWH compared with UFH. In vivo, it could be demonstrated that LMWH caused less blood loss but showed greater antithrombin activity than UFH.[38]

The effect of all the studied LMWHs and UFH on the aPTT and the thrombin clotting time was completely (99.8%) neutralized by protamine sulfate independently of the

Apparent inhibition velocity	MRT Anti-Xa (hours)	t₁ anti-Xa hours	Clearance (ml/min)	Bioavailability (%)
7.3 ± 2 60 3.6 11.8 ± 6.5	5.26 ± 1.15	2.81 ± 0.84* 2.31 ± 0.06**	33.3 ± 11.8	86
70	6.68 ± 0.94*	3.95 ± 0.65*	16.7 ± 5.5*	91
	6.7 ± 1.8*** 7.38 ± 0.74*	4.28 ± 1.06** 4.37 ± 0.47	13.8 ± 3.17*	
6.77 55 ml/kg 3.31	7.10 ± 0.99*	3.74 ± 0.68*	21.5 ± 7*	89–98
—	6.4 ± 1.0	3.3 ± 1	19.2 ± 3.8	
	6 to 7.6	2.97 ± 1.01	22 ± 0.5	85

administered dose; whereas, in contrast to UFH, the anti-Xa activity of LMWHs was only partially inhibited (20–40%).[39 41] Protamine sulfate neutralized about 80% of the anti-Xa activity of tinzaparin administered intravenously.[36–40] After subcutaneous injection of tinzaparin, protamine sulfate inhibited only 60% of the anti-Xa activity. Three hours after the neutralization peak, prolongation of APTT and a gradual reversion of the neutralized anti-Xa and anti-IIa activities was observed. This phenomenon is probably due to the continuous absorption of tinzaparin from its subcutaneous pool. This phenomenon was not observed after subcutaneous injection of reviparin.[42] An excess of protamine sulfate does not have an additional inhibitory effect on residual anti-Xa activity in plasma.[40]

Moreover, after neutralization by

protamine sulfate the ex vivo activity of LMWHs does not seem to be correlated with blood loss, and this suggests that an ex vivo reversal of the basal level is not necessary in order to affirm that the hemorrhagic effect is neutralized.[40–43] Interestingly, the efficacy of protamine in preventing bleeding in patients undergoing extracorporeal circulation with LMWH was clearly suggested by an early clinical work of our group.[44]

Comparing the hemorrhagic profile of intravenously injected LMWHs, Fareed et al[45] demonstrated that nadroparin, enoxaparin and dalteparin have a relatively weak hemorrhagic effect. Parnaparin, ardeparin, tinzaparin and certoparin induce a bleeding tendency similar to that of UFH at equivalent anti-Xa doses.

Affinity for antithrombin

During the depolymerization process of LMWH production, the binding sites for AT may be modified and this probably results in reduced antithrombotic activity. About 25% of heparin molecules in LMWH preparations contain the pentasaccharide sequence and possess an affinity for antithrombin. This percentage may vary from one LMWH to another. Thus, the mechanism of production, their pharmacological activity, efficacy and their tolerance must be further studied.[45] At a circulating plasma concentration of 20 µM/ml LMWHs saturate almost all the AT and HCII

binding sites and no difference among the various LMWHs could be demonstrated. After injection of tinzaparin, the plasma concentration of AT remained unmodified.[45]

Effect on platelet activity, lipids and bone metabolism

LMWHs influence platelet activity. UFH enhances platelet aggregation induced by ADP or platelet activating factor (PAF) in human plasma as demonstrated 20 years ago by Salzman et al.[46] LMWHs are less effective than UFH (at equivalent doses) at inducing platelet aggregation.

LMWHs, compared with UFH (on a gravimetric basis), induce a significantly reduced inhibition of thrombin generation in platelet-poor plasma (PPP). In platelet-rich plasma (PRP), LMWHs are more effective than UFH. LMWHs are less affected than UFH by the neutralizing activity of PF4. The degree of interaction varies according to the nature of LMWH. The interaction with platelets may have an important role in the in vivo activity of LMWHs.

LMWHs have a lower effect on the release of lipoprotein lipase and on the activity of hepatic lipase than UFH (50% in gravimetrically equivalent doses).[47–51]

The effect of LMWH on osteal absorption in rats is identical to the effect of UFH in equivalent anti-Xa concentrations.[52,53] Recently, Shaughnessy et al[54] have shown that

UFH accumulates in bone during the course of its administration and remains in bone for at least 56 days.[54] Monreal et al[55] have suggested that the risk of osteoporosis is lower in patients treated with LMWH than with UFH.

Effect on the liberation of TFPI

TFPI directly inhibits factor Xa and the complex factor VIIa/tissue factor. LMWHs have various effects on the vascular pool of TFPI as a consequence of their variable anionic strength. Some authors[6,45,56] have shown that the liberation of TFPI after injection of heparin follows a kinetic model similar to that of the anti-Xa activity.

The LMWH RO11 has dose-dependent kinetics for anti-Xa activity, whereas the kinetics of the TFPI are similar for all the doses administered either subcutaneously or intravenously.[57] Anti-Xa activity is present for 18 hours but TFPI liberation lasts for about 6–8 hours. The liberation of TFPI starts earlier than that of factor Xa. The two effects coincide for only a short period of time. This observation is important in clinical practice, since LMWHs are administered 2 or 12 hours preoperatively for prophylaxis. A possible difference between UFH and LMWH in therapeutic efficacy could be related to differences in TFPI release.[56–58]

For tinzaparin, Valentine et al[59] demonstrated a synergistic effect between LMWH at concentrations used in vivo and TFPI on the prolongation of different coagulation assays.

The ability of the various LMWHs to release the TFPI from the endogenous pool is variable. After a single intravenous administration at anti-Xa equivalent doses, the concentrations of TFPI in plasma vary from 110 to 150 ng/ml. Reviparin and tinzaparin induce a more significant release of TFPI, which resembles the release of TFPI induced by UFH at equivalent anti-Xa concentrations.[42,45] The lowest values of TFPI (110 ng/ml) are obtained by nadroparin and dalteparin. Enoxaparin and certoparin induce an intermediate release of TFPI.[45] Owing to a better bioavailability after subcutaneous injection in healthy volunteers, enoxaparin (at 40 mg or 4000 anti-Xa IU) induces an increase of the liberation of TFPI similar to that induced by UFH.[60]

Effect of coagulation on tissue factor pathway

Pentasaccharide, LMWHs and UFH have a concentration-dependent inhibitory effect on factor VIIa generation and activity. LMWHs inhibit factor VIIa generation by fragments that possess anti-Xa activity. The treatment with LMWHs in patients suffering from thrombosis inhibits the generation of factor VIIa during in vitro clotting of whole blood, PRP or PPP. The inhibitory effect of pentasaccharide, LMWH and UFH on factor VIIa generation is AT-dependent and it is not related to the release of TFPI from the vascular pool. The inhibitory effect of pentasaccharide on factor VIIa generation does not depend on TFPI activity.[61] Following activation of the tissue factor pathway, the inhibitory effect of LMWH and UFH on factor VIIa generation partially relies on the activity of TFPI. The interaction of LMWH and UFH with TFPI probably depends on the molecular weight of heparins.

After activation of the intrinsic clotting pathway, the inhibitory effect of LMWH and UFH is independent of TFPI activity. During clotting of human PPP initiated via tissue factor or intrinsic pathway activation the synthetic PS, LMWH and UFH downregulate factor VIIa generation by mainly inhibiting the generation and the activity of factors IXa and Xa.[62–64]

Effect on fibrin polymerization and clot stability

Unfractionated heparin, at concentrations used in clinical practice, induces a significant perturbation of clot structure and a pronounced inhibition of fibrin polymerization when studied in vitro. The effect of LMWH, at concentrations used in prophylaxis and treatment of DVT, is significantly less important than that of UFH.[65]

Pharmacokinetic properties

LMWHs cannot be regarded as an undifferentiated pharmacological group since they all have different pharmacokinetics (*Table 6.4*).[32,33,66–68]

The pharmacokinetic parameters of the LMWHs have been calculated or directly obtained from the curves of elimination of the anti-Xa activity, and sometimes the anti-IIa activity, from plasma, after either intravenous injection in doses of about 20 anti-Xa IU/kg (about 1200 anti-Xa IU for an individual of 60 kg) or 120 anti-Xa IU/kg or after subcutaneous injection of doses used in prophylaxis of DVT in patients at moderate risk (abdominal general surgery) or in patients at high risk (orthopedic or oncologic surgery). Healthy volunteers in most studies and in a few studies, patients, received either an LMWH or unfractionated heparin for comparison of the pharmacokinetics of these different heparins.

We consider the different pharmacokinetic parameters after subcutaneous injection especially since the use of the intravenous route is limited.

Maximal concentration

In humans the peak concentration (C_{max}) of the anti-Xa or anti-IIa activity is obtained 3–10 minutes after intravenous administration and 3–6 hours after subcutaneous injection.[67,68]

Intravenous injection

Following intravenous injection the maximal plasma concentration is proportional to the injected dose and independent of the LMWH used. For example, after nadroparin administration at a dose of 35 anti-Xa IU/kg (2100 anti-Xa IU/individual) the obtained maximal concentration is 0.5 to 0.7 anti-Xa IU/ml.[69] For a four-fold higher dose of dalteparin the maximal concentration of plasma anti-Xa activity is 2.2 ± 0.3 anti-Xa IU/ml.[70]

Subcutaneous injection

Following subcutaneous injection anti-Xa activity is well correlated with the dose given to healthy volunteers as shown in a study with enoxaparin used at increasing doses from 20 to 80 mg.[71]

The C_{max} for anti-Xa plasma activity for enoxaparin was measured during a randomized crossover trial. In this study enoxaparin was compared with reviparin. Both were administered by subcutaneous injections, twice daily, in clinically equivalent doses for the prevention of postoperative DVT (40 mg for enoxaparin, 4000 anti-Xa IU/individual; and 4250 anti-Xa IU/individual for reviparin).[72]

The peak anti-Xa plasma activity (C_{max}) after reviparin injection was slightly but significantly lower (0.42 ± 0.06 anti-Xa IU/ml) as compared with that observed after enoxaparin administration (0.45 ± 0.05 anti-Xa IU ml).

These different values are comparable with those obtained after administration of a single subcutaneous dose (40 mg sc) of enoxaparin, dalteparin and tinzaparin in human volunteers.[33] The injected dose of tinzaparin was lower but the C_{max} for anti-Xa (0.18 ± 0.04 anti-Xa IU/ml) was lower than in the two other LMWHs.[73] Moreover, this value of C_{max} corresponds to the C_{max} obtained after subcutaneous injection of 5000 anti-Xa IU of dalteparin (0.48 ± 0.13 anti-Xa IU/ml).[74]

Another study[66] compared dalteparin, enoxaparin and nadroparin administered subcutaneously at doses recommended for the prevention of DVT in patients with moderate thrombotic risk (i.e. abdominal surgery). The administered doses were about 2000–2500 anti Xa IU. For a mean injected dose of 1000 anti-Xa IU, the anti-Xa plasma activity measured after enoxaparin injection was 1.48-fold higher than the anti-Xa plasma activity measured after the injection of nadroparin and 2.78-fold higher than the anti-Xa plasma activity measured after the injection of dalteparin. Similarly, the amount of anti-Xa plasma activity measured after injection of nadroparin was 1.54-fold greater than that obtained after injection of dalteparin. In another study which compared the pharmacokinetic profile of dalteparin (administered subcutaneously at the dose of 2500 anti-Xa IU) to healthy young volunteers and to elderly hospitalized patients[74] the values of C_{max} were 0.20 ± 0.5 anti-Xa IU/ml. The C_{max} value was 0.6 ± 0.1 anti-Xa IU/ml after subcutaneous injection of 120 anti-Xa IU/kg (7200 anti-Xa/individual) and 0.98 ± 0.3 anti-Xa IU/ml after injection of 10 000 anti-Xa IU/individual.

T_{max}: the lag-time (in hours) to achieve C_{max}

After intravenous injection T_{max} for LMWHs is very short (3–10 minutes). It is about 3 hours after subcutaneous injection. T_{max} tends to be correlated with the amount of the injected dose. For doses of 2000 anti-Xa IU and 2500 anti-Xa IU of enoxaparin or dalteparin, T_{max} is 2.35 ± 0.56 and 2.82 ± 0.92 h respectively. For doses of 4000 anti-Xa IU and 5000 anti-Xa IU T_{max} is 3.00 ± 0.6 and 3.10 ± 0.4 h respectively (*Table 6.4*). T_{max} seems longer for nadroparin than that for enoxaparin. This difference could be due to the difference of salt type, calcium for the former and sodium for the latter. However, a similar observation has been made for tinzaparin although it too is a sodium salt.

Area under the curve

The numeric value of the area under the curve is calculated using a linear trapezoid method extrapolated to infinity by dividing the last measured value with the terminal slope of the curve, and it is expressed in anti-Xa IU/h/ml.[33] The AUC is naturally proportional to the administered doses and the clearance half-life.[71] However, significant differences are observed between different authors who studied the same LMWH at the same injected dose.

Anti-IIa activity

Among the different LMWHs, dalteparin induces the most important prolongation of APTT and the obtained C_{max} and AUC values are two-fold higher as compared to the values obtained after administration of equivalent doses of tinzaparin or enoxaparin.[32,33,67] However there is no bioequivalence between the same doses of enoxaparin, dalteparin and tinzaparin.[33]

After intravenous or subcutaneous administration of reviparin, at the dose of 80 anti-Xa IU/kg the AUC and C_{max} values, as well as the clearance and the distribution volume, are proportional to the injected doses.[76]

Monitoring of the kinetics of the plasma concentration of anti-IIa activity after LMWH injection at the doses used in prophylaxis is rather difficult since they have a very low anti-IIa activity (3–8-fold inferior compared to UFH).

Anti-Xa activity

Anti-Xa plasma activity and the AUC are positively correlated with the injected doses of LMWHs.[71] For nadroparin,[69] dalteparin,[70] and reviparin[76] the mean values of the anti-Xa plasma activity and the AUC are linearly dose-dependent for doses between 1200 and 7500 anti-Xa IU/individual. Enoxaparin and dalteparin (injected in similar doses) are bioequivalent in terms of the anti-Xa activity. However tinzaparin is not bioequivalent with the others and its AUC values are significantly lower.

Interestingly a study from our group[77] has clearly shown that the response to subcutaneous administration of similar anti-Xa doses of two different LMWH preparations to patients undergoing total hip replacement varies according to the LMWH used. Two groups of 221 and 219 patients received 4500 anti-Xa IU of tinzaparin and 4000 (40 mg) anti-Xa IU of enoxaparin. The mean peak anti-Xa activity was significantly higher with enoxaparin for instance at day 1 or 2 (0.55 versus 0.36, *P* < 0.001). A significant difference was also observed 12 hours after injection. These differences were present at day 1 or 2, day 5 or 6 and day 10 or 14 of treatment. They suggest that the clearance rate and the bioavailability of anti-Xa activity differ for these two drugs.[77]

The apparent volume of distribution

The apparent volume of distribution published for some LMWHs, is close to the plasmatic mass. This parameter, determined by the measurement of the anti-Xa activity after subcutaneous injection, varies for the same LMWH between different authors. The apparent volume of distribution for dalteparin is 40–60 ml/kg (about 3.6 litres for a normal individual of 60 kg), and about 200 ml/kg (11.8 ± 6.5 litres) for a dose of 2500–5000 anti-Xa IU.[70] These variations are probably due to underestimation of the AUC, which arises from lower measurements of the anti-Xa activity. In contrast, the same authors demonstrated that after subcutaneous injection of 10 000 anti-Xa IU the volume of distribution is 7.3 ± 2.0 litres. After intravenous injection of 120 anti-Xa IU/kg of dalteparin, the apparent volume of distribution is 3.4 ± 0.5 litres.[70]

If the apparent volume of distribution is calculated from the anti-IIa activity, as it has been done for tinzaparin (at the dose of 5000 anti-Xa IU administered subcutaneously) the apparent volume of distribution is about 10.1 litres according to a monocompartmental kinetic model, and 6.8 litres for a bicompartmental model.[73]

Metabolism and clearance

The metabolism of heparins involves depolymerization and desulfation. Heparins are cleared mainly through the kidney but also through the bile.[67,78] UFH is eliminated via a rapid dose-dependent saturable mechanism while LMWHs are eliminated by a non-saturable renal mechanism.[78–80] A study with radiolabelled enoxaparin has shown that about 10% of the dose injected was recovered in the urine.[81] In contrast to UFH, the clearance and the elimination half-life of LMWHs is not altered by the administered doses. LMWHs are principally eliminated by the kidney via a first order process.[67,79]

The values of clearance of the most frequently used LMWHs expressed as litres/hours are different. The clearance of enoxaparin is 16.7 ± 5 ml/min, the clearance of dalteparin is 33.3 ± 11.8 ml/min and the clearance of nadroparin is 21.7 ± 7.0 ml/min. The clearance of dalteparin should be distinguished from that of UFH and the other LMWHs. The heavy chains of dalteparin are relatively resistant to elimination from the circulation. Moreover these chains transport the TFPI.[12] Dalteparin, similarly to enoxaparin and nadroparin, may accumulate in the plasma of patients with renal insufficiency.[79] Thus a dose adjustment is necessary particularly when LMWHs are administered for therapeutic purposes. Biological monitoring of LMWH treatment by measuring the anti-Xa plasma activity is recommended when the clearance of creatinine is decreased.

Mean retention time

Higher values around 7 hours are observed for enoxaparin and nadroparin than dalteparin and ardeparin (about 5 hours).

Elimination half-life

The elimination half-life $(t_{\frac{1}{2}})$ of LMWHs intravenously and subcutaneously administered is different.

Intravenous route

The elimination half-life of LMWHs is different for the anti-IIa or anti-Xa specific activity. For anti-IIa activity the elimination half-life is relatively short and slightly different from one LMWH to another (for the three LMWHs widely used in France). Dalteparin and tinzaparin have the shortest elimination half-life (1.3 ± 0.2 h) whereas nadroparin has a longer one (2.16 ± 0.45 h). The clearance of enoxaparin is significantly more elevated (4.1 ± 0.1 litre/h).[32]

Subcutaneous route

After subcutaneous administration the elimination half-life of the anti-Xa activity differs from one LMWH to another. Thus, the elimination half-life of the anti-Xa activity of tinzaparin after a single subcutaneous injection of 5000 anti-Xa IU is 1.4 hours and that of enoxaparin is about 4 hours (*Table 6.4*).

Bioavailability

The bioavailability of relatively low doses of UFH (5000–15 000 IU/12h) administered subcutaneously is about 10–30%. The half-life of LMWHs at prophylactic doses (2500 to 5000 anti-Xa IV) is about 2–4 times higher than that of UFH. The bioavailability of the anti-Xa specific activity varies from 86–87% for dalteparin,[80] to 98% for nadroparin.[69] For the other LMWHs the bioavailability is situated in the range 90–98% (90% for tinzaparin, greater than 90% for parnaparin and ardeparin).[82] LMWHs injected subcutaneously are easily absorbed from the subcutaneous tissue and they probably bind to the endothelium less than UFH. Thus, the bioavailability of LMWHs reaches the 90% level and their half-lives are two times longer than that of UFH.

The bioavailability of anti-IIa seems lower than that of anti-Xa.

LMWHs are not transferred in the placenta although some anti-Xa activity has been detected in the fetal blood of the sheep.[83] However, it was not possible to demonstrate any anti-Xa activity in treated pregnant women in the first or second trimester of the pregnancy.[84–86] (See Feigin and Lourwood[87] on the use of LMWHs in obstetrics and gynecology.)

LMWHs in some special situations

LMWHs in elderly patients

The response to LMWHs of elderly patients is said to be higher than in healthy young volunteers. However, in a study[88] with nadroparin an accumulation of factor Xa activity but not of antithrombin activity in a group of 71 patients hospitalized for DVT was observed compared to healthy young volunteers.

In a recent pharmacokinetic study with tinzaparin, Siguret et al[89] found no correlation between anti-Xa and anti-IIa activity and age in 30 patients receiving 176 U anti-Xa/kg body weight during 10 days although renal function is related to age.[89]

LMWHs in liver disease

Patients with liver cirrhosis are highly sensitive to UFH. No clear recommendation has been made concerning the use of LMWHs in liver disease.

LMWHs in pregnancy and lactation

LMWHs are frequently used in pregnant women although in some countries the health authorities have not registered this indication. Several recent studies have shown a good tolerance and safety of long-term treatment with various LMWHs in pregnant women.[90–95] It is generally accepted that

LMWHs are safe and effective in pregnant women at risk of VTE.

No data are available regarding the failure of LMWHs to pass into the milk. At this time the use of LMWHs in lactating women has not been documented.[67]

Conclusion

LMWHs belong to the same family of drugs. The pharmacodynamics and pharmacokinetics have been well documented. LMWHs have a more predictable response, a greater bioavailability and a longer half-life than UFH. However, they differ from each other in manufacturing, distribution of molecular weight of their constituents and some other physicochemical and biological properties as well as their pharmacokinetics. The concept of anti-Xa/anti-IIa ratio, determined in vitro, tends to obscure the fact that the clearance of anti-IIa activity is usually faster in vivo than that of anti-Xa activity. It does not take into account the pharmacokinetics of anti-Xa and anti-IIa activity which differ from one LMWH to another. Therefore, the clinical findings associated with a given LMWH preparation cannot be extrapolated to another one or generalized to the whole family of LMWHs as stated by several authors.

References

1. Bergqvist D. Low molecular weight heparins. *J Intern Med* 1996; **240**: 63–72.

2. Weitz JI. Low molecular weight heparins. *N Engl J Med* 1997; **337**: 688–698.

3. Hirsh J, Warkentin TE, Raschke R et al. Heparin and low molecular weight heparin: mechanism of action, pharmacokinetics, dosing considerations, monitoring, efficacy, and safety. *Chest* 1998; **114**: 489S–510S.

4. Jeske W, Fareed J. In vitro studies on the biochemistry and pharmacology of low molecular weight heparins. *Semin Thromb Hemost* 1999; **25**: 27–33.

5. Samama MM, Bara L, Gerotziafas GT. Mechanisms for antithrombotic activity in man of low molecular weight heparins. *Haemostasis* 1994; **24**: 105–117.

6. Sandset M, Abildgaard U, Larsen ML. Heparin induces release of extrinsic coagulation pathway inhibitor (EPI). *Thromb Res* 1988; **50**: 803–813.

7. Holmer E, Mattsson C, Nilsson S. Anticoagulant and antithrombotic effects of heparin and low molecular weight heparin fragments in rabbits. *Thromb Res* 1982; **25**: 475–485.

8. Bara L, Trillou M, Mardiguian J, Samama M Comparison of antithrombotic activity of two heparin fragments PK 10169 (MW 5000) and EMT 680 (MW 2500) and unfractionated heparin in a rabbit experimental thrombosis model: relative importance of systemic anti-Xa and anti-IIa activities. *Nouv Rev Fr Hematol* 1986; **28**: 355–358.

9. Cade JF, Buchanan MR, Boneu B et al. A comparison of the antithrombotic and haemorrhagic effects of low molecular weight

heparin fractions: the influence of the method of preparation. *Thromb Res* 1984; **15:** 613–625.

10. Ostegaard PB, Nilsson B, Bergqvist D et al. The effect of low molecular weight heparin on experimental thrombosis and haemostasis — the influence of production method. *Thromb Res* 1987; **45:** 739–749.

11. Fareed J, Jeske W, Eschenfelder V et al. Preclinical studies on low molecular weight heparins. *Thromb Res* 1996; **81:** S1–27.

12. Brieger D, Dawes J. Production method affects the pharmacokinetic and ex vivo biological properties of low molecular weight heparins. *Thromb Haemost* 1997; **77:** 317–322.

13. Linhardt RJ, Gunay NS. Production and chemical processing of low molecular weight heparins. *Semin Thromb Hemost* 1999; **25:** 5–16.

14. Fareed J, Jeske W, Hoppensteadt D et al. Are the available low molecular weight heparin preparations the same? *Semin Thromb Hemost* 1996; **22:** 77–91.

15. Troy S, Fruncillo R, Ozawa T et al. The dose proportionality of the pharmacokinetics of ardeparin, a low molecular weight heparin, in healthy volunteers. *J Clin Pharmacol* 1995; **35:** 1194–1199.

16. Neville GA, Mori F, Racey TJ et al. Chemical composition, particle size range, and biological activity of some low molecular weight heparin derivatives. *J Pharm Sci* 1990; **79:** 339.

17. Komatsu H, Takahata T, Tanaka M et al. Determination of the molecular weight distribution of low molecular weight heparins using high-performance gel permeation chromatography. *Biol Pharm Bull* 1993; **16:** 1189–1193.

18. Horne MK. Heparin binding to normal and abnormal platelets. *Thromb Res* 1988; **51:** 135–144.

19. Horne MK, Chao ES. Heparin binding to resting and activated platelets. *Blood* 1989; **74:** 238–243.

20. Horne MK, Chao ES. The effect of molecular weight on heparin binding to platelets. *Br J Haematol* 1990; **74:** 306–312.

21. Suda Y, Marques D, Kermode JC et al. Structural characterisation of heparin's liaison domain for human platelets. *Thromb Res* 1993; **69:** 501–508.

22. Sobel M, Adelman B. Characterisation of platelet binding of heparins and other glycosaminoglycans. *Thromb Res* 1988; **50:** 815–826.

23. Kaplan KL, Broekman MJ, Chernoff A et al. Platelet alpha granule proteins: studies on release and subcellular localisation. *Blood* 1979; **53:** 604–615.

24. Horne MK. The effect of secreted heparin-binding proteins on heparin binding to platelets. *Thromb Res* 1993; **70:** 97–98.

25. Hirsh J, Levine MN. Low molecular weight heparin. *Blood* 1992; **79:** 1–17.

26. Young E, Wells P, Holloway S et al. Ex vivo and in vitro evidence that low molecular weight heparins exhibit less binding to plasma proteins than unfractionated heparin. *Thromb Haemost* 1994; **71:** 300–304.

27. Bender F, Aronson L. Bioequivalence of subcutaneous calcium and sodium heparins. *Clin Pharmacol Ther* 1980; **27:** 224–229.

28. Hemker HC, Beguin S. The activity of heparin in the presence of Ca^{2+} ions: why the anti-Xa activity of LMW heparins is about two times overestimated. *Thromb Haemost* 1993; **70:** 717–718.

29. Bara L, Samama M. The need for standardization of low molecular weight heparin (LMWH). *Thromb Haemost* 1986; **56**: 418.

30. Barrowcliffe TW, Curtis AD, Johnson EA, Thomas DP. An international standard for low molecular weight heparin. *Thromb Haemost* 1988; **60**: 1–7.

31. Dautzenberg MS, Bara L, Cornu P, Samama M. Specific anti-Xa activity of LMWH (Kabi 2165, CY 216, PK 10169) against the first international standard of LMWH: a collaborative study. *Thromb Haemost* 1990; **64**: 490–491.

32. Stiekema JC, Van Griensven JM, Van Dinther TG, Cohen AF. A cross-over comparison of the anti-clotting effects of three low molecular weight heparins and glycosaminoglycan. *Br J Clin Pharmacol* 1993; **36**: 51–56.

33. Eriksson BL, Soderberg K, Widlund L et al. A comparative study of three low molecular weight heparins (LMWH) and unfractionated heparin (UH) in healthy volunteers. *Thromb Haemost* 1995; **73**: 398–401.

34. Davis R, Faulds D. Nadroparin calcium. A review of its pharmacology and clinical use in the prevention and treatment of thromboembolic disorders. *Drugs Aging* 1997; **10**: 299–322.

35. Frampton JE, Faulds D. Parnaparin. A review of its pharmacology, and clinical application in the prevention and treatment of thromboembolic and other vascular disorders. *Drugs* 1994; **47**: 652–676.

36. Friedel HA, Balfour JA. Tinzaparin. A review of its pharmacology and clinical potential in the prevention and treatment of thromboembolic disorders. *Drugs* 1994; **48**: 638–660.

37. Woltz M, Eder M, Weltermann A et al. Comparison of the effects of different low molecular weight heparins on the hemostatic system activation in vivo in man. *Thromb Haemost* 1997; **78**: 876–879.

38. Carter CJ, Kelton JG, Hirsh J et al. The relationship between the hemorrhagic and antithrombotic properties of low molecular weight heparin in rabbits. *Blood* 1982; **59**: 1239–1245.

39. Holst J, Lindblad B, Bergqvist D et al. Protamine neutralization in intravenous and subcutaneous low molecular weight heparin (Tinzaparin, Logiparin). An experimental investigation in healthy volunteers. *Blood Coagul Fibrinolysis* 1994; **5**: 795–803.

40. Harenberg J, Gnasso A, de Vries JX et al. Inhibition of low molecular weight heparin by protamine chloride in vivo. *Thromb Res* 1985; **38**: 11–20.

41. Harenberg J, Giese C, Knodler A et al. Neutralization of low molecular weight heparin Kabi 2165 by protamine chloride. *Klin Wochenschr* 1986; **64**: 1171–1175.

42. Andrassy K, Eschenfelder V, Koderisch J, Weber E. Pharmacokinetics of Clivarin a new low molecular weight heparin in healthy volunteers. *Thromb Res* 1994; **73**: 95–108.

43. Racanelli A, Fareed J. Neutralization of the antithrombotic effects of heparin and Fraxiparin by protamine sulfate. *Thromb Res* 1992; **68**: 211–222.

44. Massonet-Castel S, Pelissier E, Bara L et al. Partial reversal of low molecular weight heparin (PK 10169) anti-Xa activity by protamine sulfate: in vitro and in vivo study during cardiac surgery with extracorporeal circulation. *Haemostasis* 1986; **16**: 139–146.

45. Fareed J, Hoppensteadt D, Jeske W et al. The available low molecular weight heparin

preparations are not the same. *Clin Appl Thromb Haemost* 1997; **3**: S38–S52.

46. Salzman EW, Rosenberg RD, Smith MH et al. Effect of heparin and heparin fractions on platelet aggregation. *J Clin Invest* 1980; **65**: 64–73.

47. Harenberg J, Stehle G, Dempfle CE et al. The pharmacological profile of the low molecular weight heparin 21–23 in man: anticoagulant, lipolytic and protamine reversible effects. *Folia Haematol Int Mag Klin Morphol Blutforsch* 1989; **116**: 967–980.

48. Persson E, Nilsson-Ehle P. Release of lipoprotein lipase and hepatic lipase activity. Effects of heparin and low molecular weight heparin fragment. *Scand J Clin Lab Invest* 1990; **50**: 43–49.

49. Barrowcliffe TW, Merton RE, Gray E, Thomas DP. Heparin and bleeding: an association with lipase release. *Thromb Haemost* 1988; **60**: 434–436.

50. Persson E. Lipoprotein lipase, hepatic lipase and plasma lipolytic activity. Effects of heparin and a low molecular weight heparin fragment (Fragmin). *Acta Med Scand* 1988; **724**: 1–56.

51. Millot F, Bara L, Etienne J et al. Activité lipolytique et anticoagulante de l'héparine et d'un de ses dérivés de faible poids moléculaire. *Nouv Rev Fr Hématol* 1987; **29**: 397–400.

52. Monreal M, Vinas L, Monreal L et al. Heparin-related osteoporosis in rats. A comparative study between unfractionated heparin and a low molecular weight heparin. *Haemostasis* 1990; **20**: 204–207.

53. Mätzch T, Bergqvist D, Hedner U et al. Effects of low molecular weight heparin and unfragmented heparin on induction of osteoporosis in rats. *Thromb Haemost* 1990; **63**: 505–509.

54. Shaughnessy SG, Hirsh J, Bhandari M et al. A histomorphometric evaluation of heparin-induced bone loss after discontinuation of heparin treatment in rats. *Blood* 1999; **93**: 1231–1236.

55. Monreal M, Lafoz E, Olive A et al. Comparison of subcutaneous unfractionated heparin with a low molecular weight heparin (Fragmin) in patients with venous thromboembolism and contraindications to coumarin. *Thromb Haemost* 1994; **74**: 7–11.

56. Hansen JB, Sandset PM, Huseby KR et al. Differential effect of unfractionated heparin and low molecular weight heparin on intravascular tissue factor pathway inhibitor: evidence for a difference in antithrombotic action. *Br J Haematol* 1998; **101**: 638–646.

57. Falkon L, Gari M, Barbanoj M et al. Tissue factor pathway inhibitor and anti-FXa kinetic profiles of a new low molecular mass heparin, Bemiparin, at therapeutic subcutaneous doses. *Blood Coagul Fibrinolysis* 1998; **9**: 137–141.

58. Hansen JB, Sandset PM. Differential effects of low molecular weight heparin and unfractionated heparin on circulating levels of antithrombin and tissue factor pathway inhibitor (TFPI): a possible mechanism for difference in therapeutic efficacy. *Thromb Res* 1998; **91**: 177–181.

59. Valentine S, Ostergaard P, Kristensen H, Nordfang O. Simultaneous presence of tissue pathway inhibitor (TFPI) and low molecular weight heparin has a synergistic effect in different coagulation assays. *Blood Coagul Fibrinolysis* 1991; **2**: 629–635.

60. Bara L, Bloch MF, Zitoun D et al. Comparative effects of enoxaparin and unfractionated heparin in healthy volunteers on prothrombin consumption in whole blood during coagulation, and release of tissue factor

pathway inhibitor. *Thromb Res* 1993; **69**: 443–452.

61. Zitoun D, Bara L, Bloch MF, Samama MM. Plasma TFPI activity after intravenous injection of pentasaccharide (PS) and unfractionated heparin in rabbits. *Thromb Res* 1994; **75**: 577–580.

62. Gerotziafas GT, Bara L, Bloch MF et al. Treatment with LMWHs inhibits factor VIIa generation during in vitro coagulation of whole blood. *Thromb Res* 1996; **81**: 491–496.

63. Gerotziafas GT, Bara L, Bloch MF et al. Comparative effects of synthetic pentasaccharide, low molecular weight heparin, unfractionated heparin and recombinant hirudin on the generation of factor VIIa and prothrombin activation after coagulation of human plasma. *Blood Coagul Fibrinolysis* 1998; **9**: 571–580.

64. Gerotziafas G. Génération de FVIIa pendant la coagulation du plasma humain. Etude du mécanisme d'inhibition de la génération et de l'activité du FVIIa induite par le pentasaccharide synthétique, une héparine de bas poids moléculaire et l'héparine non fractionnée. Comparaison avec l'hirudine. PhD Thesis. Faculty of Medicine, University Pierre et Marie Curie, Paris VI, France 1999.

65. Gerotziafas GT, Samama M. In vitro LMWH affects less than UFH the formation and the structure of normal clot. A thromboelastography study. *Haemostasis* 1994; **24**: 246 (abstract) 13th International Congress on Thrombosis, Bilbao 1994.

66. Collignon F, Frydman A, Caplain H et al. Comparison of pharmacokinetic profiles of three low molecular weight heparins: dalteparin, enoxaparin and nadroparin administered subcutaneously in healthy volunteers (doses for prevention of thromboembolism). *Thromb Haemost* 1995; **73**: 630–640.

67. Frydman A. Low molecular weight heparins: an overview of their pharmacodynamics, pharmacokinetics and metabolism in humans. *Haemostasis* 1996; **26**: 24–38.

68. Bara L, Samama M. Pharmacokinetics of low molecular weight heparins. *Acta Chir Scand* 1990; **556**: 57–61.

69. Rostin M, Montastrux JL, Houin G et al. Pharmacodynamics of CY 216 in healthy volunteers: inter-individual variations. *Fundam Clin Pharmacol* 1990; **4**: 17–23.

70. Bratt G, Törnebohm E, Widlund L, Lockner D. Low molecular weight heparin (Kabi 2165, Fragmin): pharmacokinetics after intravenous and subcutaneous administration in human volunteers. *Thromb Res* 1986; **42**: 613–620.

71. Frydman AM, Bara L, Le Roux Y et al. The antithrombotic activity and pharmacokinetics of enoxaparin, a low molecular weight heparin, in humans given single subcutaneous doses of 20–80 mg. *J Clin Pharmacol* 1988; **28**: 609–618.

72. Azizi M, Veyssier-Belot C, Alhenc-Gelas M et al. Comparison of biological activities of two low molecular weight heparins in 10 healthy volunteers. *Br J Clin Pharmacol* 1995; **40**: 577–584.

73. Pedersen PC, Ostergaard PB, Hedner U et al. Pharmacokinetics of a low molecular weight heparin, logiparin, after intravenous and subcutaneous administration to healthy volunteers. *Thromb Res* 1991; **61**: 477–487.

74. Simoneau G, Bergmann JF, Kher A et al. Pharmacokinetics of a low molecular weight heparin (Fragmin) in young and elderly subjects. *Thromb Res* 1992; **66**: 603–607.

75. Frydman AM, Bara L, Le Roux Y et al. The

antithrombotic activity and pharmacokinetics of enoxaparin, a low molecular weight heparin, in humans given single subcutaneous doses of 20–80 mg. *J Clin Pharmacol* 1988; **28**: 609–618.

76. Jeske W, Fareed J, Eschenfelder C et al. Biochemical and pharmacologic characteristics of Reviparin, a low molecular weight heparin. *Semin Thromb Hemost* 1997; **23**: 119–128.

77. Bara L, Planes A, Samama MM. Occurrence of thrombosis and haemorrhage, relationship with anti-Xa, anti-IIa activities, and D-dimer plasma levels in patients receiving a low molecular weight heparin, enoxaparin or tinzaparin, to prevent deep vein thrombosis after hip surgery. *Br J Haematol* 1999; **140**: 230–240.

78. Verstraete M. Pharmacotherapeutic aspects of unfractionated and low molecular weight heparins. *Drugs* 1990; **40**: 498–530.

79. Cadroy Y, Pourrat J, Baladre MF et al. Delayed elimination of enoxaparin in patients with chronic renal insufficiency. *Thromb Res* 1991; **63**: 385–390.

80. Howard PA, Dalteparin: a low molecular weight heparin. *Ann Pharmacol* 1997; **31**: 192–200.

81. Laforest MD, Colas Linhart N, Guiraud-Vitaux et al. Pharmacokinetics and biodistribution of technetium 99m labelled standard heparin and a low molecular weight heparin (enoxaparin) after intravenous injection in normal volunteers. *Br J Haematol* 1991; **77**: 201–208.

82. Troy S, Fruncillo R, Ozawa T. Absolute and comparative subcutaneous bioavailability of ardeparin sodium, a low molecular weight heparin. *Thromb Haemost* 1997; **78**: 871–875.

83. Andrew M, Boneu B, Cade J et al. Placental transport of low molecular weight heparin to the pregnant sheep. *Br J Haematol* 1985; **59**: 103–108.

84. Forestier F, Daffos F, Capella-Pavlowsky M. Low molecular weight heparin (PK 10169) does not cross the placenta during the second trimester of pregnancy: study by direct fetal blood sampling under ultrasound. *Thromb Res* 1984; **34**: 557–560.

85. Forestier F, Daffos F, Renaut M et al. Low molecular weight heparin (CY 219-6) does not cross the placenta during the third trimester of pregnancy. *Thromb Haemost* 1987; **57**: 234.

86. Omri A, Delaloye JF, Anderson H et al. Low molecular weight heparin NOVO (LHN-1) does not cross the placenta during the second trimester of pregnancy. *Thromb Haemost* 1989; **61**: 55–56.

87. Feigin MD, Lourwood DL. Low molecular weight heparins and their use in obstetrics and gynecology. *Obstet Gynecol Surv* 1994; **49**: 424–431.

88. Mismetti P, Laporte-Simisidis S, Navarro C et al. Aging and venous thromboembolism influence the pharmacodynamics of the anti-factor Xa and antithrombin activities of a low molecular weight heparin (nadroparin). *Thromb Haemost* 1998; **79**: 1162–1165.

89. Siguret V, Pautas E, Février M et al. Older patients treated with tinzaparin administered once daily (175 anti-Xa IU/kg): a pharmacokinetic study over 10 days. *Thromb Haemost* 1999. XVIIth Congress of the International Society on Thrombosis and Haemostasis, Washington. Abstract p. 63.

90. Ginsberg JS, Hirsh J. Use of antithrombotic agents during pregnancy. *Chest* 1998; (Suppl.) S524–S530.

91. Gillis S, Shushan A, Eldor A. Use of low molecular weight heparin for prophylaxis and

treatment of thromboembolism in pregnancy. *Int J Gynecol Obstet* 1992; **39:** 297–301.

92.   Melissari E, Parker CJ, Wilson NV et al. Use of low molecular weight heparin in pregnancy. *Thromb Haemost* 1992; **68:** 652–656.

93.   Nelson Piercy C, Letsky EA, de Swiet M. Low molecular weight heparin for obstetric thromboprophylaxis: experience of sixty-nine pregnant women at high risk. *Am J Obstet Gynecol* 1997; **176:** 1052–1068.

94.   Blombäck M, Bremme K, Hellgren M et al. Thromboprophylaxis with low molecular weight heparin, Fragrim (dalteparin) during pregnancy: longitudinal safety study? *Blood Coagul Fibrinolysis* 1998; **9:** 1–9.

95.   Sanson BJ, Lensing AWA, Prins MH et al. Safety of low molecular weight heparin in pregnancy: a systematic review. *Thromb Haemost* 1999; **81:** 668–672.

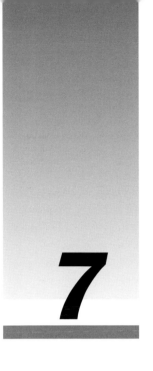

Unfractionated heparin, low molecular weight heparins and heparinoid in orthopedic and trauma surgery

André Planes and Meyer Michel Samama

7

For a long time orthopedic and trauma surgery has been recognized as giving a high risk for venous thromboembolism (VTE). In 1955, Merle d'Aubigné et al[1] presented the results of a clinical survey of 2220 operated patients at his University Department of Orthopedic and Trauma surgery in Paris. In his presentation, he stressed some points of interest. The rates of symptomatic manifestations of VTE were 15% in hip surgery, 22% in hip arthroplasties, and 32% after hip arthrodesis. However, they were only 4.4% after spinal surgery and practically nil after upper limb surgery. Moreover, the diagnosis of VTE, based on clinical manifestations, led to three consequences: an elevated number of severe peripheral manifestations of *phlegmatia alba dolens*; pulmonary embolism in 30% of the cases; and a significant frequency of late sequelae of phlebitis that was related to delayed therapy. He proposed systematic prevention by oral anticoagulants, with a dosage adjusted by the prothrombin time, and the treatment to be prolonged 1 month after elective hip surgery and 3 months after hip arthrodesis. These clinical observations were confirmed later, emphasizing the morbidity of this disease.

In 1959, Sevitt and Gallagher[2] stressed the point of fatal pulmonary embolism. They performed the first orthopedic prospective, randomized clinical trial on 300 patients with fractured neck of the femur. Only half of their patients were protected by adjusted doses of oral anticoagulant. Clinical manifestations of VTE were observed in 28.7% of unprotected patients with 10% dying from fatal pulmonary embolism, which was confirmed by autopsy, versus 2.7% and 1.3% in the group of protected patients. Thus, this group demonstrated that systematic prophylaxis with adjusted doses of oral anticoagulant, not only protected against clinical manifestations of VTE but also saved lives.[2]

In 1962, Sharnhoff[3] introduced a 'plan of heparinization' for surgical patients to prevent deep-vein thrombosis. It may be considered, with an interval of 37 years, that his method of adjusted regimen was too advanced for his time because of the lack of a simple and reliable assay to determine the plasma heparin levels — he proposed the standard Lee–White clotting test, which is insensitive and no longer in use.

In the late 1960s the radioactive fibrinogen uptake test was introduced. It demonstrated an increased risk of asymptomatic deep-vein thrombosis for lower limbs in orthopedic and trauma patients. Thus prospective, randomized, double-blind trials on two parallel groups of patients were then possible with smaller samples of patients, allowing an easier determination of the efficacy of an antithrombotic drug.

In 1975 Kakkar et al[4] published the results of an international multicentre trial. They demonstrated, mainly in general surgery, that fixed mini-doses of calcium heparin 5000 U three times daily were statistically effective in protecting the patients against radioisotopic and clinical deep-vein thrombosis, as well as against clinical and fatal pulmonary embolism. The first injection was given 2 hours before surgery, followed every 8-hourly postoperatively.

In the orthopedic field, and especially after total hip replacement, a controversy appeared concerning the efficacy and safety of Kakkar's method of heparin administration. Favorable results were reported[5–10] however this was strongly contested by Mannucci et al who found a hemorrhagic tendency and moreover by the Groote Schuur Hospital Thromboembolism study group and Hampson who found that this method only delayed the onset of deep-vein thrombosis.[11–13]

Using this method, opinion leaders such as Sir John Charnley in England[14] and William Harris in the USA[15], observed a huge hemorrhagic tendency and in these countries the use of heparin did not become popular. In the USA, prophylaxis remained focused on warfarin under the direction of the Mayo Clinic[16] in spite of the efforts of Sharnhoff.[17]

In 1977, a round table organized by the French Orthopedic Society, introduced to

France the use of heparin at doses adjusted according to the activated partial thromboplastin time (APTT) in orthopedics.[18] The need for phlebography was also stressed to improve the detection of deep-vein thrombosis of lower limbs in hip surgery as demonstrated by Evarts in 1971.[19] Similarly pulmonary angiography was considered the 'gold standard' in the diagnosis of pulmonary embolism. Thus, fixed mini-doses of heparin were then considered insufficient against VTE and even dangerous, favoring, by unstable anticoagulation, the formation of the floating proximal clot (the 'widow makers'). From that time the regimen of adjusted doses of heparin was popularized in France.[20,21] In 1983 it was made official internationally by Leyvraz et al.[22] It must be noted that the controversy on the safety and efficacy of fixed mini-doses of heparin was only considered solved by the Oxford meta-analysis of Collins et al.[23] In 1988 they stated that such a regimen halved the absolute risk of venographic deep-vein thrombosis and subsequently decreased the risk of pulmonary embolism, especially that of fatal pulmonary embolism ($P < 0.0001$). The price to pay was an increased bleeding tendency. As pointed out by Collins et al 'although excessive bleeding or need for transfusion appeared to be increased by about one-half to two-thirds, the absolute excess was small (about 2%)'.[23]

In 1986 the first American Consensus Conference took place under the auspices of the National Institutes of Health.[24] The need for systematic prophylaxis was stressed in the high-risk group of orthopedic and trauma patients. Among other methods of prophylaxis, adjusted doses of unfractionated heparin were recommended. Also, venographically proven deep-vein thrombosis was considered as a reliable marker of VTE disease. The clinical relevance of such asymptomatic deep-vein thrombosis was and is still debatable, the rationale behind this position is that eradication of deep-vein thrombosis would ultimately result in a reduction of non-fatal and fatal pulmonary embolism and late sequelae of postthrombotic syndrome.

Systematic use of phlebography allowed the description of the risk for deep venous thrombosis in orthopedic and trauma patients. The figures may be found in recent books and consensuses.[25–32] Risks are generally high and the great majority of these patients is considered at high or at very high risk of VTE disease. We try later to discriminate between these patients.

In the late 1980s the era of low molecular weight heparins (LMWHs) began. By fractionation of commercial grade unfractionated heparin (UFH) new compounds were obtained. They differ according to the methods of preparation (see Chapter 7.) These new heparin preparations with low molecular weight exhibited new properties that rapidly led to them being regarded as belonging to a new family of drugs but as separate compounds inside this family.

Being more or less devoid of the long polysaccharide chains of UFH responsible mainly for the anti-IIa activity, they possess an increased anti-Xa activity, leading to different anti-Xa/anti-IIa ratios. Moreover they showed excellent absorption after subcutaneous administration leading to an almost complete bioavailability. Also, lesser binding to the vascular wall and to platelets resulted in an increased half-life after subcutaneous administration and a more stable heparinization. These differences were rapidly considered an important improvement in the management of heparin. Moreover, it was demonstrated in 1986 that twice daily postoperative administration of enoxaparin resulted in a 70% relative risk reduction of venographic deep-vein thrombosis after total hip replacement in comparison with placebo.[33] In 1988 it was demonstrated that enoxaparin could be administered as a once daily fixed dose with no laboratory monitoring of blood coagulation. This mode of administration decreased the relative risk of venographic deep-vein thrombosis by 50% after total hip replacement in comparison with Kakkar's regimen of administration of unfractionated heparin.[34] These trials were rapidly followed by a large number of others that demonstrated the efficacy and safety of different LMWHs. *Table 7.1* shows the names and the dosages recommended by the manufacturers for approved LMWHs. *Tables 7.2* to *7.7* present the main trials carried out with internationally approved LMWHs in prevention of deep-vein thrombosis after total hip replacement. Similarly *Table 7.8* presents the results for total knee replacement. We have selected trials where deep-vein thromboses was venographically demonstrated. In these tables, one may observe a great variability in the observed rates of deep-vein thrombosis with the same drug. This discrepancy is explained by variability in patient population, in centre effect, in the dosages of the drugs, and in the venographic adjudications that are more or less subjective and also do not retain the same criteria for thrombosis (intraluminal filling defects, with or without muscular vein thrombosis; non-opacification of a vein, or a segment thereof, despite repeated injection of contrast medium, or on venograms made at different times).

It is now considered, after more than 10 years of use that LMWHs belong to the same family of drugs (MM Samama, personal communication). Also the elegant expression of Barrowcliffe et al[25] that they were 'siblings and not distant cousins' was perfectly justified. At least, as they pointed out, 'if their mean molecular weight stands in the range of 4000–6000 daltons'.

With the advent of an appropriate standard for LMWHs, we are now convinced that for most actual LMWHs, a dosage between 4000 and 5000 IU anti-Xa, on a

Table 7.1
LMWH and heparinoid in orthopedics and trauma: countries and related approved dosages

	EU	USA
Enoxaparin	4000 IU*/day started 12 h preoperatively	3000 IU × 2/day started 12/24 h postoperatively
Fraxiparin	Weight-adapted dosage	—
Fragmin	5000 IU/day started 12 h preoperatively or 2500 IU × 2/day	2500 IU 2 h preoperatively then 5000 IU/day
Tinzaparin	4500 IU/day or weight-adapted started 12 h preoperatively	—
Reviparin	4200 IU/day started 12 h preoperatively	—
Ardeparin	—	50 IU/kg × 2/day started 12/24 h postoperatively
Danaparoid	Only for HIT†	750 IU 1–2 h preoperatively and twice daily after
Parnaparin	Italy	—
Bemiparin	Spain 3500 IU/day 6 h postoperatively	—
Certoparin	Germany	

* IU = anti-factor Xa IU
† HIT = heparin-induced thrombocytopenia

once daily basis is appropriate. However, for each compound the correct dosage must be determined, although two recent comparative studies have demonstrated that the results obtained with these dosages led to clinically similar results.[35,36] Also these drugs are not considered interchangeable. Interestingly they have a special efficacy against proximal deep-vein thrombosis, with a once or twice daily administration at fixed dose with no need for coagulation monitoring apart from platelet counts, which should be monitored. This led to an improved compliance, and resulted in a generalization of their use.

Successive European, International and American consensus conferences contributed to the large audience found by these LMWHs in this group of high risk patients.[26–32] Practically, all successive meta-analyses concluded the same way,[37–41] but they also

Table 7.2
Prophylaxis with LMWH in patients operated on for total hip replacement

Enoxaparin European dosage 40 mg/day begun 12 h preoperatively		Number of patients randomized		Number of patients evaluated		All deep-vein thrombosis	
First author (Reference)	Year	LMWH	Control	LMWH	Control	LMWH Number	%
			UFH 5000 × 3		UFH		
Planès (34)	1988	124	113	120	108	15	(12.5)
			Dextran		Dextran		
Danish Group (42)	1991	108	111	108	111	7	(6.5)
			Desirudin		Desirudin		
Eriksson (43)	1997	785	802	785	768	196	(25.5)
			Foot pump		Foot pump		
Warwick (44)	1998	143	147	138	136	18	(13)
			Reviparin		Reviparin		
Planès (35)	1998	251	247	209	207	18	(9)
			Tinzaparin		Tinzaparin		
Planès (36)	1999	248	251	219	221	44	(20.1)

UFH: unfractionated heparin

	Proximal deep-vein thrombosis					Major bleeding	
Control Number	%	LMWH Number	%	Control Number	%	LMWH %	Control %
27	(25)	9	(7.5)	20	(18.5)	1.6	0
24	(22)	2	(2)	6	(5.4)	0	0
142	(18.4)	59	(7.5)	36	(4.5)	2	1.9
24	(18)	12	(9)	17	(13)	0	0
21	(10)	13	(6)	12	(6)	0.7	0.4
48	(21.7)	23	(10.5)	21	(9.5)	1.6	0.7

Table 7.3
Prophylaxis with LMWH in patients operated on for total hip replacement

Enoxaparin North American dosage 30 mg × 2/day begun 12/24 h postoperatively				Number of patients evaluated		All deep-vein thrombosis	
First author (Reference)	Year	LMWH	Control	LMWH	Control	LMWH Number	%
Turpie (33)	1986	50	Placebo 50	37	Placebo 39	4	(10.8)
Levine (45)	1994	333	UFH 7500 × 2 332	258	263	50	(19.4)
Colwell Jr (46)	1994	194	UFH 5000 × 3 207	136	142	8	(6)
Spiro (47)	1994	Eno-xaparin 30 × 2 post-operatively 208	Eno-xaparin 10 mg post-operatively 161	149	116	16	(11)
		Enoxaparin 40 mg postoperatively 199		143		21	(14)

UFH: unfractionated heparin

		Proximal deep-vein thrombosis				Major bleeding	
Control Number	**%**	**LMWH Number**	**%**	**Control Number**	**%**	**LMWH %**	**Control %**
20	(51.3)	2	(5.4)	9	(21.3)	2	4
61	(23.2)	14	(5.4)	17	(6.5)	3.3	5.7
21	(15)	4	(3)	10	(7)	4	6
36	(31)	9	(6)	16	(14)	5	2
		8	(6)			4	

Table 7.4
Prophylaxis with LMWH in patients operated on for total hip replacement

Dalteparin 2500 IU 2 h preoperatively and 5000 IU/ day after or 2500 IU: 2/day				Number of patients randomized		Number of patients evaluated		All deep-vein thrombosis	
First author (Reference)	Year	LMWH	Control	LMWH	Control			LMWH Number	%
Eriksson (48)	1988	49	Dextran 49	49	49			10	(20)
Dechavanne (49)	1989	82	UFH 40	82	40			5	(6)
Eriksson (50)	1991	63	UFH 5000 × 3 59	63	59			19	(30)
Francis (51)	1997	271	Warfarin 279	192	190			28	(15)
Pineo (52) 2500 IU 2 h preoperatively 2500 IU 12 h postoperatively then 5000 U/day or 2500 IU 6 h postoperatively then 5000 U/day	1999	414 414	Warfarin 414	337 336	338			36 44	(10.7) (13.1)

UFH: unfractionated heparin; IU: anti-factor Xa IU.

	Proximal deep-vein thrombosis					Major bleeding	
Control Number	%	LMWH Number	%	Control Number	%	LMWH %	Control %
22	(45)	?		?		?	?
4	(10)	2	(3)	3	(7.5)	?	?
25	(42)	6	(10)	18	(31)	?	?
49	(26)	10	(5)	16	(8)	2	1
81	(24)	3	(0.8)	11	(3)	8.9	4.5
		3	(0.8)			?	

Table 7.5
Prophylaxis with LMWH in patients operated on for total hip replacement

Fraxiparin		Number of patients randomized		Number of patients evaluated		All deep vein thrombosis	
First author (Reference) Dose	Year	LMWH	Control	LMWH	Control	LMWH Number	%
Leyvraz (53) 41 IU/kg/day for 3 days then 62 IU/kg/day from day 4 to day 10	1991	205	UFH Adjusted APTT 204	174	175	22	(12.6
GHAT Group (54) 4166 IU/day	1992	169	UFH 5000 U × 3/day 172	137	136	45	(33.3
Hamulyak (55) <60 kg–0.3 ml (3075 IU) 60–80 kg–0.4 ml (4100 IU) >80 kg–0.5 ml (6150 IU)	1994	?	OAC INR = 2–3 ?	195	196	27	(13.8

UFH: unfractionated heparin; IU: anti-factor Xa IU; OAC: oral anti-coagulant (acenocoumarol).

	Proximal deep vein thrombosis					Major bleeding	
Control Number	*%*	*LMWH Number*	*%*	*Control Number*	*%*	*LMWH %*	*Control %*
28	(16)	5	(2.9)	23	(13.1)	0.5	1.4
47	(34.3)	14	(10.3)	26	(19)	1.2	1.2
27	(13.8)	12	(6.2)	9	(4.6)	1.5	2.3

Table 7.6
Prophylaxis with LMWH in patients operated on for total hip replacement

Tinzaparin		Number of patients randomized		Number of patients evaluated		All deep-vein thrombosis	
First author (Reference) Dose	Year	LMWH	Control	LMWH	Control	LMWH Number	%
Lassen (56) 50 IU/kg/day	1991	105	Placebo 105	93	Placebo 97	30	(32)
Hull (57) 75 IU/kg/day begun 12/24 h postoperatively	1993	398	Warfarin 397	330	335	69	(20.8)
Planès (36) 4500 IU/day begun 12 h preoperatively	1999	251	Enoxaparin 248	221	219	48	(21.7)
IU: anti-factor Xa IU.							

	Proximal deep-vein thrombosis					Major bleeding	
Control		**LMWH**		**Control**		**LMWH**	**Control**
Number	**%**	**Number**	**%**	**Number**	**%**	**%**	**%**
45	(46)	24	(25)	35	(36)	?	?
79	(23.2)	16	(4.8)	13	(3.8)	2.8	1.5
44	(20.1)	23	(10.5)	21	(9.5)	0.8	1.6

Table 7.7
Prophylaxis with LMWH in patients operated on for total hip replacement

Reviparin and lomoparan		Number of patients randomized		Number of patients evaluated		All deep-vein thrombosis	
First author (Reference) Dose	Year	LMWH	Control	LMWH	Control	LMWH Number %	
Reviparin Planès (35) 4200 IU: day begun 12 h preoperatively	1998	247	Enoxaparin 251	207	Enoxaparin 209	21	(10)
Lomoparan org 10172 Leyvraz (58) 750 IU × 2/day	1992	154	UFH + DHE 155	145	139	25	(17)

UFH: unfractionated heparin; IU: anti-factor Xa IU; DHE: Dihydroergotamin.

	Proximal deep-vein thrombosis						Major bleeding	
Control Number	%	LMWH Number	%	Control Number	%		LMWH %	Control %
18	(9)	12	(6)	13	(6)		0.4	0.8
44	(32)	7	(5)	9	(6)		0.6	0.6

Table 7.8
Prophylaxis with LMWH in patients operated on for total knee replacement

First author (Reference) Dose	Year	Number of patients randomized		Number of patients evaluated		All deep-vein thrombosis	
		LMWH	Control	LMWH	Control	LMWH Number	%
Leclerc (59) Enoxaparin 30 mg × 2	1992	66	Placebo 65	41	54	8	(20)
Hull (57) Tinzaparin	1993	317	Warfarin 324	249	268	116	(47)
Faunø (60) Enoxaparin 40 mg	1994	108	UFH 116	92	93	21	(23)
Hamulyak (55) Nadroparin	1994	?	Acenocoumarol ?	65	61	16	(25)
RD Heparin Group (61)	1994	344	Warfarin 180	299	147	78	(26)
Colwell (62) Enoxaparin 30 mg × 2	1995	228	UFH 225	143	145	56	(39)
Fitzgerald (63) Enoxaparin 30 × 2	1995	?	Warfarin ?	176	176	44	(25)
Leclerc (64) Enoxaparin 30 mg × 2	1996	336	Warfarin 334	206	211	76	(37)
Levine (65) RD Heparin	1996	122	Elastic stockings 124	96	103	28	(29)
Heit (66) RD Heparin	1997	277	Warfarin 279	232	222	63	(27)

UFH: unfractionated heparin.

		Proximal deep-vein thrombosis				Major bleeding	
Control		**LMWH**		**Control**		**LMWH**	**Control**
Number	**%**	**Number**	**%**	**Number**	**%**	**%**	**%**
35	(65)	0	(0)	11	(20)	0	2
152	(57)	20	(8)	34	(13)	3	1
25	(27)	3	(3)	5	(5)	0	0
25	(38)	5	(8)	6	(10)	2.3	1.5
60	(41)	16	(5)	15	(10)	?	?
77	(53)	5	(3)	22	(15)	1.0	1.0
79	(45)	3	(2)	20	(11)	5	2
109	(52)	24	(12)	22	(10)	2	2
60	(58)	2	(2)	16	(16)	2.5	2.4
85	(38)	15	(6)	15	(7)	?	?

failed generally to demonstrate a lesser bleeding tendency when these compounds were used instead of unfractionated heparin. The consensus on this observation remains based on the conclusions of Collins[23] concerning unfractionated heparin as mentioned above.[23]

Some important points of interest still require further investigations. Do all orthopedic and trauma patients require mandatory systematic prophylaxis? Although, to our knowledge, no venographic study of upper limb surgery exists, this type of surgery has been considered for a long time to be at very low risk of VTE and does not need systematic prophylaxis if an intravenous catheter has not been used or if there is no cancer treatment.

Spinal surgery is associated with a comparable risk to general surgery when the patient is able to walk rapidly following the surgery and in the absence of paralysis. In this group of patients the risk of bleeding must always be kept in mind. In current practice, prophylaxis, when deemed justified, is often begun after surgery when the risk of intraspinal bleeding is over, as in neurosurgery.[67]

The risk in trauma patients has been clearly demonstrated by a large venographic study of Geerts et al.[68] Unexpected incidences of venographic deep-venous thrombosis were found in face, chest, abdominal, spinal and in lower limb trauma patients. Moreover when

these trauma were associated the risk was higher. In major articular replacements, the hip has been commonly used as a model because of the relative standardization and frequency of the operation, and allows for easier group comparisons. It now appears that knee replacement is more resistant to prophylaxis. This point has recently been studied in detail.[69]

Femoral neck fractures represent a difficult problem. In the elderly population, these fractures happen frequently, often spontaneously and a short time before the end of the life. In clinical research, it is impossible to assemble homogeneous cohorts of patients having the same life expectancy and seen rapidly after fracture. These patients come often to the hospital hours or days after fracture and the rate of preoperative deep-vein thrombosis may be as high as 10–15%. Objectively, in this type of surgery the main outcome endpoint is survival at 90 days. As pointed out by the East Anglian audit, lower mortality is the result of the cumulative effect of several aspects of the organization of treatment and management includes pharmaceutical prophylaxis, antibiotic prophylaxis and early mobilization.[70]

To summarize, LMWHs have demonstrated a relatively good clinical effectiveness and safety when used as prophylaxis in all these types of surgery. The point is now to consider whether it is necessary to completely clear the veins of all residual intraluminal filling defects. It seems necessary to balance this point with the clinical protection afforded to patients and to weight the real clinical benefit afforded by new more effective (and expensive) compounds.

Concomitant use of LMWHs and spinal or epidural anesthesia is a problem. In some countries, such as Scandinavian countries the risk of intraspinal bleeding is considered minimal and LMWHs are begun 12 hours preoperatively in association with the once daily dosing. In many other countries, a warning has been given by the administrative health authorities or by legal jurisprudence. This risk is maximal when an epidural catheter is used and moreover left in situ for some days. In such cases caution must be taken to remove the catheter at trough level of heparin and to administrate an LMWH at least 2 or 3 hours after removal of the catheter. A reasonable position seems afforded by the fact that spinal anesthesia by itself affords a protection against VTE, which may be equal to that of unfractionated heparin. Thus it seems redundant to combine heparin with major conduction anesthesia and its concurrent use could be considered contraindicated. Then comes the 'key question needing an answer' pointed out by the last International Consensus Statement of 1997:[31] 'The hypothesis that low molecular weight heparin twice daily subcutaneously is necessary if commenced postoperatively instead of the same dose once daily requires

further investigations by randomized controlled trials for each individual agent separately.'

A recent trial comparing pre- and postoperative administration of LMWH has demonstrated an almost equivalent clinical efficacy of the same dose of LMWH administered either 2 hours pre- or 6 hours postoperatively.[52] An increase in bleeding tendency was observed with the preoperative administration. This verification leads to the concept of perioperative administration of the LMWH and is in accordance with the results of a previous trial.[71] Thus it now appears that a consensus is possible on the postoperative administration of LMWH as a single shot administered daily begun 6 ± 2 hours after surgery.

A point of debate is the choice between an adjusted LMWH dosage according to the body weight or to the time of administration. Adapted weight dosages have not demonstrated a superior efficacy or safety in various studies of prophylaxis. The actual tendency, with these so different dosages, is to simplify the work of the nurses by applying dosages adapted by cross-sections of body-weight (generally three different dosages).[55] This method is less and less used, remains complicated and is no more effective than the simplified one. Thus adaptation of a fixed dosage by the first time of administration seems the best way, as pointed out above. However, it has to be considered that obesity, as defined by the body mass index is a risk factor for thrombosis. Obesity, rather than increased body weight may require a higher dose of LMWH. (MM Samama, personal communication.)

A burning point is the problem of prolongation of prophylaxis after discharge of the patient from the hospital. Five studies have demonstrated a persistence and new formation of radiologic asymptomatic deep-vein thrombosis after total hip replacement.[72–76] Prolonged prophylaxis for 1 month with LMWHs afforded a mean relative risk reduction of the risk of deep-vein thrombosis of 50%. The persistence of a notable rate of proximal DVT through these studies constitutes the rationale for prolonged prophylaxis in these high-risk patients. Nevertheless the type of prophylaxis that may be proposed (LMWH or oral antivitamin K), the problem of residual mortality and morbidity after a 10–12 days course of prophylaxis as compared with that observed after a prolonged course of LMWH, the problem of the exact duration of this prolongation, and of its cost-effectiveness, need further investigation. It is interesting to note that these problems, which were raised by Merle d'Aubigné in 1955, are still awaiting a solution in our modern era of evidence-based medicine.

Postthrombotic syndrome is always a pending problem. Its exact rate is now unknown in the patients who receive in-hospital prophylaxis. Studies based on a prolonged survey of patients presenting an asymptomatic radiologic deep-vein thrombosis are possible, but they are biased by the fact that these patients are usually treated. Thus, late reviews of these patients detect only the result of these treatments and not the natural history of this late complication. Nevertheless a high rate of early postthrombotic syndrome has been found after clinically symptomatic deep-vein thrombosis, 22.8% at 2 years, 29.1% at 8 years.[77]

Finally, it appears that LMWHs have progressively replaced unfractionated heparin in the prophylaxis of patients in orthopedics and trauma. They have really improved the safety and the efficacy of prophylaxis. However, this success, with its linked commercial advantage, has greatly stimulated research in this field. Now, very low LMWH (with mean molecular weight 3000 anti-Xa IU) and pure synthetic anti-Xa inhibitor is thought promising and under development. Among them pentasaccharide is already used in several clinical trials, as well as an anti-IIa inhibitor, desirudin (r-hirudin), which has been demonstrated to be more effective than and as safe as unfractionated heparin and an LMWH when administered subcutaneously twice daily and begun preoperatively.[43,78,79]

Other anti-IIa inhibitors, such as Melagatran (Astra Zeneca, Mölndal, Sweden), which could be administered orally are under development and some opportunities are appearing for orally administered heparin.[80] Thus a great challenge is open and the future of prophylaxis for the next decade in this type of surgery is very promising. However a robust cost-effectiveness approach to these new strategies will become more and more important.[81]

References

1. Merle d'Aubigné R, Tubiana R, Duparc J. Les complications thromboemboliques en chirurgie orthopédique et en traumatologie. Leur fréquence et leur prévention. Bull Acad Chir Scéance du 14 décembre 1955; 1011–1022.

2. Sevitt S, Gallagher NG. Prevention of venous thrombosis and pulmonary embolism in injured patients. A trial of anticoagulant prophylaxis with phenindione in middle-aged and elderly patients with fractured neck of the femur. Lancet 1959; 2: 981–989.

3. Sharnhoff JG, Kass HH, Mistica BA. A plan of heparinization of the surgical patient to prevent postoperative thromboembolism. Surg Gynecol Obstet 1962; 2: 75–79.

4. Prevention of fatal postoperative pulmonary embolism by low doses of heparin, an international multicentre trial. Lancet 1975; ii: 45–51.

5. Gallus AS, Hirsh J, Tuttle RJ et al. Small subcutaneous doses of heparin in prevention of venous thrombosis. N Engl J Med 1973; 288: 545–551.

6. Morris GK, Henry APJ, Preston BJ. Prevention of deep-vein thrombosis by low-dose heparin in patients undergoing total hip replacement. Lancet 1974; ii: 797–799.

7. Dechavanne M, Saudin F, Viala JJ et al. Prevention des thromboses veineuses. Nouv Presse Méd 1974; 20: 1317–1319.

8. Nicolaides A, Dupont P, Parsons D et al. Small dose subcutaneous heparin in preventing deep venous thrombosis after elective hip surgery. Surg Res Soc 1974; 61: 320.

9. Venous Thrombosis Clinical Study Group. Small doses of subcutaneous sodium heparin in the prevention of deep vein thrombosis after elective hip operations. Br J Surg 1975; 62: 348–350.

10. Sagar S, Stamatakis JD, Higgins AF et al. Efficacy of low-dose heparin in prevention of extensive deep-vein thrombosis in patients undergoing total-hip replacement. Lancet 1976; ii: 1151–1154.

11. Mannucci PM, Citterio LE, Panajotopoulos N. Low-dose heparin and deep-vein thrombosis after total hip replacement. Thromb Haemost 1976; 36: 157–164.

12. Groote Schuur Hospital Thromboembolus study group. Failure of low-dose heparin to prevent significant thromboembolic complications in high risk surgical patients: interim report of prospective trial. Br Med J 1979; i: 1447–1450.

13. Hampson WGJ, Keith Lucas H, Harris FC, Roberts PH. Failure of low-dose heparin to prevent deep vein thrombosis after hip-replacement arthroplasty. Lancet 1974; ii: 795–797.

14. Crawford WJ, Hillmann F, Charnley J. A clinical trial of prophylactic anticoagulant therapy in elective hip surgery. Internal publication, Wrightington Centre for Hip Surgery 1968; 14: 1–11.

15. Harris WH, Salzman EW, Athanasoulis C et al. Comparison of warfarin, low-molecular-

weight dextran, aspirin, and subcutaneous heparin in prevention of venous thromboembolism following total hip replacement. *J Bone Joint Surg* 1974; **56A:** 1552–1562.

16. Coventry JG, Declan RN, Beckenbaugh RD. 'Delayed' prophylactic anticoagulation: a study of results and complications in 2012 total hip arthroplasties. *J Bone Joint Surg* 1973; **55A:** 1487–1492.

17. Sharnhoff JG, Rosen RL, Sadler AH, Ibarra-Isunza GC. Prevention of fatal pulmonary embolism by heparin prophylaxis after surgery for hip fractures. *J Bone Joint Surg* 1976; **58A:** 913–918.

18. Groulier P, Barsotti J, Bousignon JP et al. Le risque thrombo-embolique et sa prevention en chirurgie orthopedique. *Rev Chir Orthop* 1978; **64** (Suppl II): 143–155.

19. Evarts CM, Feil EJ. Prevention of thromboembolic disease after elective surgery of the hip. *J Bone Joint Surg* 1971; **53A:** 1271–1280.

20. de Mourgues G, Pagnier F, Clermont N et al. Etude de l'efficacité de l'heparine sous-cutanée utilisée selon deux protocoles dans la prevention de la thrombose veineuse post-operatoire après prothèse totale de la hanche. *Rev Chir Orthop* 1979; **65** (Suppl II): 74–76.

21. Planes A, Vochelle N, Fagola M et al. Phlebographie apres prothèse totale. Action de l'héparine sodique sous-cutanée dans la prévention de la maladie thrombo-embolique. *Rev Chir Orthop* 1984; **70:** 11–20.

22. Leyvraz PF, Richard J, Bachmann F et al. Adjusted versus fixed-dose subcutaneous heparin in the prevention of deep-vein thrombosis after total hip replacement. *N Engl J Med* 1983; **309:** 954–958.

23. Collins R, Scrimgeour A, Yusuf S, Peto R. Reduction in fatal pulmonary embolism and venous thrombosis by perioperative administration of subcutaneous heparin. *N Engl J Med* 1988; **318:** 1162–1173.

24. Consensus Conference. Prevention of venous thrombosis and pulmonary embolism. *JAMA* 1986; **256:** 744–749.

25. Barrowcliffe TW, Johnson EA, Thomas DP. *Low Molecular Weight Heparin.* John Wiley: Chichester, UK; 1992.

26. First ACCP-NHLBI National Conference on antithrombotic therapy. *Chest* 1986; **89** (Suppl): 1S–106S.

27. Second ACCP Conference on antithrombotic therapy. *Chest* 1989; **95** (Suppl): 1S–169S.

27a. Conférence de Consensus. Prophylaxie des thromboses veineuses profondes et des embolies pulmonaires postopératoires (chirurgie générale, gynécologique et orthopédique). AP-HP, 8 mars 1991, Paris, *Annales françaises d'anesthésie et de réanimation* 1991; **10:** 417–421.

28. European Consensus Statement. 1–5 November 1991. Prevention of venous thromboembolism. *Int Angiol* 1992; **11:** 151–159.

29. Third ACCP Consensus conference on antithrombotic therapy. *Chest* 1992; **102** (Suppl): 1S–549S.

30. Fourth ACCP Consensus conference on antithrombotic therapy. *Chest* 1995; **108** (Suppl): 1S–522S.

31. International Consensus Statement (guidelines according to scientific evidence). Prevention of venous thromboembolism. *Int Angiol* 1997; **16:** 3–38.

32. Fifth ACCP Consensus Conference on antithrombotic therapy. *Chest* 1998; **114** (Suppl): 1S–769S.

33. Turpie AGG, Levine MN, Hirsh J et al. A randomized controlled trial of a low-molecular-weight heparin (enoxaparin) to prevent deep-vein thrombosis in patients undergoing elective hip surgery. *N Engl J Med* 1986; **315**: 925–929.

34. Planes A, Vochelle N, Mazas F et al. A randomized trial comparing unfractionated heparin with low molecular weight heparin in patients undergoing total hip replacement. *Thromb Haemost* 1988; **60**: 407–410.

35. Planes A, Vochelle N, Fagola M et al. Comparison of two low-molecular-weight heparins for the prevention of postoperative venous thromboembolism after elective hip surgery. *Blood Coagul Fibrinolysis* 1998; **9**: 499–505.

36. Planes A, Samama MM, Lensing AWA et al. Prevention of deep vein thrombosis after hip replacement. Comparison between two low-molecular-weight heparins, tinzaparin and enoxaparin. *Thromb Haemost* 1999; **81**: 22–25.

37. Leizerowicz A, Haugh MC, Chapuis FR et al. Low-molecular-weight heparin in prevention of perioperative thrombosis. *Br Med J* 1992; **305**: 913–920.

38. Nurmohamed MT, Rosendaal FR, Büller HR et al. Low-molecular-weight heparin versus standard heparin in general and orthopaedic surgery: a meta-analysis. *Lancet* 1992; **ii**: 152–156.

39. Jorgensen LN, Wille-Jorgensen P, Hauch O. Prophylaxis of postoperative thromboembolism with low molecular weight heparins. *Br J Surg* 1993; **80**: 689–704.

40. Imperiale TF, Speroff T. A meta-analysis of methods to prevent venous thromboembolism following total hip replacement. *JAMA* 1994; **271**: 1780–1785.

41. Koch A, Bouges S, Ziegler S et al. Low molecular weight heparin and unfractionated heparin in thrombosis prophylaxis after major surgical intervention: update of previous meta-analysis. *Br J Surg* 1997; **84**: 750–759.

42. The Danish Enoxaparin Study Group. Low-molecular-weight heparin (enoxaparin) vs Dextran 70. *Arch Intern Med* 1991; **151**: 1621–1624.

43. Eriksson BI, Wille-Jorgensen P, Kälebo P et al. A comparison of recombinant hirudin with a low-molecular-weight heparin to prevent thromboembolic complications after total hip replacement. *N Engl J Med* 1997; **337**: 1329–1335.

44. Warwick D, Harrison J, Glew D et al. Comparison of the use of a foot pump with the use of low-molecular-weight heparin for the prevention of deep-vein thrombosis after total hip replacement. *J Bone Joint Surg* 1998; **80A**: 1158–1166.

45. Levine MN, Hirsh J, Gent M et al. Prevention of deep vein thrombosis after elective hip surgery. *Ann Intern Med* 1994; **114**: 545–551.

46. Colwell CW Jr, Spiro TE, Trowbridge AA et al. Use of enoxaparin, a low molecular-weight heparin, and unfractionated heparin for the prevention of deep venous thrombosis after elective hip replacement. *J Bone Joint Surg* 1994; **76A**: 3–14.

47. Spiro TE, Johnson GJ, Christie MJ et al. Efficacy and safety of enoxaparin to prevent deep venous thrombosis after hip replacement surgery. *Ann Intern Med* 1994; **121**: 81–89.

48. Eriksson BI, Zachrisson BE, Teger-Nilsson AC, Risberg B. Thrombosis prophylaxis with low molecular weight heparin in total hip replacement. *Br J Surg* 1988; **75**: 1053–1057.

49. Dechavanne M, Ville D, Berruyer M et al.

Randomized trial of a low-molecular-weight heparin (Kabi 2165) versus adjusted-dose subcutaneous standard heparin in the prophylaxis of deep-vein thrombosis after elective hip surgery. *Haemostasis* 1989; **1**: 5–12.

50. Eriksson BI, Kälebo P, Anthmyr BA et al. Prevention of deep-vein thrombosis and pulmonary embolism after total hip replacement. *J Bone Joint Surg* 1991; **73A**: 484–493.

51. Francis CW, Pellegrini VD, Totterman S et al. Prevention of deep-vein thrombosis after total hip anthroplasty. Comparison of warfarin and dalteparin. *J Bone Joint Surg* 1997; **79A**: 1365–1372.

52. Pineo GF, Hull RD for the NAFT investigators. A comparison of pre-operative dalteparin with post-operative dalteparin and with warfarin sodium for prophylaxis against deep vein thrombosis after total hip replacement during the hospital stay. *Thromb Haemost* 1999 (Abst Suppl): A 1194.

53. Leyvraz PF, Bachmann F, Hoek J et al Prevention of deep vein thrombosis after hip replacement: randomised comparison between unfractionated heparin and low molecular weight heparin. *Br Med J* 1991; **303**: 543–548.

54. The German Hip Arthroplasty Trial (GHAT) group. Prevention of deep vein thrombosis with low molecular-weight heparin in patients undergoing total hip replacement. *Arch Orthop Trauma Surg* 1992; **111**: 110–120.

55. Hamulyak K, Lensing AWA, van der Meer J et al. Subcutaneous low-molecular weight heparin or oral anticoagulants for the prevention of deep-vein thrombosis in elective hip and knee replacement? *Thromb Haemost* 1994; **74**: 1428–1431.

56. Lassen MR, Borris LC, Christiansen HM et al. Prevention of thromboembolism in 190 hip arthroplasties. *Acta Orthop Scand* 1991; **62**: 33–38.

57. Hull R, Raskob G, Pineo G et al. A comparison of subcutaneous low-molecular-weight heparin with warfarin sodium for prophylaxis against deep-vein thrombosis after hip or knee implantation. *N Engl J Med* 1993; **329**: 1370–1376.

58. Leyvraz P, Bachmann F, Bohnet J et al. Thromboembolic prophylaxis in total hip replacement: a comparison between low molecular weight heparinoid lomoparan and heparin-dihydroergotamine. *Br J Surg* 1992; **79**: 911–914.

59. Leclerc JR, Geerts WH, Desjardins L et al. Prevention of deep vein thrombosis after major knee surgery: a randomized, double-blind trial comparing a low molecular weight heparin fragment (enoxaparin) to placebo. *Thromb Haemost* 1992; **67**: 417–423.

60. Fauno P, Suomalainen AO, Rehnberg V et al. Prophylaxis for the prevention of venous thromboembolism after total knee replacement. *J Bone Joint Surg* 1994; **76A**: 1814–1818.

61. The RD Heparin arthroplasty group. RD Heparin compared with warfarin for prevention of venous thromboembolic disease following total hip and knee arthroplasty. *J Bone Joint Surg* 1994; **76A**: 1174–1185.

62. Colwell Jr CW, Spiro TE, Trowbridge AA et al. Efficacy and safety of enoxaparin versus unfractionated heparin for prevention of deep venous thrombosis after elective knee arthroplasty. *Clin Orthop* 1995; **321**: 19–27.

63. Fitzgerald RH Jr. Preventing deep vein thrombosis following total knee replacement:

a review of recent clinical trials. *Orthopedics* 1995; **18** (Suppl): 1–10.

64. Leclerc JR, Geerts WH, Desjardins L et al. Prevention of venous thromboembolism after knee arthroplasty. *Ann Intern Med* 1996; **124**: 619–626.

65. Levine MN, Gent M, Hirsh J et al. Ardeparin (low-molecular-weight heparin) vs graduated compression stockings for prevention of venous thromboembolism. A randomized trial in patients undergoing knee surgery. *Arch Intern Med* 1996; **156**: 851–856.

66. Heit JA, Berkowitz SD, Bona R et al. Efficacy and safety of low molecular weight heparin (ardeparin sodium) compared to warfarin for the prevention of venous thromboembolism after total knee replacement surgery: a double-blind, dose-ranging study. *Thromb Haemost* 1997; **77**: 32–38.

67. Agnelli G, Piovella F, Buoncristiani P et al. Enoxaparin plus compression stockings compared with compression stockings alone in the prevention of venous thromboembolism after elective neurosurgery. *N Engl J Med* 1998; **339**: 80–85.

68. Geerts W, Code KI, Jay RM et al. A prospective study of venous thromboembolism after major trauma. *N Engl J Med* 1994; **331**: 1601–1606.

69. Planes A, Vochelle N, Fagola M. Venous thromboembolic prophylaxis in orthopedic surgery· knee surgery. *Semin Thromb Hemost* 1999; (Suppl): 73–77.

70. Todd CJ, Freeman CJ, Camilleri-Ferrante C et al. Differences in mortality after fracture of hip: the East Anglian audit. *BMJ* 1995; **310**: 904–908.

71. Planes A, Vochelle N, Fagola M et al. Prevention of deep vein thrombosis after total

hip replacement. *J Bone Joint Surg* 1991; **73B**: 418–422.

72. Planes A, Vochelle N, Darmon JY et al. Risk of deep venous thrombosis after hospital discharge in patients having undergone total hip replacement: double blind randomized comparison of enoxaparin versus placebo. *Lancet* 1996; **348**: 224–228.

73. Bergqvist D, Benoni G, Björgell O et al. Low-molecular-weight heparin (enoxaparin) as prophylaxis against venous thromboembolism after total hip replacement. *N Engl J Med* 1996; **335**: 696–700.

74. Dahl O, Andreassen G, Aspelin T et al. Prolonged thromboprophylaxis following hip replacement surgery. Results of a double-blind, prospective, randomised, placebo-controlled study with dalteparin (Fragmin). *Thromb Haemost* 1997; **77**: 26–31.

75. Lassen MR, Borris LC, Anderson B et al. Efficacy and safety of prolonged prophylaxis with a low molecular weight heparin (dalteparin) after total hip arthroplasty: the Danish Prolonged Prophylaxis (DaPP) study. *Thromb Res* 1998; **89**: 81–87.

76. Hull RD, Brant RF, Pineo GF et al. Preoperative vs postoperative initiation of low-molecular-weight heparin prophylaxis against venous thrombolism in patients undergoing elective hip replacement. *Arch Intern Med* 1999; **159**: 137–141.

77. Prandoni P, Lensing AWA, Cogo A et al. The long-term clinical course of acute deep venous thrombosis. *Ann Intern Med* 1996; **125**: 1–7.

78. Eriksson BI, Ekman S, Kälebo P et al. Prevention of deep-vein thrombosis after total hip replacement: direct thrombin inhibition

with recombinant hirudin, CGP 39393. *Lancet* 1996; **347**: 635–639.

79. Eriksson BI, Ekman S, Lindbratt S et al. Prevention of thromboembolism with use of recombinant hirudin. *J Bone Joint Surg* 1997; **79A**: 326–333.

80. Berkowitz SD, Kosutic G, Marder VJ et al. Heparin administered orally via a novel carrier system (SNAC) is comparable to sc heparin when used to prevent venous thromboembolic events following elective total hip arthroplasty. *Thromb Haemost* 1999; (Abst Suppl): A 1553.

81. Doubilet P, Weinstein MC, McNeil BJ. Use and misuse of the term 'cost effective' in medicine. *N Engl J Med* 1986; **314**: 253–256.

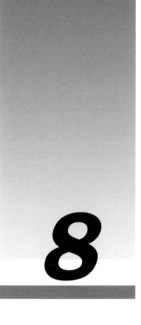

Efficacy and safety of low molecular weight heparins in the prevention of venous thromboembolism in general surgery

Grigoris T Gerotziafas and

Meyer Michel Samama

Introduction

The risk of postoperative venous thromboembolism (VTE) is well established in surgical patients. Prophylaxis with low-dose heparin has contributed significantly to the reduction in thromboembolic complications in surgery. Without prophylaxis, the rate of deep-vein thrombosis (DVT) is about 30% in patients undergoing general surgery, rising up to 70% in orthopedic and trauma surgery. The efficacy of unfractionated heparin (UFH) treatment for the prevention of VTE in surgical and orthopedic patients is accepted worldwide. According to Collins et al[1] and Clagett and Reisch[2], heparin prevented at least 60% of DVT.

During the last decade a large number of clinical trials and several meta-analyses proved that the various preparations of LMWHs are at least as effective and safe as unfractionated heparin (UFH) in the prophylaxis of VTE in surgical patients.[3,4] LMWHs gained the predominant role in the prevention of VTE as a result of their proven efficacy and safety, established by the above-mentioned clinical trials and meta-analyses but also as a consequence of their pharmacological properties, which have been reviewed in

Chapter 6. Some trials and one meta-analysis demonstrated that aspirin also contributes to the prevention of venous thromboembolism in surgical patients.[1,5] However the interpretation of these results is rather difficult since the trials are quite heterogeneous. On the other hand, the use of LMWHs in the prophylaxis of venous thromboembolism in surgical patients is now included in the guidelines issued from the American Consensus of Chest Physicians.[6] This chapter focuses on trials on the prophylaxis against venous thromboembolism in surgical patients published during the last 5 years.

The 'new generation' of this type of clinical trial verifies the efficacy and safety of LMWH administration for VTE prophylaxis in surgical patients. However, some other important issues are more systematically approached. Thus, a classification of surgical patients according to the risk for VTE derived either by their disease or by the type of the surgical procedure, the optimal duration and the optimal dosage of LMWH prophylactic regimen, and the need for adaptation of LMWH dosage according to the thromboembolic risk are the most relevant topics of these recent clinical trials. The trials presented in this review are classified in six categories: (a) surgical out-patients and long-term prophylaxis; (b) low-risk surgical patients; (c) moderate-risk patients; (d) high-risk patients; (e) patients undergoing specialized surgical procedures (neurosurgery or vascular surgery); (f) a study of the safety of LMWH prophylactic regimen. The duration of the treatment, the health economics and the side-effects are also discussed.

Surgical out-patients and long-term prophylaxis with LMWH

The incidence of VTE in surgical and orthopedic out-patients has not been sufficiently studied (*Table 8.1*). The efficacy and safety of the prophylactic regimen with LMWHs in this group of patients, is unknown. One recent study presented by Harenberg et al, evaluated the feasibility (in terms of efficacy and safety) of LMWH reviparin 1750 anti-Xa IU in prophylaxis of thromboembolic complications in surgical and orthopedic out-patients who were not operated, compared with a group of operated out-patients who also received a regimen with LMWH.[7] The LMWH regimen was administered for a long period (1–4 weeks; mean 17 days). The incidence of clinically diagnosed venous thromboembolism was rather low in both groups: 11/1604 (0.7%) in operated and 8/1017 (0.8%) in non-operated patients receiving LMWH. Pulmonary embolism occurred twice in operated patients (0.1%) and in none of the non-operated patients. However, since the only criterion for the diagnosis of VTE was the clinical symptoms, the absolute value of these data is questionable although the studied groups included a large number of patients. It is important to notice that in both operated and non-operated surgical and orthopedic patients, LMWH regimen in a long-term prophylactic administration is a safe regimen since minor bleeding complications were rare and major bleeding complications did not occur.

Lausen et al, in a randomized, controlled, open trial, with blinded evaluation studied the incidence of late DVT, and evaluated a regimen of prolonged thromboprophylaxis with LMWH (tinzaparin) after general surgery in 118 consecutive patients undergoing major elective abdominal or non-cardiac thoracic operations.[8] The effect of long-term administration of tinzaparin (one subcutaneous injection per day, given for 4 weeks; $N - 58$), was compared with that of short-term administration of the same dose of tinzaparin (one week administration; control group, $N = 60$). The presence of DVT was established by bilateral venography 4 weeks after the operation. This trial did not demonstrate any significant favourable effect of prolonged LMWH prophylactic administration although the incidence of late DVT in the long-term prophylaxis group (3/58 or 5.2%, 95% confidence interval (CI): 1–14%) was somewhat lower as compared to the control group (6/60 or 10%, 95% CI: 4–21%; $P = 0.49$).

Prophylaxis of VTE in low-risk surgical patients

The incidence of VTE and the benefit of prophylaxis with LMWH in patients undergoing minimal surgical procedures have not been studied. A recent prospective, randomized, controlled clinical trial was performed with such a patient group.[9] The 718 selected patients underwent laparoscopic cholecystectomy and other types of minimally invasive surgery. The authors included patients at low risk for VTE. All patients received graduated elastic stockings. The LMWH group ($N = 359$) received one subcutaneous injection of reviparin sodium per day, and the control group ($N = 359$) received placebo injection. Diagnosis for DVT was suboptimal using duplex scan and when positive a phlebography was performed. Only one patient (0.1%) in the overall population experienced DVT (phlebographically confirmed). There was also only one patient (0.1%) with pulmonary embolism, confirmed by scintigraphy. The use of reviparin for prevention of venous thromboembolism was safe and convenient, the rate of postoperative bleeding complications was 2.3% in the LMWH group, even lower than in the control group (3.2%). In low risk patients undergoing minimal surgical procedures the incidence of VTE is rather low and physical preventive measures are sufficient enough for the prophylaxis of VTE.

Table 8.1
Prophylaxis with LWMH in low-risk or surgical out-patients

First author	Type of surgery	Type of study	Treatment
Harenberg 1998[7]	Operated patients, ambulatory surgical patients, unoperated surgical		Reviparin
Lausen 1998[8]	Major elective abdominal or non-cardiac thoracic surgery	Randomized, controlled, open trial with blinded evaluation	Tinzaparin
Baca 1997[9]	Minimal invasive abdominal surgery	Prospective, randomized, controlled trial	Reviparin/GES (N = 359) Placebo/GES† (N = 359)

GES: graduated elastic stocking.

Another prospective trial presented by Catheline et al assessed the thromboembolic risk in patients undergoing laparoscopic digestive surgery.[10] A total of 2384 patients were enrolled in the study. All patients received perioperative LMWH prophylaxis until the patients resumed ambulatory activity. Eight cases of DVT (0.33%) were observed but no pulmonary embolism was noted. Although there was no control group, the incidence of VTE episodes presented in this study is very low and comparable to that reported in the previous study.[9] Reverse Tredelenburg position, pneumoperitoneum and long duration of the surgical procedure are regarded as predisposing factors for venous thromboembolic episodes.

Thus, a regimen with LMWH in low-risk surgical patients, although it is safe, is not more beneficial than the physical preventive measures. The use of physical preventive measures, the rapid mobilization of the patients and the control of predisposing risk factors during the surgical procedure could be sufficient measures for an efficient prevention of venous thromboembolism.

Duration	DVT	Haemorrhage	Diagnosis
1–4 weeks (mean 17 days)	11/1604 (0.7%) in operated patients 8/1017 (0.8%) in non-operated patients	4%	Clinical examination
4 weeks (N = 58) versus 1 week (N = 60) (control group)	3/58 (5.2%) 6/60 (10%) P = 0.49		Bilateral venography 4 weeks postoperatively
5 days	0.1%	2.3%	Duplex scanning
	0%	3.2%	

Prophylaxis of VTE in moderate-risk surgical patients

Moreno et al carried out a prospective, multicenter, double-blind, controlled randomized trial, in two groups of patients (including 100 patients in each group) with a low or moderate risk of VTE, who underwent elective abdominal surgery (*Table 8.2*).[11] They evaluated the efficacy and safety of RO-11 at a daily subcutaneous injection (2500 anti-Xa IU per day), compared with UFH administered as subcutaneous injection of 5000 IU twice daily for 7 days. There were no cases of DVT, pulmonary embolism (PE) or death in any group. The requirement of transfusion, reoperation because of bleeding, and the frequency of wound hematoma were higher in the UFH group. RO-11 at a single subcutaneous dose of 2500 anti-Xa IU is as efficient as, and safer than, UFH in the prevention of VTE in moderate- and low-risk surgical patients.

An interesting study was presented by Bergqvist et al who carried out a prospective randomized double-blind placebo controlled study on the efficacy of postoperative VTE

Table 8.2
Prophylaxis of venous thromboembolism with LWMH in moderate-risk surgical patients

First author	Type of surgery	Type of study	Treatment
Moreno 1996[11]	Elective abdominal surgery	Multicenter double-blind, randomized controlled trial. (N = 200)	RO-11 (N = 100) UFH (N = 100)
Bergqvist 1996[12]	Emergency abdominal surgery	Prospective, randomized, double-blind, controlled trial. (N = 80)	Tinzaparin, placebo
Limmer 1994[13]	Elective abdominal surgery	Randomized controlled trial (N = 203)	LMWH 21–23 (Braun) (N = 103) UFH (N = 100)

prophylaxis. Tinzaparin (one daily injection) was compared with placebo.[12] The study enrolled 80 patients undergoing emergency abdominal surgery allocated to two groups. The fibrinogen uptake test was used for the diagnosis of VTE but because of withdrawal of the labeled fibrinogen from the market the calculated number of patients was not reached. The frequency of deep-vein thrombosis was reduced with prophylaxis from 22% in the placebo group (95% CI: 11–38%) to 8% in the tinzaparin group (95% CI; 2–21%), revealing a risk reduction of 65%, which is however, not significant. Although the difference was not significant,

prophylaxis with LMWH tends to reduce the frequency of VTE in this category of surgical patients, where the incidence of VTE is not negligible.

A prospective, randomized, controlled clinical trial was performed by Limmer et al comparing the antithrombotic efficacy of the low molecular weight heparin LMWH 21–23 (Braun) administered once daily, with UFH twice daily in 203 elective general surgical patients over an observation period of 7 postoperative days.[13] About 50% of the patients were operated for malignant disease. None of the patients died due to fatal pulmonary embolism. In the LMWH group,

Duration	DVT	Haemorrhage	Diagnosis
7 days	0	Non-significant	?
	0		
Postoperative ?	8%		Fibrinogen uptake test
	22% $P > 0.05$		
7 days	4/103 (3.9%)	No	Fibrinogen uptake test
	5/100 (5%)	No	

four patients revealed a positive ^{125}I-labeled fibrinogen uptake test (3.9%). In the UFH group, five patients displayed a positive fibrinogen uptake test (5%). In this trial as well, the prophylactic regimen with LMWH is at least as effective and safe as UFH.

Prophylaxis of VTE in high-risk surgical patients undergoing major surgery

Prophylaxis for VTE in patients undergoing major surgical procedures with either UFH or LWMH is widely used and it is considered unethical not to give prophylaxis (*Table 8.3*).

Thus, there are few placebo controlled trials in patients undergoing major surgery reviewed by Bergqvist in 1994 and the international consensus report some years later.[14,15] These studies demonstrated that the frequency of VTE was 15.9% in the placebo group and the LMWHs reduced the frequency of VTE to 4.2%. The subgroup analysis revealed that the frequency of VTE was even higher in patients operated for malignant disease, being rather low in non-cancer patients. During the 1990s, the efficacy and safety of LMWHs in the prophylaxis of VTE in high-risk patients undergoing major surgery has been established by numerous trials reviewed by several

Table 8.3
Prophylaxis of venous thromboembolism with LWMH in high-risk surgical patients

First author	Type of surgery	Type of study	Treatment	Duration
ENOXACAN study 1997[16]	Elective abdominal or pelvic cancer surgery	Prospective, double-blind, randomized controlled multicenter trial.	Enoxaparin (N = 315) UFH (N = 316)	
Von Tempelhoff 1997[17]	Major abdominal cancer surgery (ovarian malignancy)	Prospective, double-blind, randomized trial.	Certoparin (N = 28) UFH (N = 32)	8 days
Azorin 1997[18]	Lung cancer surgery	Multicenter, open randomized dose finding trial	Nadroparin	8 days
Kakkar 1997[19]	Abdominal surgery	Double-blind, randomized controlled multicenter trial.	Reviparin (N = 655) UFH (N = 677)	
Nurmohamed 1995[20]	Major general surgery	Multicenter double-blind randomized controlled trial.	Enoxaparin (N = 718) UFH (N = 709)	?
Wiig 1995[21]	Elective abdominal surgery (gastrointestinal operations)	Multicenter, randomized double-blind, controlled trial. (N = 329)	Enoxaparin, dextran	10 days
Bergqvist 1995[22]	Elective general surgery	Multicenter double-blind, randomized controlled trial. Dose-finding study	Dalteparin (N = 1957)	?

DVT	Haemorrhage	Diagnosis
14.7%	Similar outcome in bleeding episodes; 1 patient in UFH group developed HIT	Bilateral phlebography and/or pulmonary scintigraphy; 3 months follow-up
18.2%		
4/28 (6.7%)		Impedance plethysmography (IPG), physical examination. Phlebography when IPG positive. Ventilation lung scanning when clinical symptoms of PE
0/32 (0%)		
P < 0.05		
0/75	2/75 (2.6%)	Doppler ultrasound (D0 and D8) and bilateral phlebography when positive doppler
0/75	6/75 (8%)	
4.7%	8.3%	
4.3%	11.8%	
P > 0.05	P < 0.05	
58/718 (8.1%)	11/718 (1.5%)	Fibrinogen uptake test
45/709 (6.3%)	18/709 (2.5%)	
P > 0.05	P > 0.05	
33/101 (33%) in high risk patients		Phlebography
2/27 (7%) in moderate risk patients		
6/49 (12%) in high risk patients		
31/107 (31%) in high risk patients		
5/27 (19%) in moderate risk patients		
13.8%	2.7%	Fibrinogen uptake test
6.8%	4.7%	
P < 0.001	P = 0.02	

authors. Recent meta-analysis concludes that LMWHs are at least as effective and safe as UFH. Some more recent studies examining the efficacy and safety of newer LMWH preparations in this category of surgical patients confirm the primary conclusion.

Two recent trials demonstrated that LMWH (enoxaparin 4000 anti-Xa IU and certoparin 3000 anti-Xa IU), administered in one daily injection in cancer patients undergoing therapeutic surgical procedures, was as effective and safe as UFH administered three times daily, for the prevention of VTE.[16,17] A third multicenter open randomized dose-finding trial performed in lung cancer patients undergoing thoracic surgery demonstrated that administration of a single fixed dose of nadroparin (3075 anti-Xa IU daily) is as effective and safe as the administration of a single weight-adjusted dose (4100–6150 anti-Xa IU daily).[18] Similarly low-dose reviparin (1750 anti-Xa IU daily) is as effective as, and safer than UFH administered in high-risk surgical patients undergoing major abdominal surgery.[19] Low-dose enoxaparin (2000 anti-Xa IU administered in a single daily injection) to surgical patients undergoing major abdominal surgery is as effective and slightly safer than low dose UFH.[20] However, contradictory results were presented by Wiig et al.[21] In this study, the frequency of VTE in high-risk surgical patients undergoing elective gastrointestinal surgery receiving low-dose

enoxaparin (2000 anti-Xa IU daily) was rather high (33%) whereas only 7% of moderate risk patients receiving the same dose of enoxaparin experienced VTE.

In a third group of high-risk patients receiving enoxaparin, 4000 anti-Xa IU daily the frequency of VTE was significantly reduced (12%). In the former study, phlebography was used for the diagnosis of VTE. In the same line are the data from an interesting trial carried out by Bergqvist et al on high-risk surgical patients.[22] This study demonstrated that a higher prophylactic dose of dalteparin (5000 anti-Xa IU once daily) is more effective than a lower dose of dalteparin (2500 anti-Xa IU once daily). The frequency of VTE was 6.8% in the former and 13.8% in the latter group. However, the frequency of important bleeding increases with high doses of LMWH but interestingly, the increased bleeding was observed only in non-cancer patients. The overall frequency of PE with dalteparin is extremely low in this high-risk group of surgical patients.

Prophylaxis in neurosurgery, vascular surgery and laparoscopic surgery
Neurosurgery

Although in general surgery LMWHs have proven to be effective for prophylaxis of VTE when administered postoperatively, with the advantage of lower bleeding risk during surgery, anticoagulant prophylaxis in neurosurgical patients has not gained wide acceptance due to the fear of intracranial bleeding. Physical methods give a worthwhile reduction of postoperative VTE but there still remains a substantial residual incidence.

Agnelli et al, in a multicenter, randomized, double-blind trial, assessed the efficacy and safety of enoxaparin in conjunction with the use of compression stockings in the prevention of venous thromboembolism in patients undergoing elective neurosurgery.[23] Enoxaparin (40 mg once daily) or placebo was given subcutaneously for not less than 7 days beginning within 24 hours after the completion of surgery. The primary end-point was symptomatic, objectively confirmed venous thromboembolism or deep-vein thrombosis assessed by bilateral venography. One patient in the placebo group died before venography of autopsy-confirmed pulmonary embolism. In this analysis, 42 patients given placebo (32%) and 22 patients given enoxaparin (17%) had DVT (relative risk in the enoxaparin group: 0.52; 95% CI: 0.33–0.82; $P = 0.004$). The rates of proximal DVT were 13% in patients receiving placebo and 5% in patients receiving enoxaparin (relative risk reduction in the enoxaparin group: 0.41, 95% CI: 0.17–0.95; $P = 0.04$). Two patients in the placebo group died of autopsy-confirmed pulmonary embolism on days 9 and 16. Major bleeding occurred in four patients receiving placebo

(intracranial bleeding in all four) and four patients (intracranial bleeding in three) receiving enoxaparin (3% of each group). Thus enoxaparin combined with compression stockings is more effective than compression stockings alone for the prevention of venous thromboembolism after elective neurosurgery and does not increase the frequency (rate) of bleeding complications.

Dickinson et al, in a randomized controlled trial investigated the efficacy and safety of enoxaparin in preventing DVT in patients with brain tumours.[24] A retrospective analysis of patients undergoing neurosurgical procedures demonstrated a high incidence (14%) of postoperative DVT among patients with intracranial neoplasms treated with sequential compression device (SCD) prophylaxis alone. The goal of the study was to compare SCD, enoxaparin, and combined SCD/enoxaparin prophylaxis among patients requiring surgery for treatment of intracranial neoplasms. A total of 68 patients was randomized to SCD, enoxaparin, or combined therapy. Treatment was initiated before the induction of anesthesia and was continued throughout the hospital stay. Patients were screened for DVT, using duplex imaging, on four occasions in the first month after surgery. Postoperative DVT occurred in three of 22 (13.6%) SCD-treated patients, one of 23 (4.3%) enoxaparin-treated patients, and four of 23 (17.4%) SCD/enoxaparin-treated patients. Differences were not statistically significant. Postoperative intracranial hemorrhage did not occur in patients in the SCD-treated group, whereas five of 46 (10.8%) patients receiving LMWH suffered clinically significant intracranial hemorrhage. The study was terminated because of the increased incidence of adverse events in the enoxaparin-treated groups. Enoxaparin therapy initiated at the time of anesthesia induction increases postoperative intracranial hemorrhage.

Nurmohamed et al performed a multicentre, randomized, double-blind trial in neurosurgical patients to investigate the efficacy and safety of adding nadroparin, initiated postoperatively, to graduated compression stockings in the prevention of VTE. DVT was detected by mandatory venography.[25] Bleeding was determined according to predefined objective criteria for major and minor episodes. A total of 31 of 166 LMWH patients (18.7%) and 47 of 179 control patients (26.3%) had VTE up to day 10 postoperatively ($P = 0.047$). The relative risk reduction was 28.9%. The rates for proximal DVT/pulmonary embolism were 6.9% and 11.5% for the two groups, respectively (relative risk ratio: 40.2%; $P = 0.065$). Major bleeding complications, during the treatment period, occurred in six LMWH-treated patients (2.5%) and in two control patients (0.8%; $P = 0.87$). A higher mortality was observed in the LMWH group over the 56-day follow-up period (22 versus 10; $P = 0.026$). However, none of these deaths judged by a blinded adjudication committee was related to the studied drug. In conclusion, this study demonstrated that nadroparin, added to graduated compression stockings is beneficial for the prevention of VTE without increasing the bleeding risk.

Harris et al retrospectively analyzed the efficacy and safety of LMWH prophylactic administration in spinal injured patients.[26] Enoxaparin (3000 anti-Xa IU) was injected subcutaneously once daily. From a total of 105 patients no one developed clinical evidence of thromboembolism, and none of the 60 venous ultrasound examinations showed a deep-vein thrombus. Eleven patients had evidence of hemorrhage, but the LMWH was considered to have contributed to the bleeding in only three patients. This additional experience with enoxaparin reinforces the opinion that LMWHs are safe and effective thromboprophylactic agents in spinal injured patients.

Vascular surgery

There have been few studies investigating LMWH in the prophylaxis of arterial thrombosis in vascular surgery. A search using MEDLINE revealed only four clinical trials comparing LMWH administration versus unfractionated heparin in the prophylaxis of arterial thrombosis. One of these trials which included only 42 patients will not be discussed here.

One open randomized multicenter study presented by Samama et al enrolled 201 consecutive patients scheduled for femorodistal reconstructive surgery under general anesthesia.[27] This study showed that enoxaparin was more effective and as safe as UFH when used for the prevention of early graft thrombosis in patients undergoing femorodistal reconstructive surgery.

Similarly McMillan et al compared the efficacy and safety of subcutaneous LMWH with intravenously infused UFH for perioperative anticoagulation in patients who underwent infrageniculate bypass procedures with polytetrafluoroethylene grafts.[28] A total of 68 patients were enrolled with 69 bypass procedures for study. Patients were allocated to receive either LMWH or intravenous unfractionated heparin. The morbidity and mortality rates in both groups were similar. There were no significant differences in the number of grafts that failed before discharge and the incidence of bleeding complications was also not significantly different although it was slightly decreased in the LMWH group (15% in the UFH group versus 7% in the LMWH group). The mean number of postoperative hospital days was significantly lower in the LMWH group (9.5 days in the UFH group and 7.2 days in the LMWH group; $P < 0.009$).

In a multicenter randomized controlled trial 94 patients were randomized to receive a daily injection of 2500 anti-Xa IU LMWH, and 106 patients received 300 mg aspirin with 100 mg dipyridamole 8 hourly for 3 months and were followed up for 1 year.[29] No major bleeding events occurred in either group. LMWH is better than aspirin and dipyridamole in maintaining femoropopliteal-graft patency in patients with critical limb ischemia undergoing salvage surgery in this small group of patients.

Pre- or postoperative initiation of LMWHs?

This question is still debated. The safety of enoxaparin started preoperatively versus postoperatively as prophylaxis against venous thromboembolism for digestive surgery was studied in a play-the-winner (PTW) designed trial.[30] A total of 316 patients was included. In a PTW-designed study the treatment of any next patient depends on the outcome of the previous patient. If successful, the next patient receives the same treatment, if not, the comparative regimen is given. Excessive bleeding according to specified criteria, severe adverse reactions, clinically detected deep venous thrombosis, or pulmonary embolism were criteria for classification as 'loser'. The PTW design allocates most patients to the superior treatment. The main variable in PTW studies is the number of consecutive patients receiving the same treatment. In this study 163 patients were allocated to postoperatively started and 153 to preoperatively started prophylaxis with enoxaparin. The frequency of 'winners' was found to be 82.8% and 78.4% in the post- and preoperatively treated groups, respectively. No significant differences were found between the groups with regard to frequency of 'winners' or the number of consecutive patients before change of treatment. The percentile of survival distribution did not detect superiority of any group. Prophylaxis against postoperative venous thromboembolism for digestive surgery using enoxaparin can safely be started preoperatively. Moreover, in the national French consensus in 1991, although preoperative initiation of heparin was recommended it was noted that many surgeons start the injections 12–24 hours after surgery.[31] However, in an old study of our group in 1981, in cancer patients undergoing thoracic surgery we compared pre- and postoperative initiation of prophylactic treatment with low dose of UFH.[32] Deaths from PE were significantly more frequent when subcutaneous calcium heparin was started postoperatively rather than preoperatively.

Duration of the treatment

Although there is some evidence of late postoperative thrombosis, the generally recommended duration is around 7 days. Because of the shortening of hospitalization duration, home treatment should be considered.

Health economic aspects

They are of increasing importance in this category of patients. Most experts have shown that the use of LMWHs leads to a net saving per patient.[33,34]

Side-effects

Perioperative bleeding must be studied in a double-blind fashion to avoid bias. There is a rather weak relationship between the dose of injected LMWH and bleeding risk at the doses recommended in this population of patients. No correlation between anti-Xa activity and bleeding could be evidenced.[35]

An open question is related to the increase in wound hematomas in patients receiving aspirin or anti-inflammatory drugs possessing inhibitory effects on platelet function. The increased risk attributed to such a combination of drugs is expected but not well documented. According to Bergqvist the use of aspirin in low doses (325 mg) is safe.[36]

Allergic reactions are very rare. Skin necrosis has been reported in extremely rare patients.[31]

Transient elevations of transaminases are seen after both UFH and LMWH administration. The mechanism is not well understood. A decreased clearance of these enzymes has been reported (J Hirsh, personal communication).

Finally, heparin-induced thrombocytopenia type II (HIT) although less frequent with LMWH than with UFH is potentially the most severe complication of heparin treatment.[37] There is no gold standard for its diagnosis and laboratory diagnosis has some limitations. Treatment with danaparoid is well tolerated and has been widely used. In rare cases cross-reactivity with danaparoid/heparin has been observed. Thus, platelet count should be monitored regularly in LMWH-treated patients. Another drug that has also been studied is hirudin as an alternative to heparin in HIT.

The peak frequency of HIT is between 5 and 14–21 days of treatment. This observation led to the recommendation of monitoring platelet count before the first injection, then 5 days later and twice a week until heparin interruption.

Conclusion

The primary conclusion from the presented trials is that LMWH prophylactic administration in surgical patients is at least as efficient and slightly safer than the regimen

with UFH. A stratification of surgical patients according to the risk for VTE allows a more beneficial outcome of the LMWH prophylactic regimen and might also improve the cost/benefit ratio.

In low-risk patients the use of physical preventive measures such as elastic compression stockings and rapid mobilization is sufficient for the prevention of VTE. In this case LMWH administration is probably not cost-effective.

In moderate-risk patients a preventive regimen with LMWH seems to be beneficial for the patients. The efficacy and safety of LMWH and UFH are similar. Low dose LMWH is proven to be sufficient for adequate prevention of VTE. This conclusion is in good agreement with the recent results of Haas et al[38] who have studied the efficacy of subcutaneous heparins in 23 078 patients over the age of 40 years scheduled for any type of surgery lasting longer than 45 minutes. The frequency of fatal PE frequently confirmed by autopsy was around 0.17% suggesting that the rate of fatal PE in comparison with that of previous heparin trials significantly decreased since it ranges from 0.62 to 1.1% in the meta-analysis of Clagett and Reisch in 1988.[2]

In high-risk patients prophylaxis with one subcutaneous injection of LMWH per day, is at least as efficient and slightly safer than the regiment with UFH (two or three injections per day) as mentioned previously. Higher doses of LMWH are required for adequate prevention in very high-risk patients. The appropriate dose of LMWH in this group seems significantly higher than the one used in patients with moderate risk of VTE but this difference is not mentioned for some LMWH preparations.

In patients undergoing general surgical procedures, long-term prophylactic administration of LMWH does not seem to be beneficial compared with the effect of the administration during the 7–10 postoperative days. However, long-term administration of LMWH is not associated with increased hemorrhagic risk. Still, the financial cost/benefit ratio is not favorable for long-term prophylaxis with LMWH.[39] It is necessary to define the groups of patients which need to receive prolonged prophylaxis with LMWH. These groups should include patients such as those with hereditary thrombophilia or VTE antecedents. The duration could be prolonged to 4–6 weeks in these patients. A LMWH or an oral anticoagulant drug could be used. Clinical trials comparing these two strategies are being completed.

Prophylaxis with LMWH is more convenient than UFH for both nurses and patients since it consists frequently of a single injection per day. LMWHs are less frequently responsible for heparin-induced thrombocytopenia[37] and have a more predictable response than UFH.

The data presented verify that there is no need for laboratory monitoring of the LMWH regimen since the incidence of serious hemorrhages is low. However, the risk of bleeding increases when high doses of LMWH are used. This conclusion is also supported by a recent meta-analysis, which demonstrated a higher incidence of bleeding complications in high-risk surgical patients receiving LMWH.[3] In neurosurgical patients, the benefit of LMWH is still unclear because of the high incidence of severe hemorrhages. Laboratory monitoring of the LMWH regimen might be beneficial in patients undergoing procedures associated with a high hemorrhagic risk. However there is no reliable biological assay for the monitoring of the anticoagulant effect of LMWH treatment. The relation between anti-Xa plasma level and the risk of bleeding is weak. It is likely that the hemorrhagic risk arising from the patient's characteristics or arising from the type of surgical procedure should be considered when the prophylactic regimen is planned.

References

1. Collins R, Scrimgeour A, Yusuf S, Peto R. Reduction in fatal pulmonary embolism and venous thrombosis by perioperative administration of subcutaneous heparin. Overview of results of randomized trials in general, orthopedic, and urologic surgery. *N Engl J Med* 1988; **318**: 1162–1173.

2. Clagett GP, Reisch JS. Prevention of venous thromboembolism in general surgical patients.

Results of meta-analysis. *Ann Surg* 1988; **208**: 227–240.

3. Koch A, Bouges S, Ziegler S et al. Low molecular weight heparin and unfractionated heparin in thrombosis prophylaxis after major surgical intervention: update of previous meta-analyses. *Br J Surg* 1997; **84**: 750–759.

4. Palmer AJ, Schramm W, Kirchhof B, Bergemann R. Low molecular weight heparin and unfractionated heparin for prevention of thrombo-embolism in general surgery: a meta-analysis of randomised clinical trials. *Haemostasis* 1997; **27**: 65–74.

5. Antiplatelet Trialists' Collaboration. Collaborative overview of randomized trials of antiplatelet therapy III. Reduction in venous thrombosis and pulmonary embolism by antiplatelet prophylaxis among surgical and medical patients. *Br Med J* 1994; **308**: 235–246.

6. Clagett G, Anderson FA, Geerts W et al. Prevention of venous thromboembolism. *Chest* 1998; **114 (Suppl 5)**: 531S–560S.

7. Harenberg J, Piazolo L, Misselwitz F. Prevention of thromboembolism with low-molecular-weight heparin in ambulatory surgery and in operated surgical and orthopedic patients. *Zentralbl Chir* 1998; **123**: 1284–1287 (In German).

8. Lausen I, Jensen R, Jorgensen LN et al. Incidence and prevention of deep venous thrombosis occurring late after general surgery: randomised controlled study of prolonged thromboprophylaxis. *Eur J Surg* 1998; **164**: 657–663.

9. Baca I, Schneider B, Kohler T et al. Prevention of thromboembolism in minimal invasive interventions and brief in patient treatment. Results of a multicenter, prospective, randomized, controlled study

with a low molecular weight heparin. *Chirurg* 1997; **68**: 1275–1280 (in German).

10. Catheline JM, Gaillard JL, Rizk N et al. Risk factors and prevention of thromboembolic risk in laparoscopy. *Ann Chir* 1998; **52**: 890–895 (In French).

11. Moreno Gonzalez E, Fontcuberta J, de la Llama F. Prophylaxis of thromboembolic disease with RO-11 (ROVI), during abdominal surgery. EMRO1 (Grupo Fstudio Multicintrico RO-11). *Hepatogastroenterology* 1996; **43**: 744–747.

12. Bergqvist D, Flordal PA, Friberg B et al. Thromboprophylaxis with a low molecular weight heparin (tinzaparin) in emergency abdominal surgery. A double-blind multicenter trial. *Vasa* 1996; **25**: 156–160.

13. Limmer J, Ellbruck D, Muller H et al. Prospective randomized clinical study in general surgery comparing a new low molecular weight heparin with unfractionated heparin in the prevention of thrombosis. *Clin Invest* 1994; **72**: 913–919.

14. Bergqvist D. Low molecular weight heparins for prevention of venous thromboembolism following general surgery. In: Bounameaux (ed). *Low Molecular Weight Heparins in Prophylaxis and Therapy of Thromboembolic Diseases*. Marcel Dekker: New York, 1994: 169–185.

15. Opinions regarding the diagnosis and management of venous thromboembolic disease. ACCP Consensus Committee on Pulmonary Embolism. American College of Chest Physicians. *Chest* 1998; **113**: 499–504.

16. Enoxacan Study Group. Efficacy and safety of enoxaparin versus unfractionated heparin for prevention of deep vein thrombosis in elective cancer surgery: a double-blind randomized

multicentre trial with venographic assessment. *Br J Surg* 1997; **84**: 1099–1103.

17. Von Tempelhoff GF, Dietrich M, Niemann F et al. Blood coagulation and thrombosis in patients with ovarian malignancy. *Thromb Haemost* 1997; **77**: 456–461.

18. Azorin JF, Regnard JF, Dahan M, Pansart M. Efficacy and tolerability of fraxiparine in the prevention of thromboembolic complications in oncologic thoracic surgery. *Ann Cardiol Angiol* 1997; **46**: 341–347.

19. Kakkar VV, Boeckl O, Boneu B et al. Efficacy and safety of a low-molecular-weight heparin and standard unfractionated heparin for prophylaxis of postoperative venous thromboembolism: European multicenter trial. *World J Surg* 1997; **21**: 2–8.

20. Nurmohamed MT, Verhaeghe R, Haas S et al. A comparative trial of a low molecular weight heparin (enoxaparin) versus standard heparin for the prophylaxis of postoperative deep vein thrombosis in general surgery. *Am J Surg* 1995; **169**: 567–571.

21. Wiig JN, Solhaug JH, Bilberg T et al. Prophylaxis of venographically diagnosed deep vein thrombosis in gastrointestinal surgery. Multicentre trials of 20 mg and 40 mg enoxaparin versus dextran. *Eur J Surg* 1995; **161**: 663–668.

22. Bergqvist D, Burmark US, Flordal PA et al. Low molecular weight heparin started before surgery as prophylaxis against deep vein thrombosis: 2500 versus 5000 XaI units in 2070 patients. *Br J Surg* 1995; **82**: 496–501.

23. Agnelli G, Piovella F, Buoncristiania P et al. Enoxaparin plus compression stockings compared with compression stockings alone in the prevention of venous thromboembolism after elective neurosurgery. *N Engl J Med* 1998; **339**: 80–85.

24. Dickinson LD, Miller LD, Patel CP, Gupta SK. Enoxaparin increases the incidence of postoperative intracranial hemorrhage when initiated preoperatively for deep venous thrombosis prophylaxis in patients with brain tumors. *Neurosurgery* 1998; **43**: 1074–1081.

25. Nurmohamed MT, van Riel AM, Henkens CM et al. Low molecular weight heparin and compression stockings in the prevention of venous thromboembolism in neurosurgery. *Thromb Haemost* 1996; **75**: 233–238.

26. Harris S, Chen D, Green D. Enoxaparin for thromboembolism prophylaxis in spinal injury: preliminary report on experience with 105 patients. *Am J Phys Med Rehabil* 1996; **75**: 326–327.

27. Samama CM, Gigou F, Ill P. Low-molecular-weight heparin vs. unfractionated heparin in femorodistal reconstructive surgery: a multicenter open randomized study. Enoxart Study Group. *Ann Vasc Surg* 1995; **9** (**Suppl**): S45–S53.

28. McMillan WD, McCarthy WJ, Lin SJ et al. Perioperative low molecular weight heparin for infrageniculate bypass. *J Vasc Surg* 1997; **25**: 796–801.

29. Edmondson RA, Cohen AT, Das SK et al. Low-molecular weight heparin versus aspirin and dipyridamole after femoropopliteal bypass grafting. *Lancet* 1994; **344**: 914–918.

30. Bjerkeset O, Larsen S, Reiertsen O. Evaluation of enoxaparin given before and after operation to prevent venous thromboembolism during digestive surgery: play-the-winner designed study. *World J Surg* 1997; **21**: 584–588.

31. Chapuis Y, Augereau B, Clergue F et al. Prophylaxie des thromboses veineuses postopératoires: recommandations de

l'Assitance Publique-Hôpitaux de Paris. *STV* 1995; **7**: 119–120 (in French).

32. Le Brigand H, Morille P, Garnier B et al. Prevention of postoperative thrombo-embolic accidents following thoracic surgery by low-dose calcium heparinate: a comparative study. *Sem Hop* 1981; **57**: 972–977 (in French).

33. Bergqvist D, Lingren B, Matzsch T. Comparison of the cost of preventing postoperative deep vein thrombosis with either unfractionated or low molecular weight heparin. *Br J Surg* 1996; **83**: 1548–1552.

34. Lloyd A, Aitken JA, Hoffmeyer UK et al. Economic evaluation of the use of nadroparin calcium in the prophylaxis of deep vein thrombosis and pulmonary embolism in surgical patients in Italy. *Pharmacoeconomics* 1997; **12**: 475–485.

35. Bara L, Planes A, Samama M. Occurrence of thrombosis and haemorrhage, relationship with the anti-Xa, anti-IIa activities and D-dimer plasma levels in patients receiving a low molecular weight heparin, enoxaparin or

tinzaparin, to prevent deep vein thrombosis after hip surgery. *Br J Haematol* 1999; **104**: 230–240.

36. Bergqvist D, Bergentz SE, Fredin H. Thromboembolism in orthopaedic surgery. *Acta Orthop Scand* 1984; **55**: 247–250.

37. Warkentin TE, Levine MN, Hirsh J et al. Heparin-induced thrombocytopenia in patients treated with low-molecular-weight heparin or unfractionated heparin. *N Engl J Med* 1995; **332**: 1330–1335.

38. Haas SK, Wolf H, Encke A, Fareed J. Prevention of fatal postoperative pulmonary embolism by low molecular weight heparin: a double blind comparison of certoparin and unfractionated heparin. *Thromb Haemost* 1999 (suppl abst 1548): 491.

39. Sarasin FP, Bounameaux H. Cost-effectiveness of prophylactic anticoagulation prolonged after hospital discharge following general surgery. *Arch Surg* 1996; **131**: 694–697.

Direct, selective inhibitors of coagulation factors

Sam Schulman

Oral anticoagulant therapy has been completely dominated by vitamin K antagonists for more than half a century. These agents were introduced by three different groups in 1942[1-3] and, in spite of a multitude of interactions with other drugs and food and the necessity for frequent monitoring, better alternatives were not found. Only very recently have new anticoagulants been entered into clinical trials. Oral route of administration may not be an absolute requirement if the new agent has other advantageous properties, such as improved efficacy or safety. These new drugs are inhibitors of either factor Xa, the factor VIIa–tissue factor complex or thrombin. In general such inhibitors may be naturally occurring polypeptides, recombinant forms of the full length molecules or shorter derivatives thereof, small synthetic peptides and finally peptidomimetic molecules.

Factor Xa-inhibitors

The direct inhibitors of factor Xa are capable of exerting their effect on factor Xa in its free form as well as on phospholipid-bound molecules, by binding to the active site. Two highly selective inhibitors for factor Xa have been found in the animal world, the tick anticoagulant peptide (TAP) and antistasin.

TAP was initially purified from whole-body extracts of the soft tick *Ornithodouros moubata* and is a polypeptide consisting of 60 amino acids with $M_r = 6977$.[4] It has also now been produced in a recombinant form, which was a requirement for further characterization of the structure. The molecule has three disulphide bonds and the tertiary structure is unique. It binds reversibly to factor Xa in a competitive fashion. TAP seems to bind initially to a site separate from the active site (exosite) on factor Xa with a low affinity interaction and thereafter with high affinity to the catalytic site. Recombinant TAP has been evaluated in primates and other animals and a pronounced antithrombotic effect was observed, especially in arterial thrombosis.

Antistasin was isolated from the salivary gland of *Haementeria officinalis*, a Mexican leech, and from 150 mg of its extract 200–300 µg purified protein was obtained.[5] It was characterized as a polypeptide of 119 amino acids and $M_r = 17\ 000$.[5] Besides inhibiting factor Xa efficiently, it was also described as a potent antimetastatic agent. Recombinant antistasin has subsequently been produced. The inhibitory effect against factor Xa is located within residue 1–55 (domain I) and even shorter peptides down to seven amino acids, corresponding to residue 33–39, demonstrate such activity.[6]

The nonpeptidic factor Xa inhibitors YM-60828 and DX 9065a have a potent antithrombotic effect with minimal or no prolongation of the bleeding time in animal studies.[7,8] YM-60828 is orally active with a bioavailability of about 20%.[9] DX 9065a or APAP is a dibasic amidinoaryl propanoic acid derivative. It is also orally active and has, beside its antithrombotic effects demonstrated a protective capacity against disseminated intravascular coagulation.[10] In an animal model experiment with equipotent doses of DX 9065a and warfarin, the factor Xa inhibitor induced much less bleeding.[11]

Factor VIIa–tissue factor inhibitors

The current opinion is that basal haemostasis is initiated from the extrinsic pathway via factor VIIa and tissue factor.[12] Inhibition of this pathway has been evaluated in the prophylaxis of thrombosis.

Whereas recombinant activated factor VII (rFVIIa) is being marketed as a haemostatic agent, the active-site-inhibited counterpart (rFVIIai) has an antithrombotic effect by competing with factor VIIa for binding to a limited number of tissue factor sites induced on cells after perturbation. rFVIIai has a higher or an altered affinity for tissue factor than plasma factor VIIa. The antithrombotic effect has been demonstrated in primates[13] and other animal models on the arterial side.[14]

Tissue factor can be blocked by antibodies,

competitively inhibited by soluble mutant analogues or by peptide analogues. The complex of factor VIIa and tissue factor is naturally inhibited by tissue factor pathway inhibitor (TFPI), which binds to factor Xa. The latter becomes inactivated and the complex of the two can subsequently inactivate factor VIIa, bound to tissue factor. TFPI has been tested in models for disseminated intravascular coagulation but not in venous thrombosis.

The hookworm anticoagulant protein NAPc2 belongs to a family of 75–84 amino acid polypeptides, isolated from *Anchlostoma caninum*. It is bound to an exosite on factor X or Xa, when it reaches factor VIIa in its complex with tissue factor.[15] The mechanism of inhibition is similar to that of TFPI, except that TFPI binds to the catalytic site of factor Xa and the half-life of NAPc2 is much longer — about 50 hours.

Thrombin (factor IIa) inhibitors

Indirect thrombin inhibitors, for example unfractionated heparin, low molecular weight heparin and dermatan sulphate need to activate antithrombin or heparin cofactor II in order to inactivate thrombin. Direct inhibitors work independently of antithrombin or heparin cofactor II and are able to inhibit both fibrin-bound and free thrombin (*Figure 9.1*).

Hirudin

Haycraft described in 1884 the antithrombotic characteristic of saliva from the leech *Hirudo medicinalis*.[16] This was the only agent to prevent clotting until heparin was discovered a few decades later. In 1904 Jacoby isolated the active substance from the head of the leech and named it 'hirudin'.[17]

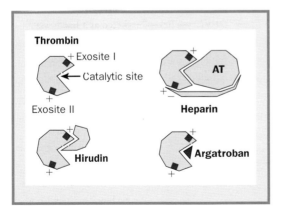

Figure 9.1
Site of action of the indirect thrombin inhibitor heparin, which acts via antithrombin, and the direct inhibitors hirudin and argatroban.

Markwardt isolated hirudin from the peripharyngeal glands of the leech, produced it in the pure crystalline form and described its action.[18] It was, however, only with recombinant hirudin that sufficient amounts became available for clinical trials. Hirudin is a polypeptide with 65 amino acids and M_r of ≈ 7000.

Desirudin

The recombinant form lacks a sulphate residue on Tyr-63, which causes a 10-fold lower affinity for thrombin. This form is called desirudin and is commercially produced in yeast, *Saccharomyces cerevisiae*, cultures and purified to a specific activity of 12 000 thrombin inhibiting units/mg protein. Desirudin has been evaluated in the prevention of venous thromboembolism after total hip replacement and was found to be safe and more effective than unfractionated heparin[19,20] and low molecular weight heparin (*Figure 9.2*).[21] Owing to a higher cost, desirudin may still not be the first choice in surgical prophylaxis of venous thromboembolism. Recombinant hirudin has also been used in the treatment of established deep-vein thrombosis. In a comparison with unfractionated heparin, recombinant hirudin, administered subcutaneously for 5 days, resulted in significantly fewer new perfusion defects on repeat lung scanning (*Figure 9.3*).[22]

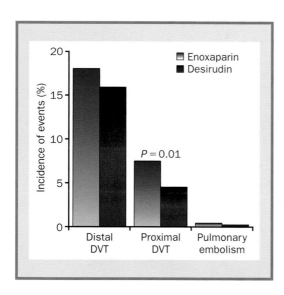

Figure 9.2

Main outcome of a comparison of recombinant hirudin with a low molecular weight heparin in the prophylaxis of venous thromboembolism after total hip replacement. The difference in total deep-vein thrombosis (DVT) was also statistically significant (P = 0.001). (Adapted from Eriksson et al.[20])

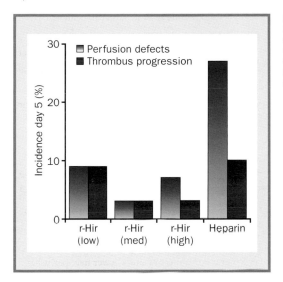

Figure 9.3
New perfusion defects and venographic extension of the thrombus in patients with deep-vein thrombosis, randomized to three different doses of r-hirudin (r-Hir) or to heparin. (Data adapted from Schiele et al.[22])

Direct inhibition of thrombin is of great theoretical interest in arterial thrombotic disease, since thrombin is the most potent platelet agonist in addition to its central role in the coagulation system and its effect on smooth muscle cell proliferation. The latter is mediated by stimulation of thrombin receptors on the surface of smooth muscle cells and the release of growth factors. This was tested in patients undergoing percutaneous transluminal coronary angioplasty (PTCA) with desirudin administered intravenously or subcutaneously or unfractionated heparin.[23] No significant difference in the primary endpoint of event-free survival at 7 months was achieved, but

hirudin was associated with a lower incidence of early coronary events.

In the GUSTO IIb trial over 12 000 patients with acute myocardial infarction or unstable angina were randomized to treatment with unfractionated heparin or recombinant hirudin intravenously.[24] Although at 24 hours there was a significant reduction of the risk of death or myocardial infarction in the hirudin group, this was not paralleled by an appreciable difference in the late results (*Figure 9.4*).

Hirugen

Several variants of recombinant hirudin with exchange of individual amino acids at the

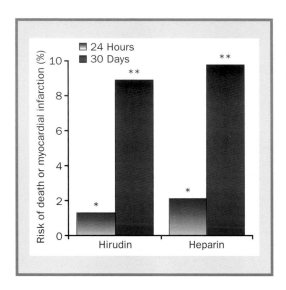

Figure 9.4
*Primary endpoints in a comparison of r-hirudin and heparin for patients with acute coronary syndromes (GUSTO IIb). *P = 0.001; **P = 0.06. Data adapted from GUSTO IIb investigators.[24]*

N-terminal or in position 47 have been studied. The carboxy-terminal 12-amino acid sequence of hirudin (residues 53–64) has been synthetically produced, including proper sulphation of tyrosine at position 63.[25] This dodecapeptide, hirugen, has a high affinity for thrombin but binds only to its exosite 1 and prevents interaction between thrombin and fibrinogen or platelets, but the active site is not blocked from cleaving low molecular weight thrombin-directed substrates.

Bivalirudin

By adding a small molecule, which reacts with the active site in thrombin — D-Phe-Pro-Arg-Pro — to the aminoterminal of hirugen a potent bivalent thrombin inhibitor is obtained. Bivalirudin binds to exosite 1 as well as to the active site on thrombin. However, thereafter the Arg-Pro bond is quickly cleaved, and affinity decreases sharply. This may explain the lower incidence of bleeding compared with heparin in patients treated during and after coronary angioplasty.[26] Bivalirudin did not appear to be more effective than heparin in this trial.

Lepirudin

Another modification of hirudin is lepirudin, (Leu1-Thr2)-63-desulfohirudin, which is produced in yeast cells with a specific activity of 16 000 000 thrombin inhibiting units/mg protein. This substance has been approved in many countries for the treatment of thrombosis in patients who have developed heparin-induced thrombocytopenia, and in whom heparin or its analogues would be contraindicated. For these patients lepirudin is an effective alternative, which allows a rapid normalization of platelet counts.[27] In the OASIS-2 trial over 10 000 patients with unstable angina or suspected myocardial infarction without ST-elevation were randomized to 72 hours infusion with unfractionated heparin or lepirudin.[28] There was a lower incidence of cardiovascular death, myocardial infarction and refractory angina in the group treated with lepirudin, but at the same time an excess of major haemorrhage, requiring transfusions (*Figure 9.5*).

PPACK

Oligopeptides that fit into the active site of thrombin and provide a selective inhibition by binding covalently there have been developed and the prototype is D-Phe-Pro-ArgCH$_2$Cl or PPACK. Several boroarginine tripeptide derivatives are being tested for potency and selectivity.[29] One tripeptide arginal inhibitor is efegatran (LY294468) and it has been evaluated in a phase II study in patients with

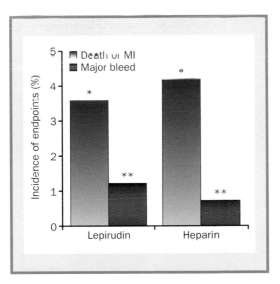

Figure 9.5
Risk of death or myocardial infarction after 7 days of major haemorrhage, requiring transfusion, in patients with acute coronary syndromes treated with lepirudin or heparin (OASIS-2). *P = 0.077;**P = 0.01. (Data adapted from OASIS-2 investigators.[28])

unstable angina. Of 87 patients treated with efegatran, four had myocardial infarction, five required revascularization procedures and one died, and among 17 treated with heparin the corresponding figures were three, zero and zero.[30]

Peptidomimetics

Further development of small size direct thrombin inhibitors has yielded nonpeptidic molecules. The first one, argatroban, is an L-arginine derivative with an M_r of 509. It is a competitive inhibitor of thrombin, and it is administered as an intravenous infusion since the half-life is only 45–65 minutes.[31] Argatroban has been evaluated in the anticoagulant therapy of patients with heparin-induced thrombocytopenia with favourable results. In a small clinical trial in patients with unstable angina, argatroban was infused for 4 hours intravenously without myocardial ischaemia during this period.[32] After discontinuation of the infusion nine of 43 patients developed recurrent unstable angina, paralleled by laboratory evidence that thrombin formation had not been suppressed.

Napsagatran (Ro 46-6240) is a highly selective, potent competitive thrombin inhibitor with a half-life of 40 minutes. It has been compared in two doses with unfractionated heparin in the treatment of proximal deep-vein thrombosis in the ADVENT trial.[33] No differences in efficacy or safety were detected. Napsagatran at the higher dose level (9 mg/h) lowered the thrombin–antithrombin complex level more effectively than heparin, indicating a more potent thrombin inhibition of the former, but reduced the prothrombin fragment 1 + 2 less than heparin, suggesting a less effective inhibition of thrombin generation.[34]

Inogatran and melagatran, 439 and 430 Da, respectively, nonpeptide molecules, are also selective active site inhibitors of thrombin. In an open pilot study inogatran in three different doses was infused during 4 hours in patients with unstable angina or non-Q wave myocardial infarction, and a suppression of thrombin generation was seen. After discontinuation, however, there were episodes of ischaemia and rebound thrombin activity.[35] In a subsequent study (TRIM-trial) of patients with the same acute coronary syndromes three doses of inogatran infused during 74 hours were compared with heparin.[36] During the infusion there were fewer composite events in the heparin group, but after 7 or 30 days there were no statistically significant differences between any of the groups. Inogatran is not being studied in current clinical trials. Its successor, melagatran, is instead being developed for oral administration.[37] It is well tolerated by intravenous administration, the clearance has a low interpatient variability, correlating linearly to the creatinine clearance, the effect on the activated partial thromboplastin time

(APTT) appears less pronounced than that of heparin, and the effect in patients with acute deep-vein thrombosis, as assessed by Marder score, is comparable to that of heparin.[38] Both inogatran and melagatran have a less steep dose-response curve than warfarin and heparin, with the slopes 1.1, 1.2, 3.6 and 1.8, respectively,[39] which indicates wider therapeutic ranges for the thrombin inhibitors.

Reversal of effect

These new, highly selective anticoagulants have one disadvantage in common. There is no antidote in case rapid reversal is required. For some of the agents with short half-life and intravenous administration this will not be a problem. According to a case report of a patient who was treated with recombinant hirudin and developed multiple-site haemorrhage, desmopressin, fresh frozen plasma and red cell transfusions were ineffective.[40] However, prothrombin complex concentrated at a dose of 25 U/kg proved useful and, if confirmed by other cases, could be considered in case of life-threatening bleeding. In a pig model the effect of recombinant hirudin on the skin bleeding time could be reversed by a factor VIII-von Willebrand factor concentrate.[41] This possibility should be evaluated in humans since the thrombogenicity of such a concentrate is probably lower than that of prothrombin complex concentrate.

References

1. Allen EV, Barker NW, Waugh JM. A preparation from spoiled sweet clover (3.3'-methylene-bis-(4-hydroxycoumarin)) which prolongs coagulation and prothrombin time of the blood: a clinical study. *JAMA* 1942; **120:** 1009–1015.

2. Butsch WC, Stewart JD. Clinical experience with dicoumarin, 3.3'-methylene-bis-(4-hydroxycoumarin). *JAMA* 1942: **120:** 1625–1626.

3. Lehmann J. Hypoprothrombinaemia produced by methylene-bis-(hydroxycoumarin), its use in thrombosis. *Lancet* 1942; **i:** 318.

4. Vlasuk GP. Structural and functional characterization of tick anticoagulant peptide (TAP): a potent and selective inhibitor of blood coagulation factor Xa. *Thromb Haemost* 1993; **70:** 212–216.

5. Tuszyuski G, Gasic TB, Gasic GJ. Isolation and characterization of antistasin *J Biol Chem* 1987; **262:** 9718–9723.

6. Ohta N, Brush M, Jacobs JW. Interaction of antistasin-related peptides with factor Xa: identification of a core inhibitory sequence. *Thromb Haemost* 1994; **72:** 825–830.

7. Sato K, Kawasaki T, Hisamichi N et al. Antithrombotic effects of YM-60828 in three thrombosis models in guinea pigs. *Eur J Pharmacol* 1998; **350:** 87–91.

8. Morishima Y, Tanabe K, Terada Y et al. Antithrombotic and hemorrhagic effects of DX-9065a, a direct and selective factor Xa inhibitor: comparison with a direct thrombin inhibitor and antithrombin III-dependent anticoagulants. *Thromb Haemost* 1997; **78:** 1366–1371.

9. Taniuchi Y, Sakai Y, Hisamichi N et al.

Biochemical and pharmacological characterization of YM-60828, a newly synthesized and orally active inhibitor of human factor Xa. *Thromb Haemost* 1998; **79**: 543–548.

10. Yamazaki M, Asakura H, Aoshima K et al. Protective effects of DX-9065a, an orally active, novel synthesized and selective inhibitor of factor Xa, against thromboplastin-induced experimental disseminated intravascular coagulation in rats. *Semin Thromb Hemost* 1996; **22**: 255–259.

11. Tanabe K, Morishima Y, Shibutani T et al. DX-9065a, an orally active factor Xa inhibitor, does not facilitate haemorrhage induced by tail transection or gastric ulcer at the effective doses in rat thrombosis model. *Thromb Haemost* 1999; **81**: 828–834.

12. Bauer KA, Mannucci PM, Gringeri A et al. Factor IXa–factor VIIIa-cell surface complex does not contribute to the basal activation of the coagulation mechanism in vivo. *Blood* 1992; **79**: 2039–2047.

13. Harker LA, Hanson SR, Wilcox JN, Kelly AB. Antithrombotic and antilesion benefits without hemorrhagic risks by inhibiting tissue factor pathway. *Haemostasis* 1996; **26**: 76–82.

14. Sørensen BB, Rao LVM. Interaction of activated factor VII and active site-inhibited activated factor VII with tissue factor. *Blood Coagul Fibrinolysis* 1998; **9** (suppl 1): S67–S71.

15. Stassens P, Bergum PW, Gansemans Y et al. Anticoagulant repertoire of the hookworm *Ancylostoma caninum. Proc Natl Acad Sci USA* 1996; **93**: 2149–54.

16. Haycraft JB. On the action of a secretion obtained from the medicinal leech on the coagulation of the blood. *Proc R Soc Lond* 1884; **36**: 478.

17. Jacoby C. Über Hirudin. *Dtsch Med Wochenschr* 1904; **30**: 1786.

18. Markwardt F. Die Isolierung und chemische Charakterisierung des Hirudins. *Hoppe Seyler's Z Physiol Chem* 1957; **308**: 147–156.

19. Eriksson BI, Ekman S, Kälebo P et al. Prevention of deep-vein thrombosis after total hip replacement: direct thrombin inhibition with recombinant hirudin, CGP 39393. *Lancet* 1996; **347**: 635–639.

20. Eriksson BI, Ekman S, Lindbratt S et al. Prevention of thromboembolism with use of recombinant hirudin: results of a double-blind, multicenter trial comparing the efficacy of desirudin (Revasc) with that of unfractionated heparin in patients having a total hip replacement. *J Bone Joint Surg Am* 1997; **79**: 326–333.

21. Eriksson BI, Whille-Jørgensen P, Kälebo P et al. A comparison of recombinant hirudin with a low-molecular-weight heparin to prevent thromboembolic complications after total hip replacement. *N Engl J Med* 1997; **337**: 1329–1335.

22. Schiele F, Lindgaerde F, Eriksson H et al. Subcutaneous recombinant hirudin (HBW 023) versus intravenous sodium heparin in treatment of established acute deep vein thrombosis of the legs: a multicentre prospective dose-ranging randomized trial. *Thromb Haemost* 1997; **77**: 834–838.

23. Serruys PW, Herrman JP, Simon R et al. A comparison of hirudin with heparin in the prevention of restenosis after coronary angioplasty. Helvetica Investigators. *N Engl J Med* 1995; **333**: 757–763.

24. The Global Use of Strategies to Open Occluded Coronary Arteries (GUSTO) IIb investigators. A comparison of recombinant hirudin with heparin for the treatment of

acute coronary syndromes. *N Engl J Med* 1996; **335**: 775–782.

25. Maraganore JM, Chao B, Joseph ML et al. Anticoagulant activity of synthetic hirudin fragments. *J Biol Chem* 1989; **264**: 8692–8698.

26. Bittl JA, Strony J, Brinker JA et al. Treatment with bivalirudin (Hirulog) as compared with heparin during coronary angioplasty for unstable or postinfarction angina. Hirulog Angioplasty Study Investigators. *N Engl J Med* 1995; **333**: 764–769.

27. Greinacher A, Völpel H, Janssens U et al. Recombinant hirudin (lepirudin) provides safe and effective anticoagulation in patients with heparin-induced thrombocytopenia: a prospective study. *Circulation* 1999; **99**: 73–80.

28. Organisation to Assess Strategies for Ischemic Syndromes (OASIS-2) investigators. Effects of recombinant hirudin (lepirudin) compared with heparin on death, myocardial infarction, refractory angina, and revascularisation procedures in patients with acute myocardial ischaemia without ST elevation: a randomised trial. *Lancet* 1999; **353**: 429–438.

29. Rupin A, Mennecier P, Lila C et al. Selection of S18326 as a new potent and selective boronic acid direct thrombin inhibitor. *Thromb Haemost* 1997; **78**: 1221–7.

30. Jackson CV, Satterwhite J, Roberts E. Preclinical and clinical pharmacology of efegatran (LY294468): a novel antithrombin for the treatment of acute coronary syndromes. *Clin Appl Thromb Hemost* 1996; **2**: 258–267.

31. Schwarz RP, Becker J-CP, Brooks RL et al. The preclinical and clinical pharmacology of Novastan (argatroban): a small-molecule, direct thrombin inhibitor. *Clin Appl Thromb Haemost* 1997; **3**: 1–15.

32. Gold HK, Torres FW, Garabedian HD et al. Evidence for a rebound coagulation phenomenon after cessation of a 4-hour infusion of a specific thrombin inhibitor in patients with unstable angina pectoris. *Am Coll Cardiol* 1993; **21**: 1039–1047.

33. Bounameaux H, Ehringer H, Hulting J et al. An exploratory trial of two dosages of a novel synthetic thrombin inhibitor (Napsagatran, Ro 46-6240) compared with unfractionated heparin for treatment of proximal deep-vein thrombosis. Results of the European multicenter ADVENT trial. *Thromb Haemost* 1997; **78**: 997–1002.

34. Bounameaux H, Ehringer H, Gast A et al. Differential inhibition of thrombin activity and thrombin generation by a synthetic direct thrombin inhibitor (napsagatran, Ro 46-6240) and unfractionated heparin in patients with deep vein thrombosis. *Thromb Haemost* 1999; **81**: 498–501.

35. Andersen K, Dellborg M, Emanuelsson H et al. Thrombin inhibition with inogatran for unstable angina pectoris: evidence for reactivated ischaemia after cessation of short term treatment. *Coron Artery Dis* 1996; **7**: 673–681.

36. Thrombin Inhibition in Myocardial Ischaemia (TRIM) study group. A low molecular weight, selective thrombin inhibitor, inogatran, vs heparin, in unstable coronary artery disease in 1209 patients. *Eur Heart J* 1997; **18**: 1416–1425.

37. Gustafsson D, Antonsson T, Bylund R et al. Effects of melagatran, a new low-molecular-weight thrombin inhibitor, on thrombin and fibrinolytic enzymes. *Thromb Haemost* 1998; **79**: 110–118.

38.   Eriksson H, Eriksson UG, Frison L et al.
      Pharmacokinetics and pharmacodynamics of
      melagatran, a novel synthetic LMW thrombin
      inhibitor, in patients with acute DVT.
      Thromb Haemost 1999; **81**: 358–63.

39.   Elg M, Gustafsson D, Carlsson S.
      Antithrombotic effects and bleeding time of
      thrombin inhibitors and warfarin in the rat.
      Thromb Res 1999; **94**: 187–97.

40.   Irani MS, White HJ, Sexon RN. Reversal of
      hirudin-induced bleeding diathesis by
      prothrombin complex concentrate. *Am J
      Cardiol* 1995; **75**: 422–423.

41.   Dickneite G, Nicolay U, Friesen H-J, Reers
      M. Development of an anti-bleeding agent
      for recombinant hirudin induced skin
      bleeding in the pig. *Thromb Haemost* 1998;
      80: 192–198.

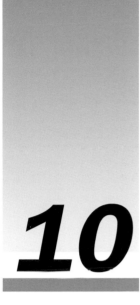

The role of antithrombotic agents in ischemic heart disease: platelet inhibitors

Marc Cohen

10

Hemostasis is established by interaction of three main components: circulating platelets, plasma coagulation proteins, and the vessel wall. The maintenance of blood fluidity under normal circumstances is dependent upon an intact and healthy endothelium. The response of all components to vascular injury is rapid and precise, working in a coordinated manner to stop bleeding and repair damage. The relatively fragile platelet plug formed by vascular damage is anchored by the insoluble protein meshwork of fibrin to achieve stable hemostasis.

The endothelial lining of all blood vessels possesses a remarkable resistance to thrombosis. In fact, the cascade of coagulation events is triggered only when blood comes into contact with any surface other than healthy endothelium. These nonendothelial surfaces can include components of damaged blood vessels, artificial surfaces, or extravascular tissues. When the endothelial surface is damaged, circulating platelets attach in a monolayer to the vessel wall. This platelet–vessel wall interaction ('adhesion') is stimulated both by the loss of endothelial thromboresistant activities, and by the exposure of platelet activating subendothelial structures such as collagen. Adhesion of platelets is mediated primarily by the adhesive macromolecule, von Willebrand factor (vWF).[1] Examples of substances with endothelial thromboresistant activities are prostacyclin, a potent agent that prevents platelet aggregation and has vasodilator properties, and endothelium-dependent relaxing factor.[2]

Role of platelets in thrombus formation and mechanism of platelet aggregation

Thrombosis within the circulatory system is responsible for significant cardiovascular morbidity and mortality. In vivo, coagulation is initiated by the release of tissue factor after endothelial damage. The release of tissue factor leads to the activation of factor X, which produces the prothrombinase complex. The prothrombinase complex plays a fundamental role in the pathogenesis of thrombi by catalysing the conversion of prothrombin to thrombin[3] and thereby generating a potent activator of platelets.

Along with the coagulation and fibrinolytic systems, platelets participate in the maintenance and regulation of hemostasis. Platelets do not interact with normal, intact endothelium but readily adhere to damaged vascular tissue. When stimulated by exposure to damaged endothelium, platelets release the contents of their intracytoplasmic granules and produce thromboxane A_2 (TXA$_2$). The production of TXA$_2$ and release of adenosine

diphosphate (ADP) lead to the recruitment of additional platelets and the formation of aggregates at the site of vessel wall damage. These platelet aggregates provide a surface for the localization and interaction of coagulation factors enhancing the conversion of prothrombin to thrombin. Therefore, platelets and the coagulation system are intricately involved in the formation of a thrombus.[3]

The distinguishing pathological lesion defining the acute coronary artery syndromes of unstable angina and non-Q wave myocardial infarction is the platelet-rich, nonocclusive thrombus, which overlays the fissured or active plaque.[4] In acute myocardial infarction (MI), thrombi are red and fibrin-rich; complete occlusion is a more common finding in acute MI. Preventive and acute treatment of unstable coronary artery disease, logically, has focused on methods to prevent platelet activation and aggregation. Such initial management efforts can ultimately reduce the likelihood of patients with unstable coronary artery disease developing acute MI.

As a result of endothelial injury, platelets adhere to the subendothelium until a single layer of these cells has covered the damaged site. The process of platelet adherence is dependent on the interaction of platelet membrane receptors, adhesive glycoproteins, and the substrate formed by subendothelial microfibrils of collagen and other proteins. The platelet membrane receptor, glycoprotein

(GP) Ib, serves as the binding site for vWF at high shear rates and is essential for the initial contact of the platelets with the subendothelial surface. Another platelet membrane receptor, GPIIb/IIIa, binds fibrinogen during platelet aggregation and is important in the process of adhesion by serving as an additional binding site for vWF. After platelets have adhered to the subendothelium, they spread over the surface of the injury.

When a vessel sustains a deep injury (e.g. after the rupture of an atherosclerotic plaque), fibrillar collagen from the deeper layers of the arterial structures is exposed (type I). This injury also leads to the exposure of the surface platelet receptor, GPIIb/IIIa, plus the subsequent binding of fibrinogen, vWF, and fibronectin. The process of aggregation is directly governed by these essential adhesive macromolecules, which form links between the platelets. Once platelets have been activated by various stimulants (i.e. collagen, thrombin, epinephrine, TXA$_2$), calcium is released from the intracellular tubular system into the cytoplasm, where it produces cellular contraction and results in the secretion of its granular contents. The metabolically active products of platelet secretion include ADP, serotonin (5-hydroxytryptophan or 5-HT), TXA$_2$, fibronectin, fibrinogen, vWF, and platelet derived growth factor (PDGF). In addition to the presence of thrombin and collagen, the release of 5-HT, ADP and TXA$_2$

contribute to the activation of neighboring platelets through three metabolic pathways.[5]

The first pathway is dependent on the release of ADP and 5-HT from the dense granules within the cytoplasm of the platelets. Both ADP and 5-HT are powerful inducers of platelet aggregation by promoting the exposure of the platelet binding site (GPIIb/IIIa) for fibrinogen and vWF. The second pathway depends on the release of TXA$_2$ via the interaction of cyclo-oxygenase and thromboxane synthase on arachidonic acid and prostaglandin (PG) endoperoxide intermediates (i.e. PGH$_2$ and PGG$_2$). A third pathway in the process of platelet aggregation is governed by collagen and thrombin, both of which may stimulate the release of a platelet-activating factor. It may be this platelet-activating factor that favors the interaction of fibrinogen and vWF with the GPIIb/IIIa receptor.[5]

The GPIIb/IIIa receptor is therefore frequently referred to as the fibrinogen receptor. Agonist macromolecules convert platelets from a latent state to an activated state capable of binding soluble ligands. In the final process step, fibrinogen links adjacent platelets to one another and facilitates the process of aggregation. Specificity of the GPIIb/IIIa receptor is defined by two amino acid sequences in the fibrinogen molecule, which forms the 'molecular glue' for platelet aggregation. One sequence, RGD (arginine-glycine-aspartic acid), is found in the extracellular adhesive macromolecules (i.e. fibrinonectin, vitronectin, vWF, and fibrinogen). The second sequence that binds fibrinogen to the GPIIb/IIIa receptor, lysine-glutamine-alanine- glycine-aspartic acid-valine, is present only on the fibrinogen macromolecule, constituting the major binding site. *Table 10.1* summarizes the surface membrane receptors that participate in both adhesion and aggregation of platelets.[6]

An understanding of the pathophysiology of acute coronary syndromes (ACS) and the role that platelets play in this process is important in determining the best antithrombotic approach to these high-risk patients.[5] In this regard, patients with unstable coronary artery disease without ST elevation or in which only transient elevation is present, comprised primarily of unstable angina and non-Q wave myocardial infarction, have been considered together in many of the studies evaluating antithrombotic therapies. This review is focused on recent antithrombotic studies for ACS without ST elevation or with only transient deviations.

Pharmacology of platelet inhibitors and results of clinical trials

Meta-analyses of several, large scale, randomized, clinical trials demonstrated that

Table 10.1
Surface membrane glycoprotein receptors governing the adhesion and aggregation of platelets[7]

Platelet receptor	Ligand	Biological action	Receptors per platelet	Amino acid sequence recognized
GP Ib	vWF	Adhesion	25 000	Not a short sequence
GP Ia/IIa $\alpha_2\beta_1$	Collagen	Adhesion	~1000	DGEA*
GP Ic/IIa $\alpha_5\beta_1$	Fibronectin	Adhesion	~1000	RGD
GPIIb/IIIa $\alpha_{IIb}\beta_3$	Fibrinogen, vWF, Fibronectin, Vitronectin	Aggregation, Adhesion	50 000	RGD, K_{QAGDV}
$\alpha_v\beta_3$	Vitronectin, Fibrinogen, Fibronectin, vWF	Adhesion	~100	RGD

GP = Glycoprotein; vWF = von Willebrand factor.
*Other amino acid sequences may also be involved.

treatment with platelet inhibitors, specifically agents that prevent the activation of platelets, reduces the risk of nonfatal MI and stroke by 25–30%, and the rate of vascular death by about 15%.[7] These statistics substantiate the role of activated platelets as significant determinants of arterial thrombus formation and morbidity resulting from blood vessel occlusion. These events can be successfully blocked by appropriate agents that prevent the activation of platelets. The ideal agent that should prevent platelet activation would block thrombogenic platelet-dependent processes in vascular diseases without interfering with normal platelet function in hemostasis and wound healing. This ideal agent should be free of any serious adverse effects and have a duration of action easily adjustable to the therapeutic needs of the patient.[8]

Agents that interfere with secondary activation of platelets

Aspirin

The major cyclo-oxygenase product in platelets is TXA_2. Aspirin blocks the production of TXA_2 by acetylating a serine residue near the active site of cyclo-oxygenase (cyclo-oxygenase 1 or 2), the enzymes producing the cyclic endoperoxidase precursor to TXA_2. The action of aspirin on platelet cyclo-oxygenase is permanent (lasting the life of the platelet, from 7 to 10 days) because of the platelet, from 7 to 10 days) because platelets do not synthesize proteins. Therefore, repeated doses of aspirin produce a cumulative effect on platelet function.[9]

The landmark Second International Study of Infarct Survival (ISIS-2), which studied more than 17 000 patients with acute MI, demonstrated that aspirin monotherapy (160 mg/day) reduced vascular mortality by 21% at 5 weeks post-MI with benefit maintained at the 15-month follow-up.[10] When aspirin was given concurrently with streptokinase, a 40% drop in mortality rate was recorded. The ISIS-2 study also found that aspirin reduced reinfarction and stroke by approximately one half in this group of patients. *Table 10.2* summarizes the results of the ISIS-2 clinical trial.[10] Based on the results of this important trial, it was determined that aspirin dosed at 160–325 mg/day can be recommended to patients with acute MI, whether or not thrombolytic therapy is used.[3] For patients with unstable angina, aspirin dosed at 75–1300 mg/day was shown to decrease the progression to MI or death.[11–13]

Dipyridamole

This is a vasodilator agent that may interfere with platelet function by increasing the intracellular concentration of cyclic adenosine 3′,5′-monophosphate (cAMP). This effect may be governed by inhibition of cyclic nucleotide phosphodiesterase and/or by the blockade of adenosine, which stimulates

Table 10.2
ISIS-2 clinical trial results studying mortality reduction in acute myocardial infarction[10]

| Treatment regimen | Mortality reduction (%) | | | |
	0–4* (hours)	5–12 (hours)	13–24 (hours)	Overall reduction (%)
ASA	25	21	21	23
SK	35	16	21	25
ASA + SK	53	32	38	42

ASA = acetylsalicylic acid (aspirin); SK = streptokinase.
*Mortality reduction (%) per interval between onset and therapy (hours).

platelet adenyl cyclase by acting at A_2 receptors for adenosine.

There is some evidence that the aspirin/dipyridamole combination is more effective than aspirin alone in reducing the rate of the progression of peripheral vascular disease[14] and in preventing occlusion following coronary artery bypass graft (CABG) surgery.[15] However, because clinical results with this agent, by itself, have not been encouraging, dipyridamole is currently recommended for use only in high-risk patients with prosthetic heart valves and prosthetic vascular grafts when given concurrently with warfarin.[5,7]

Ticlopidine

Ticlopidine, chemically unrelated to either aspirin or dypiridamole, acts by inhibiting the effects of ADP via ADP receptor blockade,

prolongs bleeding time, and normalizes shortened platelet survival.[16–18] Clinical trials have shown that it is effective for the prevention of MI and cardiovascular death in patients with unstable angina.[19] It has also been shown that ticlopidine reduces vein graft closure after CABG surgery.[20] This agent is currently used for the prevention of thrombosis in cerebrovascular and coronary artery disease. More recent reports have demonstrated that ticlopidine reduced the incidence of acute thrombotic occlusion after coronary angioplasty with intracoronary stents.[21,22] For a while, aspirin plus ticlopidine appeared to be the best treatment strategy for patients undergoing coronary stenting. However, an unacceptable side-effect profile exists for ticlopidine, with diarrhea occurring most frequently (20%). The most serious side-effect is neutropenia occurring in 2.4% of patients, with severe neutropenia

($<0.45 \times 10^9$ cells/l) occurring in 0.85% of patients.[8] The neutropenia is generally reversible following discontinuation of this drug. Recently, ticlopidine has also been implicated in several cases of thrombotic thrombocytopenic purpura.[23]

Clopidogrel

Clopidogrel is a new thienopyridine derivative similar to ticlopidine but with an improved side-effect profile. The CAPRIE (Clopidogrel versus Aspirin in Patients at Risk of Ischemic Events) study assessed the relative efficacy of clopidogrel (75 mg/day) and aspirin (325 mg/day) in reducing the risk of a composite outcome of ischemic stroke, MI, or vascular death over a period of 1–3 years. The overall safety profile of clopidogrel was as good as that of medium-dose aspirin. The frequency of severe rash and severe diarrhea was higher with clopidogrel than with aspirin, but the frequency of neutropenia and severe neutropenia was similar in both groups. Long-term administration of clopidogrel to patients with atherosclerotic vascular disease was more effective than aspirin in reducing the combined risk of ischemic stroke, MI, or vascular death; intention-to-treat analysis of this composite outcome showed a relative-risk reduction of 8.7% with clopidogrel ($P = 0.043$).[24] In the CAPRIE study, clopidogrel provided the most benefit to those patients with peripheral vascular disease

compared with those with either stroke or MI. Clopidogrel can be used in patients with unstable coronary artery disease who cannot tolerate aspirin.[24] Currently, clopidogrel is being substituted for ticlopidine as the standard adjunct to aspirin for percutaneous coronary intervention with stents. The recent CLASSICS study randomized 1020 patients to combination aspirin plus clopidogrel versus aspirin plus ticlopidine. Adverse safety endpoints and drug discontinuation occurred less frequently with clopidogrel (4.6 versus 9.1%, $P = 0.005$).[25]

Glycoprotein IIb/IIIa receptor blockers

After platelets adhere to sites of vascular injury, they undergo activation and express functional GPIIb/IIIa receptors for circulating adhesive ligand proteins (primarily fibrinogen). These GPIIb/IIIa receptors mediate the recruitment of local platelets by forming fibrinogen bridges between platelets (i.e. 'platelet cohesion'). Functional GPIIb/IIIa receptors bind with other circulating adhesive molecules in plasma (e.g. vWF, fibronectin, vitronectin, and thrombospondin), but because of its relatively high concentration, fibrinogen is the predominant ligand. The blockade of GPIIb/IIIa receptors upon which platelet recruitment is dependent became a viable therapeutic strategy for several logical reasons.

Since GPIIb/IIIa is specific for platelets, platelet recruitment is mediated almost exclusively during the final phase of GPIIb/IIIa-dependent platelet aggregation. Furthermore, GPIIb/IIIa is the most abundant platelet membrane protein, with about 50 000–80 000 receptors per platelet.[6]

Abciximab, a chimeric monoclonal antibody to the IIb/IIIa receptor, has been shown to be effective in both the prevention of platelet-mediated arterial thrombosis and in the lysis of platelet-rich thrombi. To overcome the problems of the monoclonal antibody, such as prolonged platelet inhibitory action accompanied by increased bleeding and antigenicity, various peptides (e.g. eptifibatide) and small molecules (e.g. tirofiban) that mimic the RGD sequence and compete with fibrinogen for binding to the GPIIb/IIIa receptor were developed.[5]

The GPIIb/IIIa receptor is a member of the integrin family. It possesses a 136-kDa subunit molecule made of a heavy chain and a light chain. Its light chain component has a short cytoplasmic tail, a transmembrane region, and a short extracellular domain. The heavy chain, on the other hand, is completely extracellular.[26] *Figure 10.1* is a schematic

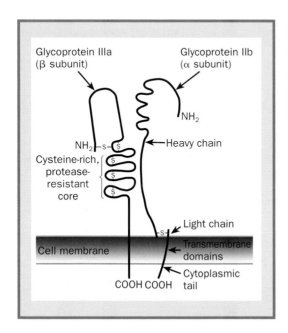

Figure 10.1
Schematic representation of a typical GPIIb/IIIa receptor as found on the platelet surface membrane. The RGD binding sites are located in the pocket enclosed by the folds occupied by disulfide (—S—) bonds and the subunit. Binding of adhesive proteins requires that calcium be displaced from the binding sites. The amino groups (NH$_2$) occupy the terminal of the heavy chain molecule. (Reprinted from Lefkovits J et al[26] with permission.)

representation of a typical platelet GPIIb/IIIa receptor.

The new class of agents, the GPIIb/IIIa blockers (unlike aspirin), prevents the binding of fibrinogen to these platelet receptors. This blockade inhibits platelet aggregation without regard to the metabolic pathway ultimately responsible for initiating the aggregation. These GPIIb/IIIa blockers have a potentially wide range of clinical uses, which include the prevention of coronary events in patients at high risk, and as antithrombotic therapy during and following percutaneous coronary interventions (PTCA), or before CABG surgery.[26]

Clinical studies with GPIIb/IIIa receptor blockers

Several important clinical trials have been conducted to evaluate the role of the GPIIb/IIIa inhibitors in the prevention of complications related to percutaneous coronary interventions, and as adjunctive therapy for patients with non-ST segment elevation acute coronary syndromes.[27]

Abciximab

Abciximab (ReoPro: Centecor, Malvern, PA) was the first GPIIb/IIIa receptor blocker to be tested in a large scale trial, the EPIC study (Evaluation of c7E3 in Preventing Ischemic Complications).[28] After a bolus injection of

0.25 mg/kg of abciximab, 85–90% of GPIIb/IIIa receptor sites are blocked. Receptor blockade can be maintained by an infusion of 10 μg/min for up to 12 hours. Receptor blockade can be detected as long as 2 weeks after a bolus injection of abciximab, but profound inhibition (greater than 80% inhibition of platelet aggregation) persists for only 6–12 hours after termination of the infusion.[28] The EPIC trial evaluated 2099 patients at high risk for complications following PTCA or directional atherectomy. Patients were enrolled and randomly assigned to one of three treatment groups: (1) placebo; (2) a bolus injection of c7E3 (0.25 mg/kg); or (3) an identical bolus followed by a 12-hour infusion (10 μg/min). All patients were given aspirin plus 10 000–12 000 units of heparin before intervention. An infusion of heparin was continued following the angioplasty procedure.[28] The most important findings of the EPIC clinical trial were the 35% marked reduction ($P = 0.008$) at 30 days in the frequency of the composite clinical endpoint (12.8% placebo versus 8.3% abciximab bolus and 12-hour infusion). This endpoint included: death, nonfatal MI, repeat revascularization (e.g. PTCA or CABG), and procedural failure requiring stent or intra-aortic balloon pump placement. Second, the frequency of major bleeding complications in the bolus plus infusion group was double that of the placebo group (14% versus 7%, $P = 0.001$).[28]

Several conclusions were drawn from the EPIC trial. The clinical trial validated the GPIIb/IIIa hypothesis that blockade of this platelet integrin during angioplasty significantly improved both short-term and long-term outcomes in patients at high risk for ischemic complications. In addition, the EPIC trial concluded that brief GPIIb/IIIa blockade (with the single bolus injection regimen) appeared to be ineffective, whereas a bolus plus a 12-hour infusion of abciximab is required for clinical efficacy.

The EPILOG trial (Evaluation of PTCA to Improve Long-Term Outcome by c7E3 GPIIb/IIIa Receptor Blockade) included 2792 patients and was designed to assess long-term outcome of treatment with abciximab and lower-dose heparin during PTCA. The intent of the study was to evaluate the efficacy and safety of abciximab in patients at all levels of risk undergoing PTCA. The trial was terminated at the first interim analysis because of positive results. There was a 56% reduction in the composite endpoint at 30 days (death, MI, or urgent revascularization) in the abciximab plus low-dose heparin compared with placebo plus standard-dose heparin (5.2 versus 11.7%, $P = 0.001$). The rates of major bleeding were equivalent in all groups, although minor bleeding was greatest in the abciximab plus standard-dose heparin group.[29]

Data from the CAPTURE trial (c7E3 Fab Antiplatelet Therapy in Unstable Refractory Angina) supported the use of abciximab in patients with refractory unstable angina who were candidates for PTCA within 24 hours. Patients already on aspirin and unfractionated heparin therapy were randomized to receive either additional placebo or abciximab for 18–24 hours before and 1 hour after the PTCA procedure: 1265 patients were enrolled and followed for 6 months. The primary endpoint of the study was a composite of death, MI, or urgent intervention within the first 30 days. There was a 29% reduction in the primary endpoint in the abciximab-treated group compared with placebo (11.3 versus 15.9%, $P = 0.012$). Major bleeding rates were more common in the abciximab group than the control group (3.8 versus 1.9%, $P = 0.043$), and there was also a higher rate of thrombocytopenia (5.6 versus 1.3%).[30]

Eptifibatide

The IMPACT II trial (Integrilin to Minimize Platelet Aggregation and Prevent Coronary Thrombosis II), investigated eptifibatide (Integrilin) in the setting of coronary intervention. This was a multicenter clinical study that enrolled 4010 patients from all risk criteria undergoing any interventional procedure. Eptifibatide is a synthetic cyclic heptapeptide with a short half-life (1.5–2.0 hours) and a high affinity and specifity for the GPIIb/IIIa receptor due to a lysine-glycine-aspartate (KGD) sequence. Patients were randomized to 24-hour treatment with placebo or one of two different doses of eptifibatide (0.50 or 0.75 g/kg per min for 20–24 hours following a 135 g/kg bolus injection) and followed for 30 days and 6 months to assess their effectiveness and safety.[31]

At the end of the 24-hour period, there was a relative reduction in the composite endpoint (death, MI, CABG surgery, repeat or urgent coronary intervention, or stent placement), with both eptifibatide strategies compared with placebo. On an intent-to-treat basis, the reduction in composite endpoint was 19% (9.2 versus 11.4%, $P = 0.06$) for low-dose eptifibatide versus placebo, and 13% (9.9 versus 11.4%, $P = 0.22$) for the high-dose eptifibatide group. Rates of major bleeding were similar in all treatment groups.[31] Conclusions drawn from both the EPIC and the IMPACT II trials confirm that short-term outcome appears to be defined by a critical period of platelet inhibition (i.e. the first 6 hours) when the majority of clinical events occur.[27]

The PURSUIT trial (Platelet Glycoprotein IIb/IIIa in Unstable Angina: Receptor Suppression Using Integrilin Therapy) trial assessed the efficacy of eptifibatide as primary management of acute coronary syndromes.[32] A total of 10 948 patients with rest unstable angina or non-Q wave myocardial infarction were randomized to receive either placebo or eptifibatide along with heparin and aspirin. At 30 days, patients receiving eptifibatide experienced a 1.5% absolute reduction in death and MI compared with placebo (14.2 versus 15.7%, $P = 0.04$). This 10% relative reduction in the endpoint was reached by 4 days and maintained for 30 days. Patients receiving eptifibatide experienced a higher rate of major bleeding compared with those patients in the placebo group (10.6 versus 9.1%) and they also required more blood transfusions (11.6 versus 9.2%).[32]

Tirofiban

The RESTORE trial (Randomized Efficacy Study of Tirofiban for Outcomes and Restenosis), was a multicenter, double-blind, randomized, study that evaluated the GPIIb/IIIa receptor antagonist, tirofiban (Aggrastat: Merck, West Pt, PA), during coronary intervention. The purpose of the RESTORE trial was to determine whether tirofiban, a nonpeptide tyrosine derivative, would improve clinical outcomes following PTCA. Study patients included those who were at increased risk for abrupt arterial closure because of unstable angina, recent MI, or direct angioplasty during an acute MI. Drug infusion in this study was extended to 36 hours postprocedure. A total of 2139 patients were randomized to either placebo or tirofiban (10 µg/kg bolus followed by

0.15 g/kg per min infusion for 36 hours). At day 2 postPTCA there was a statistically significant relative reduction (38%, $P = 0.005$) in the composite endpoint (8.7% placebo versus 5.4% tirofiban). The relative reduction at 7 days postPTCA was 27% ($P = 0.022$) in the composite endpoint (10.4% placebo versus 7.6% tirofiban); however, at 30 days, the relative reduction was 16% ($P = 0.16$). Nevertheless, effects were consistent across all components of the composite endpoint, including all subgroups of patients treated.[33]

While the EPIC trial, which assessed the use of abciximab, an anti-GPIIb/IIIa antibody, demonstrated a greater late (30-day) reduction in adverse cardiovascular events following PTCA, it is important to note that the endpoint definitions differ between the EPIC and the RESTORE trials. When a common definition of endpoints is used (i.e. CABG or PTCA for urgent/emergency indications only), the difference in outcomes between the two studies narrows: the RESTORE trial showed a relative risk reduction of 24% with tirofiban (8.0% tirofiban versus 10.5% placebo).[33] Thus, the risk reduction in the composite endpoints of death, MI, or urgent revascularization, in particular, is more significant in the tirofiban group.

The PRISM (Platelet Receptor Inhibition in Ischemic Syndrome Management)[34] and PRISM-PLUS (Platelet Receptor Inhibition in Ischemic Syndrome Management in Patients Limited by Unstable Signs and Symptoms)[35] trials examined tirofiban in patients with unstable angina. PRISM enrolled all types of unstable angina patients whereas PRISM-PLUS only enrolled patients with unstable angina who were at high risk for subsequent events. PRISM was a multicenter, double-blind study in which 3232 patients receiving aspirin were randomized to receive either tirofiban (0.6 g/kg per min for 30 minutes, followed by 0.15 g/kg per min) or heparin (5000-unit intravenous bolus followed by 1000 units/hour) for 48 hours. Treatment with tirofiban resulted in a 32% risk reduction in the composite endpoint (death, MI or refractory ischemia) at 48 hours (3.8% for tirofiban versus 5.6% for heparin, $P = 0.015$). At 30 days, the frequency of the composite endpoint was similar for both groups. However, tirofiban treatment significantly reduced the frequency of death by 39% (2.3% for tirofiban versus 3.6% for heparin, $P = 0.02$).[34]

PRISM-PLUS was a multicenter, double-blind study in which 1915 patients receiving aspirin were randomized to tirofiban plus heparin or heparin alone. Treatment with tirofiban plus heparin reduced the composite endpoint by 32% at 7 days (12.9% tirofiban plus heparin versus 17.9% heparin, $P = 0.004$). This benefit was still significant at 30 days (23% risk reduction, $P = 0.029$) and at 6 months (19% risk reduction,

$P = 0.024$).[35] In both PRISM and PRISM-PLUS, there was no excess in major bleeding compared to the control treatment groups.[34,35]

In a third treatment arm in PRISM-PLUS, patients receiving tirofiban as monotherapy were dropped as recommended by the data and safety monitoring committee because of a higher death rate. At day 7, death occurred in 4.6% of patients who received only tirofiban as compared with 1.1% in the heparin-only group. Notably, there were no adverse effects for the other endpoints (refractory ischemia and MI). Approximately 70% of patients had been receiving heparin therapy at the time of randomization and heparin rebound may have been responsible for the increase in ischemic events observed in the tirofiban monotherapy arm.[35] Subsequent analysis of the characteristics of patients in the terminated arm revealed that the incidence of ST-segment depression at time of randomization was more prevalent compared with those in the PRISM study where the tirofiban monotherapy arm was associated with a beneficial effect: 58.5% compared with 31.5%.[34] *Table 10.3* summarizes many of the clinical trials involving GPIIb/IIIa receptor blockers.[36]

Implications regarding GPIIB/IIIA blockers

Recent advances in the understanding of the role of platelet adhesion molecules in arterial thrombosis has produced a new pharmacologic era in interventional cardiology. The clinical effectiveness of the GPIIb/IIIa receptor blockers has been established and documented in numerous important studies with clinical benefits demonstrated in virtually all patient categories.[28–35] These platelet receptor blockers are effective in the short-term management of patients at very high risk for thrombotic coronary artery occlusion, such as patients undergoing thrombolysis for acute MI or during coronary intervention (e.g. PTCA).[3] They are also effective in patients with unstable angina and non Q wave myocardial infarction, in combination with aspirin and heparin. In addition, recent meta-analyses suggest that the benefit of platelet IIb/IIIa receptor blockers probably extends to 6 months.[37] As the benefits of low molecular weight heparin over unfractionated heparin are now being analysed in clinical trials,[38] it may be in the near future that GPIIb/IIIa inhibitors are used in combination with aspirin and low molecular weight heparin for the treatment of unstable angina and non-Q wave myocardial infarction.

Table 10.3
GPIIb/IIIa receptor inhibitors in clinical trials partial listing[36]

Agent	Category	Route	Receptor specificity	Use in angioplasty stent	Use in unstable angina	Use in MI
Tirofiban	Peptidomimetic	IV	GPIIb/IIIa	RESTORE*	PRISM* PRISM-PLUS*	
Abciximab	Chimeric mAb	IV	GPIIb/IIIa $\alpha_v\beta_3$	EPIC*EPILOG*R APPORT CAPTURE* ERASER		TAMI TIMI 14 SPEED
Eptifibatide	Cyclic peptide	IV	GPIIb/IIIa	IMPACT II* ESPRIT	PURSUIT*	IMPACT AMI*
Lamifiban	Peptidomimetic	IV	GPIIb/IIIa		PARAGON*	PARADIGM* PARAGON*
Xemilofiban	Peptidomimetic	Oral	GPIIb/IIIa	ORBIT	ORBIT	NA
Fradafiban	Peptidomimetic	IV	GPIIb/IIIa	NA	Phase II	NA

NA = Clinical trial status not available; mAb = monoclonal antibody; UA = unstable angina.
*Clinical trial completed.

References

1. Schafer AI. Pathophysiology of thrombosis. In: Loscalzo J et al. (eds). *Vascular Medicine: A Textbook of Vascular Biology and Disease.* Boston: Little Brown, 1992: 307–333.

2. Rubanyi GM. Endothelium-derived vasoactive factors in health and disease. In: Rubanyi GM (ed). *Cardiovascular Significance of Endothelium-Derived Vasoactive Factors.* Mount Kisco, NY: Futura Publishing, 1991: xi–xix.

3. Stein B, Fuster V. Pharmacology of anticoagulants and platelet inhibitor drugs. In: Schlant RC, Alexander RW (eds). *Hurst's The Heart.* Vol I, 8th edn. New York: McGraw-Hill, 1994: 1309–1326.

4. Campbell RWF, Wallentin L, Verheught FWA et al. Management strategies for a better outcome in unstable coronary artery disease. *Clin Cardiol* 1998; **21:** 314–322.

5. Fuster V, Jang I. Role of platelet-inhibitor agents in coronary disease. In: Topol EJ (ed). *Textbook of Interventional Cardiology.* Vol I, 2nd edn. Philadelphia: WB Saunders, 1994: 3–22.

6. Becker RC. Antiplatelet therapy. *Sci Med* 1996; **July/August:** 12–21.

7. Antiplatelet Trialist Collaboration. Collaborative overview of randomized trials on antiplatelet therapy: I. Prevention of death, myocardial infarction and stroke by antiplatelet therapy in various categories of patients. *BMJ* 1994; **308:** 81–106.

8. Schrör K. Antiplatelet drugs: a comparative review. *Drugs* 1995; **50:** 7–28.

9. Majerus PW, Broze GJ, Miletich JP, Tollefsen DM. Anticoagulant, thrombolytic, and antiplatelet drugs. In: Hardman JG et al (eds). *Goodman & Gilman's The Pharmacological Basis of Therapeutics.* 9th edn. New York: McGraw-Hill, 1996: 1341–1359.

10. ISIS-2 (Second International Study of Infarct Survival) Collaborative Group: Randomized trial of intravenous streptokinase, oral aspirin, both or neither among 17 187 cases of suspected acute myocardial infarction: ISIS-2. *Lancet* 1988; **ii:** 349–360.

11. Cairns JA, Gent M, Singer J et al. Aspirin, sulfinpyrazone, or both in unstable angina. *N Engl J Med* 1985; **313:** 1369–1375.

12. Lewis HD, Davis JW, Archibald DG et al. Protective effects of aspirin against acute myocardial infarction and death in men with unstable angina. Results of a Veterans Administration Cooperative Study. *N Engl J Med* 1983; **309:** 396–403.

13. Théroux P, Ouimer H, McCans J et al. Aspirin, heparin or both to treat acute unstable angina. *N Engl J Med* 1988; **319:** 1105–1111.

14. Hess H, Mietaschk A, Deichsel G. Drug-induced inhibition of platelet function delays progression of peripheral occlusive arterial disease: a prospective double-blind arteriographically controlled trial. *Lancet* 1985; **i:** 415–421.

15. Sanz G, Pajoron A, Alegria E et al and The Groupo Espanol para el Seguimineto del Injerto Coronario (GESIC). Prevention of early aortocoronary bypass occlusion by low-dose aspirin and dipyridamole. *Circulation* 1990; **82:** 765–773.

16. Lee H, Paton RC, Roan C. The in vitro effect of ticlopidine on fibrinogen and factor VIII binding to human platelets (abstr.) *Thromb Haemost* 1981; **46:** 67.

17. Harker LA, Fuster V. Pharmacology of platelet inhibitors. *J Am Coll Cardiol* 1986; **8**(Suppl 1B): 21B–32B.

18. O'Brien JR. Ticlopidine, a promise for the prevention and treatment of thrombosis and its complications. *Haemostasis* 1983; **13:** 1–54.

19. Balsano F, Rizzon P, Violi F et al. Antiplatelet treatment with ticlopidine in unstable angina: a controlled multicenter trial. *Circulation* 1990; **82:** 17–26.

20. Limet R, David JL, Magotteaux P et al. Prevention of aorta-coronary bypass graft occlusion. *J Thorac Cardiovasc Surg* 1987; **94:** 773–783.

21. Schomig A, Neumann FJ, Kastrati A et al. A randomized comparison of antiplatelet and anticoagulant therapy after the placement of coronary stents. *N Engl J Med* 1996; **335:** 1084–1089.

22. Leon MB, Baim DS, Popma JJ et al. A clinical trial comparing three antithrombotic-drug regimens after coronary stenting. N Engl J Med 1998; **339:** 1665–1671.

23. Steinhubl SR, Tan WA, Foody JM, Topol EJ for the EPISTENT Investigators. Incidence and clinical course of thrombotic thrombocytopenic purpura due to ticlopidine following coronary stenting. *JAMA* 1999; **281:** 806–810.

24. CAPRIE Steering Committee. A randomized, blinded trial of clopidogrel versus aspirin in patients at risk of ischemic events (CAPRIE). *Lancet* 1996; **348:** 1329–1339.

25. The CLASSICS Trial results. Presented by M Bertrand at the 48th Annual Scientific Sessions of the American College of Cardiology, 1999, New Orleans.

26. Lefkovits J, Plow EF, Topol EJ. Platelet glycoprotein IIb/IIIa receptors in cardiovascular medicine. *N Engl J Med* 1995; **332:** 1553–1559.

27. Tcheng JE. Glycoprotein IIb/IIIa receptor inhibitors: putting the EPIC, IMPACT II, RESTORE, and EPILOG trials into perspective. *Am J Cardiol* 1996; **78:** 35–40.

28. EPIC Investigators. Use of monoclonal antibody directed against the platelet glycoprotein IIb/IIIa receptor in high-risk coronary angioplasty. *N Engl J Med* 1994; **330:** 956–961.

29. The EPILOG Investigators. Platelet glycoprotein IIb/IIIa receptor blockade and low-dose heparin during percutaneous coronary revascularization. *N Engl J Med* 1997; **336:** 1689–1696.

30. The CAPTURE Investigators. Randomized placebo-controlled trial of abciximab before and during coronary intervention in refractory unstable angina: the CAPTURE study. *Lancet* 1997; **349:** 1429–1435.

31. The IMPACT-II Investigators. Randomized placebo-controlled trial of effect of eptifibatide on complications of percutaneous coronary intervention: IMPACT-II. *Lancet* 1997; **349:** 1422–1428.

32. The PURSUIT Trial Investigators. Inhibition of platelet glycoprotein IIb/IIIa with eptifibatide in patients with acute coronary syndromes. *N Engl J Med* 1998; **339:** 436–443.

33. The RESTORE Investigators. Effects of platelet glycoprotein IIb/IIIa blockade with tirofiban on adverse cardiac events in patients with unstable angina or acute myocardial infarction undergoing coronary angioplasty. *Circulation* 1997; **96:** 1445–1453.

34. PRISM Study Investigators. A comparison of aspirin plus tirofiban with aspirin plus heparin for unstable angina. *N Engl J Med* 1998; **338:** 1498–1505.

35. PRISM-PLUS Investigators. Inhibition of the

platelet glycoprotein IIb/IIIa receptor with tirofiban in unstable angina and non Q-wave myocardial infarction. *N Engl J Med* 1998; **338**: 1488–1497.

36. Coller BS, Anderson KM, Weisman HF. The anti-GPIIb-IIIa agents: fundamental and clinical aspects. *Haemostasis* 1996; **26** (Suppl 4): 285–293.

37. Kong DF, Califf RM, Miller DP et al. Clinical outcomes of therapeutic agents that block the platelet glycoprotein IIb/IIIa integrin in ischemic heart disease. *Circulation* 1998; **98**: 2829–2835.

38. Cohen M, Demers C, Gurfinkel EP et al. A comparison of low-molecular weight heparin with unfractionated heparin for unstable coronary artery disease. Efficacy and safety of subcutaneous enoxaparin non-Q-wave coronary events study group. *N Engl J Med* 1997; **337**: 447–452.

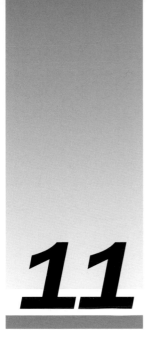

The role of antithrombotic agents in ischemic heart disease: anticoagulants

Marc Cohen

Atherosclerotic plaque erosion or disruption within the coronary arteries results in activation of the coagulation cascade and thrombin generation, as well as platelet adhesion and aggregation. The coagulation cascade is triggered by the exposure of tissue factor to circulating factor VII. The subsequent thrombus formation is the central event in the pathogenesis of the acute coronary syndromes including unstable angina and non-Q wave myocardial infarction.[1,2] Historically, inhibition of thrombin generation and activity using continuous intravenous unfractionated heparin, and oral aspirin were felt to be better than placebo in reducing recurrent ischemic events.[3-7] However, unfractionated heparin has several significant drawbacks that may limit its effectiveness.[8-10] Significant progress has been made in the field of antithrombotic therapy for patients with acute coronary syndromes, especially with direct antithrombins and the low molecular weight heparins.

Unfractionated heparin

Heparin sulfate on the surface of vascular endothelial cells or in the subendothelial extracellular matrix interacts with circulating antithrombin and provides a natural antithrombotic mechanism. The anticoagulant effect of heparin is mediated by an endogenous component of plasma (i.e. heparin cofactor or antithrombin). Antithrombin is a glycolysated polypeptide that rapidly inhibits thrombin only in the presence of heparin.[11,12] Antithrombin is homologous to the serine protease inhibitors (serpins), and is synthesized in the liver. Heparin accelerates the formation of a molecular complex between antithrombin and several serine proteases. These proteases include thrombin, coagulation factors (i.e. IXa, Xa, XIa, XII), kallikrein, and plasmin. Heparin also binds to lysine sites on antithrombin and produces a structural change in the molecule at the arginine reactive center, thus accelerating inhibitory activity on coagulation factors by 1000-fold.[13] Heparin functions by inhibiting factor Xa in the coagulation cascade. There is also evidence that the anticoagulant effect of heparin may be mediated through the inhibition of factor IXa and by promoting the release of tissue factor pathway inhibitor protein from endothelial cells.[14]

Clinical testing has established the value of heparin in the treatment of patients with acute coronary syndromes. In a meta-analysis of 20 trials, it was suggested that heparin monotherapy reduces mortality and reinfarction by about 20%.[15] Another recent study demonstrated that subcutaneous heparin at a dosage of 12 500 U twice daily reduced mortality in patients with acute infarction, whether or not a thrombolytic agent was used concurrently.[16] Because patients with myocardial infarction (MI) were at high risk for reocclusion, particularly in the first few days after thrombolysis, antithrombotic therapy with both intravenous heparin and oral aspirin seemed justified.[17] In addition, other studies have demonstrated a substantial benefit from the administration of intravenous heparin plus low-dose aspirin in patients with unstable angina or non-Q wave myocardial infarction.[3–7] Intravenous heparin, in combination with aspirin was associated with lower rates of subsequent MI and recurrent ischemia in these patients.

In spite of widespread use, unfractionated heparin has several significant drawbacks that limit its effectiveness.[8–10] It exhibits significant nonspecific binding to many circulating proteins and cells, leaving very little heparin to bind to antithrombin.[14] Young et al,[9] reported results of an animal study that shed light on why it was so difficult to maintain therapeutic antithrombotic levels with unfractionated heparin in patients with significant inflammatory processes like acute non-Q wave myocardial infarction, or malignancy. The investigators gave animals endotoxin or turpentine to induce an acute phase reaction. At different time intervals blood was withdrawn and anti-Xa activity was measured to assess antithrombotic activity, after unfractionated heparin was administered. After 24 hours, a large amount of acute phase reactant proteins in their circulation that bound the heparin was released. This resulted in hardly any detectable anti-Xa levels in the blood. These findings clearly illustrated the biologic and clinical impact of the strong nonspecific protein binding of unfractionated heparin. Patients, in whom the level of acute phase reactant proteins varies, will therefore exhibit varying levels of antithrombotic activity after administration of unfractionated heparin.

These two issues among others prompted the search for other agents more effective and reliable than conventional unfractionated heparin. For example, low molecular weight heparins were found to exhibit much less nonspecific protein binding, and therefore have much more predictable antithrombotic activity.[18,19] A second important distinction between low molecular weight heparin and unfractionated heparin is the significantly lower incidence of heparin-induced thrombocytopenia seen after administration of low molecular weight heparin.[10] In addition, the direct antithrombins like hirudin were developed and evaluated in the acute coronary syndromes.

Direct thrombin inhibitors

Thrombin plays a key role in coagulation. In addition, and critically important in the acute coronary syndromes, thrombin is a most potent trigger of platelet aggregation. Several selective thrombin inhibitors have been studied for their antiplatelet and antithrombotic activity and potential clinical use.

Hirudin is a specific and direct thrombin inhibitor that was isolated from the salivary glands of the medicinal leech, *Hirudo medicinalis*.[20,21] Recently, it has been mass produced via recombinant DNA technology.[22] Hirudin acts by stoichiometrically coupling with molecules of thrombin and powerfully inhibiting thrombin activity (not formation). This prevents the activation of clotting factors II, V, VIII, and XIII, and also prevents thrombin-mediated platelet activation.[23] More recent experimental work in an animal model has demonstrated the beneficial effect of long-acting PEG (polyethylene glycol)-hirudin in preventing thrombin-mediated platelet activation.[24]

A pilot trial of hirudin found angiographic improvement in patients with unstable angina and as evidenced by a reduction in coronary lesions. In this trial, a trend towards a lower incidence of MI was observed in these patients compared with heparin.[25] Hirudin was compared with intravenous heparin in several additional studies to further evaluate its antithrombotic efficacy in the treatment of acute coronary syndromes. In the international GUSTO (Global Use of Strategies to Open Occluded Coronary

Arteries) IIa trial, there was little difference in outcomes (death or nonfatal MI) between hirudin (11.7%) and heparin (11.0%), although hirudin was associated with a higher risk of hemorrhagic stroke compared with heparin (1.3 versus 0.7%, $P = 0.11$).[26] This is believed to be due to the higher target activated partial thromboplastin time (APTT) and therefore higher doses of hirudin and heparin. Subsequently, the GUSTO IIb trial,[27] adjusted the dose of heparin and hirudin downward to the same levels as used in GUSTO I, and a reduction in the incidence of hemorrhagic stroke (0.3% hirudin versus 0.2% heparin, $P = 0.24$) was observed. In GUSTO IIb, there was an 11% risk reduction in the primary endpoint of death or nonfatal MI reported with hirudin compared with heparin (8.9% hirudin versus 9.8% heparin, $P = 0.06$).[27] Although rates of severe bleeding were comparable in both groups, hirudin therapy was associated with a higher incidence of moderate bleeding (8.8 versus 7.7%, $P = 0.03$).[27]

The recently completely OASIS-2 study,[28] was a study of over 10 141 patients with unstable angina. At 3 days, a significant difference favoring hirudin and aspirin over unfractionated heparin was observed. However, by day 7 and at 30 days posttreatment, the difference in the rate of death or MI between the groups attenuated and was no longer statistically significant. The GUSTO IIb and the OASIS studies, suggest

that direct antithrombins have a beneficial effect in the early phase (while the hirudin is actually being infused). Unfortunately there is no sustained significant beneficial effect. Why does the effect fade? The direct antithrombins are solely involved in neutralizing thrombin. In contrast, low molecular weight heparins have multiple effects including antithrombin (IIa), antiactivated factor X (Xa), and they antagonize tissue factor by triggering the release of tissue factor pathway inhibitor from the endothelial cells.[29,30]

Small molecule, direct thrombin inhibitors, have also been evaluated. Argatroban has been shown to maintain vessel patency in animal models by preventing occlusive platelet-rich thrombosis. Vessel patency was maintained with the drug even when its effect had disappeared from the circulation, suggesting an alteration in the thrombogenicity of the endothelial surface even after 1 hour postinfusion.[31] Hirulog (bivalirudin), was used instead of heparin in order to assess the risk of ischemic or hemorrhagic complications in patients undergoing coronary angioplasty. The study concluded that bivalirudin was at least as effective as high-dose heparin in preventing ischemic complications in patients who underwent angioplasty for unstable angina, and was associated with a lower risk of bleeding.[32]

A larger clinical trial, TIMI 7 (Thrombin Inhibition in Myocardial Ischemia), evaluated hirulog used in conjunction with aspirin in patients with unstable angina. At higher doses, hirulog not only prevented the final outcome measurement (death or MI after 6 weeks), but achieved this with minimal hemorrhagic episodes. Only 3% of patients receiving the highest doses of hirulog experienced death or MI versus 13% in the low-dose group ($P < 0.06$). Hemorrhagic events occurred in 0.5% of patients.[33] Results from TIMI 7 and other studies such as Hirulog Early Reperfusion/Occlusion (HERO),[34] provide strong evidence for the improved clinical efficacy of hirulog over heparin particularly in patients with previous MI. Furthermore, in contrast to hirudin, hirulog is associated with significantly reduced major bleeding events suggesting that direct thrombin inhibition with hirulog may be a good alternative to heparin to improve clinical outcome in acute coronary syndromes.

Low molecular weight heparins

The last decade has seen the introduction of low molecular weight heparin into clinical practice.[19,35] Standard unfractionated heparin is a heterogeneous mixture of sulfated polysaccharides with an average molecular weight of 12–15 kDa and range of 5–30 kDa. Low molecular weight heparin is composed of molecules averaging 4–6.5 kDa, depending on the preparation.[8,18,36] Importantly, heparin

molecules less than 5.4 kDa lack the ability to bind thrombin and antithrombin simultaneously. Therefore, its predominant effect is the inactivation of factor Xa rather than IIa. As such, the anti-Xa to antithrombin ratio of low molecular weight heparin ranges from 1.5 to 3.9 depending on the preparation.[36] Low molecular weight heparin has several clear advantages over standard heparin. First, its effective half-life is approximately 4–6 hours which allows 12-hourly dosing. Because it does not bind to plasma proteins such as platelet factor 4 and von Willebrand factor, it cannot be neutralized and its anticoagulant response is much less erratic than that of heparin and therefore, laboratory monitoring is not required. Furthermore, low molecular weight heparin remains active in a platelet-rich environment as it can bind platelet-bound factor Xa. Unlike heparin, it does not increase vascular permeability and inhibit platelet function.[36] Finally, heparin-induced thrombocytopenia occurs much less frequently with low molecular weight heparin.[10] These properties make the low molecular weight heparins a very appealing group with which to treat the acute coronary syndromes of unstable angina or non-Q wave myocardial infarction.[8,18,19] However, not all low molecular weight heparins are the same.[29,30,37] They differ not just in their molecular weights, but also in their rate of plasma clearance and spectrum of antifactor Xa and antithrombin activity. For example, dalteparin has a lower ratio of antifactor Xa to antithrombin activity (2:1) than enoxaparin (3:1).[29,36]

Several low molecular weight heparins have been evaluated for use in unstable coronary artery disease in several large clinical trials. Historically, the first published trial of low molecular weight heparin in patients with unstable angina, was reported by Gurfinkel et al in 1995.[38] He compared nadroparin (Fraxiparin, Sanofi, France) and aspirin therapy to unfractionated heparin and aspirin, versus aspirin alone in unstable angina. A total of 219 patients with unstable angina or non-Q wave myocardial infarction were randomized to aspirin alone, aspirin plus APTT-adjusted heparin, and aspirin plus low molecular weight heparin nadroparin (214 UIC/kg anti-Xa) twice daily subcutaneously for 5–7 days after presentation. The combination of aspirin plus low molecular weight heparin was superior to the aspirin-only group with respect to recurrent angina ($P = 0.03$), nonfatal MI ($P = 0.01$), and urgent revascularization ($P = 0.01$). This combination was also superior to aspirin and unfractionated heparin with respect to recurrent angina ($P = 0.002$) and myocardial ischemia ($P = 0.04$). Additionally, patients receiving low molecular weight heparin were less likely to suffer hemorrhagic complications than those receiving intravenous heparin ($P = 0.01$).[38]

A more recent, much larger scale, blinded,

clinical trial of the low molecular weight heparin nadroparin, the FRAXIS study, was recently completed and presented.[39] The FRAXIS study group evaluated a cohort of about 3500 patients. Patients were randomized to receive aspirin and unfractionated heparin, versus aspirin and either short-term nadroparin (6 days), or longer-term nadroparin (14 days). Nadroparin was found to be equivalent to unfractionated heparin at 14 days and at 3 months with regard to the incidence of the triple composite endpoint of death, myocardial infarction or refractory angina.[39]

The FRISC (Fragmin During Instability in Coronary Artery Disease) study[40] examined the efficacy of low molecular weight heparin dalteparin in 1506 patients with unstable angina/non-Q wave myocardial infarction. It was a double-blinded, randomized, parallel group, multicenter trial comparing aspirin alone (75 mg daily) with aspirin plus dalteparin (120 IU/kg twice daily) for 5–7 days, followed by dalteparin (7500 IU subcutaneously daily) for the next 35–45 days. The primary endpoint of death and new MI was decreased by 48% (an absolute decrease of 3%) in the first 6 days by dalteparin. The rates of urgent revascularization also decreased significantly. At 40 days, the benefit of low molecular weight heparin persisted but subgroup analysis showed that the benefit only extended to nonsmokers. In addition, there was evidence of a rebound in ischemic events when the dose was lowered from twice to once daily.[40] Overall, the FRISC study suggested that the combination of aspirin plus low molecular weight heparin was better than aspirin alone.

The FRIC study (Fragmin in Unstable Coronary Artery Disease[41] compared aspirin plus low molecular weight heparin dalteparin to aspirin plus APTT-adjusted intravenous heparin. A total of 1482 patients with unstable angina/non-Q wave myocardial infarction were assigned randomly in an open label fashion to receive either twice daily subcutaneous dalteparin (120 IU/kg) or APTT-adjusted intravenous heparin, in addition to aspirin. In the second phase, patients in both groups were randomized to receive one daily injection of dalteparin (7500 IU) or placebo in a double-blinded fashion. The composite endpoint rate of death, MI, or recurrent angina was similar in the two treatment arms, 9.3% in the dalteparin group, and 7.6% in the standard unfractionated heparin group. The combined endpoint of death and MI for the two groups was 3.9 versus 3.6%, respectively. In the prolonged treatment phase, there was no difference in composite endpoint of death, MI, or recurrent angina (12.3% in both groups). These data suggest that dalteparin is roughly equivalent in its clinical antithrombotic effects compared to standard heparin in patients with unstable angina/non-Q wave myocardial infarction.[41]

The ESSENCE trial (Efficacy and Safety of Subcutaneous Enoxaparin in Non-Q-Wave Coronary Events),[42] studied 3171 patients with rest unstable angina or non-Q wave myocardial infarction. Patients were randomly assigned to subcutaneous enoxaparin (1 mg/kg) twice daily, or continuous APTT adjusted intravenous standard heparin for 2–8 days in a double-blinded, placebo-controlled fashion. After 14 days of therapy the risk of death, MI, or recurrent angina was significantly lower in patients assigned to enoxaparin compared to heparin (16.6 versus 19.8%, $P = 0.019$). This difference remained significant at 30 days (19.8 versus 23.3%, $P = 0.016$; see ***Figure 11.1***). The secondary endpoint of death or MI was reached at 14 days in 4.9% of the enoxaparin group versus 6.1% of the unfractionated heparin group ($P = 0.13$) and at 30 days by 6.2% of the enoxaparin group versus 7.7% of the unfractionated heparin group ($P = 0.08$). Furthermore, at 30 days the need for coronary revascularization with either percutaneous coronary angioplasty or coronary bypass surgery, was significantly lower in patients assigned to enoxaparin (27.1 versus 32.2%, $P = 0.001$). With regard to major hemorrhagic complications, there was no difference between the two groups.

Low molecular weight heparin enoxaparin appears to benefit different types of patients.[43] In a subanalysis of the ESSENCE study the point estimates of the odds ratios favored

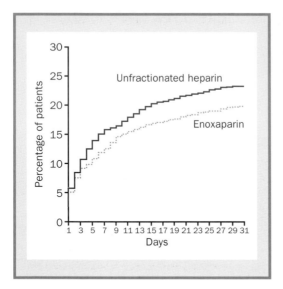

Figure 11.1
Kaplan-Meier plots of time to first event in the ESSENCE study. Reprinted with permission from Cohen MC, Demers C, Gurfinkel EP et al. N Engl J Med 1997; **337:** *447–452.*

enoxaparin over unfractionated heparin, irrespective of gender, age, diabetes, or prior aspirin use. Furthermore, patients with ST-segment depression or ECG changes in the emergency room who were considered 'high risk,' demonstrated the greatest benefit in the ESSENCE study from enoxaparin relative to unfractionated heparin. Specifically, patients with ST-segment depression, had a relative risk reduction in endpoints of almost 40% if treated with enoxaparin compared to standard unfractionated heparin. This provides strong evidence that a 'medical therapy' (enoxaparin and aspirin) can reduce recurrent ischemia in the highest risk patients. This reduction in recurrent ischemia and in revascularization procedures is the underpinning for the major savings in resource expenditures seen by giving low molecular weight heparin (enoxaparin).[44] Patients randomized to enoxaparin demonstrated a cost savings of about US $1000 per patient.[44] Another dramatic finding from the ESSENCE study derived from the analysis of recurrent ischemic events 1 year after treatment in 95% of the original 3171 patients.[45] At the end of 1 year, there remained a statistically significant reduction in recurrent ischemic events, and the number of diagnostic catheterizations and revascularizations also remained significantly lower in the patients randomized to enoxaparin.

The question arises why does one low molecular weight heparin show superiority over unfractionated heparin, while others show equivalence (see *Figure 11.2*)? There are several possible explanations. There are structural differences between each of the low molecular weight heparins.[18,36] It is also possible that the level of activity against factor Xa relative to IIa is an explanation for the very high level of anti-Xa activity that is achieved with low molecular weight heparin enoxaparin. At peak, about 2 hours after the subcutaneous injection of enoxaparin, the anti-Xa level is about 1 IU/ml.[46] At trough, 12 hours later the anti-Xa activity is down to 0.5–0.6 IU/ml. The increased anti-Xa activity is achieved without an increase in major hemorrhagic complications. So the efficacy is

there but without a sacrifice in safety.[47] It is also known that some low molecular weight heparins release more, and for a longer period of time, tissue factor pathway inhibitor (TFPI) from the endothelial cells compared to other low molecular weight heparins.[29,30] More recent analyses,[48] have suggested that enoxaparin may exert a 'passivating' effect on platelets in contrast to the slight platelet activation that occurs after administration of unfractionated heparin.[49] Montalescot et al,[48] showed that von Willebrand Factor levels in patients treated with enoxaparin stabilized 48 hours after admission, as opposed to increasing in the patients treated with unfractionated heparin.

The clinical benefit of enoxaparin has recently been corroborated by a second, large,

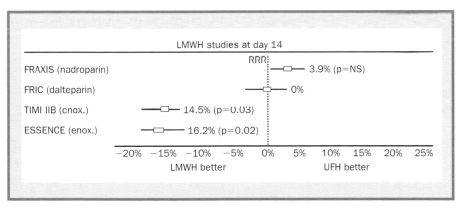

Figure 11.2
Odds ratio plots of the triple composite endpoints (death, MI, recurrent angina) for the four major low molecular weight heparin trials in unstable angina/non-Q wave myocardial infarction.

blinded three-phase clinical trial, the TIMI-11B study.[50] Patients with rest unstable angina or non-Q wave myocardial infarction ($N = 3910$) were randomly assigned to an intravenous enoxaparin bolus (30 mg), in addition to subcutaneous enoxaparin (1 mg/kg) 12 hourly, or continuous APTT-adjusted intravenous standard heparin for 2–8 days in a double-blinded, placebo-controlled fashion. After 14 days of therapy the risk of death, MI, or urgent revascularization was significantly lower in patients assigned to enoxaparin compared to heparin (15% relative risk reduction, $P = 0.04$). This difference remained significant at 43 days (12% relative risk reduction, $P = 0.049$). One of the key questions asked by the TIMI-11B study group was whether prolonging enoxaparin low molecular weight heparin therapy at home would offer additional improvement beyond that seen in the early phase. However, giving more low molecular weight heparin as an outpatient did not add any incremental benefit.[50]

A meta-analysis of the relatively similar ESSENCE and TIMI-11B databases was performed on the variables death or MI at different time points (8, 14, and 43 days). Combining 7000 patients showed that those who received aspirin and enoxaparin had a very significant reduction in death and MI (relative risk reductions of 23, 21, and 18%, respectively, $P = 0.02$).[51] This is quite dramatic relative to the loss of clinical benefit

seen over time with the direct antithrombins.[27,28] The most recent clinical trial of a low molecular weight heparin in patients with unstable angina is the FRISC II study.[52] This study had a 2×2 factorial design and looked at the role of long-term higher dose dalteparin therapy versus placebo and also an early invasive strategy versus conservative therapy in 2267 patients with unstable angina/non-Q wave myocardial infarction. Preliminary analyses suggest that at the end of 3 months there was no significant benefit of prolonged dalteparin therapy on the rate of death or MI. There did however, appear to be an advantage for the early invasive strategy over conservative therapy.[52]

Combination of anticoagulants and platelet inhibitors

There is no doubt that platelet IIb/IIIa receptor blockers have a major beneficial role not just in percutaneous coronary interventions but also as adjunctive treatment in unstable angina.[53] In general, the average point estimate of the odds ratios of relative risk for the platelet IIb/IIIa receptor blockers is about 20% in favor of these drugs over aspirin and heparin alone with placebo.[53] This degree of benefit varies depending on the IIb/IIIa receptor blocker but ironically the 20% risk reduction seen for death or MI is remarkably similar to that seen with enoxaparin based on the ESSENCE and

TIMI 11B meta-analysis,[51] (see *Figure 11.3*). In the future, appropriate studies need to be done that combine the best of the low molecular weight heparins with the best of the fibrinogen receptor antagonists or IIb/IIIa receptor blockers. Experimental work[54] showing the results in a cyclic flow reduction model of a crimped coronary artery has been done. The combination of enoxaparin and a platelet receptor blocker is dramatically superior to the combination of unfractionated heparin and the platelet receptor blocker. The best results in terms of preventing total occlusion are appreciated when low molecular weight heparin is combined with the fibrinogen receptor antagonist. When the IIb/IIIa receptor blocker, the low molecular weight heparin, or unfractionated heparin alone is administered, the number of episodes of cyclic flow reduction is reduced. However, when low molecular weight heparin and half the dose of the IIb/IIIa receptor blocker is administered together, there is a major reduction in the incidence of transient total occlusion.[54] Clinical pilot trials are now underway that evaluate combination therapy

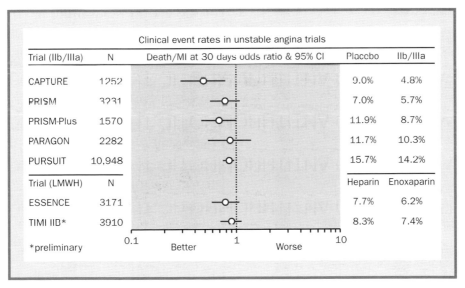

Clinical event rates in unstable angina trials					
Trial (IIb/IIIa)	N	Death/MI at 30 days odds ratio & 95% CI		Placebo	IIb/IIIa
CAPTURE	1252			9.0%	4.8%
PRISM	3231			7.0%	5.7%
PRISM-Plus	1570			11.9%	8.7%
PARAGON	2282			11.7%	10.3%
PURSUIT	10,948			15.7%	14.2%
Trial (LMWH)	N			Heparin	Enoxaparin
ESSENCE	3171			7.7%	6.2%
TIMI IIB*	3910			8.3%	7.4%
*preliminary		0.1 Better 1 Worse 10			

Figure 11.3
Odds ratio plots of the double composite endpoint (death, MI) for the two major low molecular weight heparin trials with enoxaparin, and the platelet fibrinogen receptor (IIb/IIIa) blockers in unstable angina/non-Q wave myocardial infarction.

with enoxaparin low molecular weight heparin and a platelet fibrinogen receptor blocker in patients with unstable angina.[55,56]

Thrombolytic agents

While thrombolytic therapy has demonstrated benefits for patients with acute MI, thrombolytic therapy is not recommended for patients who do not have ST-segment elevation. The TIMI IIIB trial[57] evaluated tissue plasminogen activator (t-PA) compared with placebo in patients with unstable angina or non-Q wave myocardial infarction. The incidence of death and/or MI was 54.2% in the tPA-treated patients and 55.5% in those patients treated with placebo ($P = $ NS). The lack of clinical benefit in patients with unstable angina and non-Q wave myocardial infarction, combined with a risk for intracranial hemorrhage, led to the contraindication for thrombolytic agents in patients without ST-segment elevation.

References

1. Fuster V, Badimon L, Cohen M et al. Insights into the pathogenesis of acute ischemic syndromes. *Circulation* 1988; 77: 1213–1220.

2. Davies M. The contribution of thrombosis to the clinical expression of coronary atherosclerosis. *Thromb Res* 1996; 82: 1–32.

3. Theroux P, Ouimet H, McCans J et al. Aspirin, heparin, or both to treat acute unstable angina. *N Engl J Med* 1988; 319: 1105–1111.

4. Wallentin L for the RISC Group. Risk of myocardial infarction and death during treatment with low dose aspirin and intravenous heparin in men with unstable coronary artery disease. *Lancet* 1990; 336: 827–830.

5. Cohen M, Adams PC, Parry G et al. Combination antithrombotic therapy in unstable rest angina and non-Q-wave infarction in nonprior aspirin users: primary end points analysis from the ATACS trial. *Circulation* 1994; 89: 81–88.

6. Oler A, Whooley MA, Oler J, Grady D. Adding heparin to aspirin reduces the incidence of myocardial infarction and death in patients with unstable angina: a meta-analysis. *JAMA* 1996; 276: 811–815.

7. Braunwald E, Mark DB, Jones RH et al. Unstable angina: diagnosis and management. *Clinical practice guideline number 10 AHCPR Publication No. 94–0602.* Washington DC : Agency for health care policy and research, US Department of Health and Human Services, March 1994.

8. Hirsh J, Warkentin TE, Raschke R et al. Heparin and low-molecular-weight heparin: mechanisms of action, pharmacokinetics, dosing considerations, monitoring, efficacy, and safety. *Chest* 1998; 114(Suppl): 489S–510S.

9. Young E, Podor TJ, Vemer T, Hirsch J. Induction of the acute-phase reaction increases heparin-binding proteins in plasma. *Arterioscl Thromb Vasc Biol* 1997; 17: 1568–1574.

10. Warkentin TE, Levine MN, Hirsh J. et al. Heparin-induced thrombocytopenia in patients treated with low-molecular-weight

heparin or unfractionated heparin. *N Engl J Med* 1995; **332**: 1330–1335.

11. Olson St, Björk I. Regulation of thrombin by antithrombin and heparin cofactor II. In: Berliner LJ (ed). *Thrombin: Structure and Function.* New York: Plenum Press, 1992: 159–217.

12. Majerus PW, Broze GJ, Miletich JP, Tollefsen DM. Anticoagulant, thrombolytic, and antiplatelet drugs. In: Hardman JG et al (eds). *Goodman & Gilman's The Pharmacological Basis of Therapeutics.* 9th edn. New York: McGraw-Hill, 1996: 1341–1359.

13. Rosenberg RD. The heparin–antithrombin system: a natural anticoagulant mechanism. In: Colman RW, Hirsh J, Marder VJ, Salzman EW (eds). *Hemostasis and Thrombosis: Basic Principles and Clinical Practice.* 2nd edn. Philadelphia: JB Lippincott, 1987: 1373–1392.

14. Hirsh J. Heparin. *N Engl J Med* 1991; **324**: 1565–1574.

15. MacMahon S, Collins R, Knight C et al. Reduction of major morbidity and mortality by heparin in acute myocardial infarction (abstr). *Circulation* 1988; **78**(Suppl II): II–98.

16. The SCATI (Studio sulla Caldiparin rell'Angina e rella Trombos: Ventricolare nell'Infarto) Group. Randomized controlled trial of subcutaneous calcium heparin in acute myocardial infarction. *Lancet* 1989; **ii**: 182–186.

17. Stein B, Fuster V. Pharmacology of anticoagulants and platelet inhibitor drugs. In: Schlant RC, Alexander RW (eds). *Hurst's The Heart.* Vol I, 8th edn. New York: McGraw-Hill, 1994: 1309–1326.

18. Hirsh J, Levine MN. Low molecular weight heparin. *Blood* 1992; **79**: 1–17.

19. Hirsh J. Low-molecular-weight-heparin: a review of the results of recent studies of the treatment of venous thromboembolism and unstable angina. *Circulation* 1998; **98**: 1575–1582.

20. Markwardt F. Development of hirudin as an antithrombotic agent. *Semin Thromb Hemost* 1989; **15**: 269–282.

21. Rydel TJ, Ravichandran KG, Tulinsky A et al. The structure of a complex of recombinant hirudin human alpha-thrombin. *Science* 1990; **249**: 277–280.

22. Markwardt F, Kaiser B, Nowak G. Studies on antithrombotic effects of recombinant hirudin. *Thromb Res* 1989; **54**: 377–380.

23. Heras M, Chesebro JH, Penny WJ et al. Effects of thrombin inhibition on the development of acute thrombus deposition during angioplasty in pigs: heparin versus recombinant hirudin, a specific thrombin inhibitor. *Circulation* 1989; **79**: 657–665.

24. Bossavy JP, Sakariassen KS, Rubsamen K et al. Comparison of the antithrombotic effect of PEG-hirudin and heparin in a human ex vivo model of arterial thrombosis. *Arterioscler Thromb Vasc Biol* 1999; **19**: 1348–1353.

25. Topol EJ, Fuster V, Harrington RA et al. Recombinant hirudin for unstable angina pectoris. *Circulation* 1994; **89**: 1557–1566.

26. The GUSTO IIa Investigators. Randomized trial of intravenous heparin versus recombinant hirudin for acute coronary syndromes. *Circulation* 1994; **90**: 1631–1637.

27. The GUSTO IIb Investigators. A comparison of recombinant hirudin with heparin for the treatment of acute coronary syndromes. *N Engl J Med* 1996; **335**: 775–782.

28. Organisation to Assess Strategies for Ischemic Syndromes (OASIS-2) Investigators. Effects of

recombinant hirudin (lepirudin) compared with heparin on death, myocardial infarction, refractory angina, and revascularisation procedures in patients with acute myocardial ischemia without ST elevation: a randomised trial. *Lancet* 1999; **353**: 429–438.

29. Eriksson BI, Soderberg K, Widlund L et al. A comparative study of three low-molecular weight heparins (LMWH) and unfractionated heparin (UH). *Thromb Haemost* 1995: **73**: 398–401.

30. Hoppensteadt DA, Jeske W, Fareed J, Bermes EW. The role of tissue factor pathway inhibitor in the mediation of the antithrombotic actions of heparin and low-molecular-weight heparin. *Blood Coagul Fibrinolysis* 1995; **6**: S57–S64.

31. Jang IK, Gold HK, Ziskind AA et al. Prevention of platelet-rich arterial thrombosis by selective thrombin inhibition. *Circulation* 1990; **81**: 219–225.

32. Bittl JA, Strony J, Brinker JA et al. Treatment with bivalirudin (Hirulog) as compared with heparin during coronary angioplasty for unstable or postinfarction angina. *N Engl J Med* 1995; **333**: 764–769.

33. Fuchs J, Cannon CP, the TIMI 7 Investigators. Hirulog in the treatment of unstable angina. Results of the Thrombin Inhibition in Myocardial Ischemia (TIMI) 7 trial. *Circulation* 1995; **92**: 727–733.

34. White HD, Aylward PE, Frey MJ et al. Randomized, double-blind comparison of hirulog versus heparin in patients receiving streptokinase and aspirin for acute myocardial infarction (HERO). *Circulation* 1997; **96**: 2155–2161.

35. Cohen M, Blaber R. Potential uses of a new class of low-molecular weight heparins in cardiovascular indications. *Thromb Hemost* 1996; **22**(Suppl 2): 25–27.

36. Samama M, Bara L, Gerotziafas G. Mechanisms for the antithrombotic activity in man of low molecular weight heparins. *Haemostasis* 1994; **24**: 105–117.

37. Fareed J, Jeske W, Hoppensteadt DA et al. Are the available low-molecular-weight heparin preparations the same? *Semin Thromb Hemost* 1996; **22**(Suppl 1): 77–91.

38. Gurfinkel EP, Manos EJ, Mejail RI et al. Low molecular weight heparin versus regular heparin or aspirin in the treatment of unstable angina and silent ischemia. *J Am Coll Cardiol* 1995; **26**: 313–318.

39. Leizorowicz A for the FRAXIS study group. Fraxiparine in Ischemic Syndromes. Presentation at the European Society of Cardiology, Vienna, Austria, August, 1998.

40. Instability in Coronary Artery Disease (FRISC) Study Group. Low molecular weight heparin during instability in coronary artery disease. *Lancet* 1996; **347**: 561–568.

41. Klein W, Buchwald A, Hillis SE et al. Comparison of low-molecular-weight heparin with unfractionated heparin acutely and with placebo for 6 weeks in the management of unstable coronary artery disease. Fragmin in Unstable Coronary Artery Disease Study (FRIC). *Circulation* 1997; **96**: 61–68.

42. Cohen M, Demers C, Gurfinkel EP et al for the Efficacy and Safety of Subcutaneous Enoxaparin in Non-Q-Wave Coronary Events Study Group. A comparison of low-molecular-weight heparin with unfractionated heparin for unstable coronary artery disease. *N Engl J Med* 1997; **337**: 447–452.

43. Cohen M, Stinnett S, Fromell G. Effect of low molecular weight heparin on prespecified patient subgroups with rest unstable angina or

non-Q-wave myocardial infarction. *Circulation* 1998; **98**(Suppl I): I–559.

44. Mark DB, Cowper PA, Berkowitz SD et al. Economic assessment of low molecular weight heparin (enoxaparin) versus unfractionated heparin in acute coronary syndrome patients: results from the ESSENCE randomized trial. *Circulation* 1998; **97**: 1702–1707.

45. Cohen M, Bigonzi F, Le louer V et al. One year follow-up of the ESSENCE trial (enoxaparin versus heparin in unstable angina and non Q wave myocardial infarction). *J Am Coll Cardiol* 1998; **31**(Suppl A): 79A.

46. The Thrombolysis in Myocardial Infarction (TIMI) 11a Trial Investigators. Dose ranging trial of enoxaparin for unstable angina: results of TIMI 11A. *J Am Coll Cardiol* 1997; **29**: 1474–1482.

47. Cohen M, Demers C, Frommel G et al. Hemorrhage incidence with low molecular weight heparin vs unfractionated heparin in patients with unstable angina or non-Q wave infarction (from the ESSENCE Study). *J Am Coll Cardiol* 1997; **29**(Suppl A): 410A.

48. Montalescot G, Philippe F, Ankri A et al. Early increase of von Willebrand factor predicts adverse outcome in unstable coronary artery disease: beneficial effects of enoxaparin. *Circulation* 1998; **98**: 294–299.

49. Xiao Z, Theroux P. Platelet activation with unfractionated heparin at therapeutic concentrations and comparisons with a low-molecular weight heparin and with direct thrombin inhibitor. *Circulation* 1998; **97**: 251–256.

50. Antman EM, McCabe CH, Premmereur J et al. Enoxaparin for the acute and chronic management of unstable angina/non-Q wave myocardial infarction: Results of TIMI 11B. *Circulation* 1998; **98**(Suppl I): I–504.

51. Antman EM, Cohen M, Radley D et al, for the TIMI 11 B and ESSENCE Investigators. Enoxaparin for unstable angina/non-Q wave myocardial infarction: meta-analysis of TIMI 11B and ESSENCE. *J Am Coll Cardiol* 1999; **31** (Suppl): 351A.

52. Wallentin L for the FRISC II study group. FRISC II. Presentation at the American College of Cardiology Scientific Sessions, New Orleans, USA, March, 1999.

53. Kong DF, Califf, RM, Miller DP et al. Clinical outcomes of therapeutic agents that block the platelet glycoprotein IIb/IIIa integrin in ischemic heart disease. *Circulation* 1998; **98**: 2829–2835.

54. Leadley R Jr, Kasiewski C, Bostwick J et al. Efficacy and safety of low molecular weight heparin in combination with a platelet fibrinogen receptor antagonist in a canine model of unstable angina. *Circulation* 1998; **98** (Suppl I): I–800.

55. Rhone-Poulenc Rorer Research Protocol: The safety of enoxaparin therapy in patients undergoing percutaneous coronary intervention receiving concomitant abciximab therapy (NICE-4).

56. Merck research protocol: A randomized, parallel open-label study to investigate the effect on prolongation of bleeding time by low molecular weight heparin vs. unfractionated heparin in tirofiban and aspirin treated patients with unstable angina/non-Q-wave myocardial infarction.

57. TIMI IIIB Investigators. Effects of tissue plasminogen activator and a comparison of early invasive and conservative strategies in unstable angina and non-Q-wave myocardial infarction. Results of the TIMI IIIB trial. *Circulation* 1994; **89**: 1545–1556.

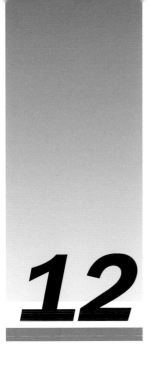

Treatment and prevention of acute ischemic stroke

12

Gilles Lugassy

*If I forget thee, oh Jerusalem, may my right hand forget its
cunning, my tongue cleave to the palate . . .*

Psalm 137

Since its first description in the Old Testament, stroke has
been perceived as a terrible threat or punishment leading to
devastating damage. Today, even more than before, stroke is
one of the leading causes of death and disability in the
modern world.[1] Hypertension and coronary heart diseases are
responsible for most of the cases of acute stroke.
Hematological disorders account for up to 8% of all ischemic
strokes.[2]

Stroke is usually classified into two categories, as follows:

- Intracerebral hemorrhage (15%)
- Ischemic stroke: atherothrombosis, 50%;
  cardioembolism, 25%; lacunes, 25%.

Prothrombotic factors in acute stroke

Pathological mechanisms of hemostasis observed in ischemic
stroke involve the activation of platelets and reduced
fibrinolysis.

Platelet activation

The activation of platelet functions, leading to hyperaggregation of platelets, has been described before and after the clinical onset of ischemic stroke. The occurrence of ischemic stroke, as a complication of primary thrombocythemia, and the effectiveness of antiplatelet agents in preventing cerebral infarction also favor the role of platelet activation in the pathogenesis of stroke.[3]

Fibrinolysis

Reduced fibrinolytic activity is considered to be a risk factor of venous and arterial thromboembolism.[4] In a recent study, Ridker et al[5] found that tissue plasminogen activator (t-PA) antigen is a predictor of the development of stroke. In a study of plasminogen activator inhibitor-1 (PAI-1) among a cohort of patients with stroke, elevated levels were found in the acute phase and 3 months after ischemic stroke.[6]

Homocysteinemia

Hyperhomocysteinemia is associated with stroke in young adults. Subjects with hereditary or acquired hyperhomocysteinemia also have a greater risk of stroke and myocardial infarction (MI) than control subjects.[7]

Antiphospholipid syndrome

Antiphospholipid antibodies (aPL), more specifically anticardiolipin antibodies, IgG_2, have been identified in 10% of unselected patients with first stroke.[8] There is a notable lack of association between activated protein C (APC) resistance, protein C or protein S deficiency and the occurrence of arterial thrombosis.[9]

Management of acute stroke

Despite the numerous trials conducted over the past decade, stroke, in contrast to myocardial infarction, has suffered from a lack of effective and safe treatments. Massive trials, recruiting thousands of patients, often lead to conflicting results and contradictory guidelines and recommendations.[10,11] Therefore, reviewing the main trials and therapies currently available for management of acute ischemic stroke is of great interest.

Thrombolytic therapy of acute ischemic stroke

The impressive results of thrombolysis in myocardial infarction,[12] have raised a considerable interest in the use of thrombolytic agents in acute stroke management. Animal studies have demonstrated that thrombolysis can reduce the extent of neuronal damage following cerebral ischemia.[13] The early human trials met with unacceptable hemorrhagic risks, partly due to the difficulty — in pre-computed tomography (CT) days — of avoiding the treatment of some patients with cerebral hemorrhage. Other reasons for the failure of early trials were delay in the onset of treatment and the lack of experience with the agents used. With the introduction of newer thrombolytic drugs and the ability to initiate early treatment after excluding hemorrhage, the interest in thrombolytic therapy of acute stroke has re-emerged. Large clinical trials present considerable organizational difficulties, often leading to conflicting interpretations.

Streptokinase in acute stroke: condemned in trial

Three randomized, controlled, symptom-based large trials of streptokinase were halted by safety committees due to high mortality and intracranial bleeding rates. Each study used a single intravenous infusion of 1.5×10^6 IU streptokinase in the active arm. The Multicenter Acute Stroke Trial Europe (MAST-E)[14] recruited patients with moderate to severe ischemia in the territory of the middle cerebral artery. They were randomized to receive streptokinase or placebo within 6 hours after the onset of stroke. Recruitment was discontinued early, after the Data Monitoring Committee reported an increased

mortality at 10 days, due to intracerebral hemorrhage: 34% in the streptokinase group versus 18.2% in the placebo group.

The Multicenter Acute Stroke Trial — Italy (MAST-I)[15] was another randomized but unblinded trial that compared outcomes among patients assigned to 1.5×10^6 units streptokinase or 300 mg aspirin daily for 10 days, or both together or control, initiated within 6 hours of stroke. Analysis of the data confirmed the increased risk of early death in the streptokinase group, with an even higher mortality at 10 days with streptokinase plus aspirin.

The Australian Streptokinase (ASK) trial[16] tested the hypothesis that there might be a difference in outcomes between acute ischemic stroke patients who received 1.5×10^6 units of streptokinase between 0 and 3 hours after occurrence of symptoms and those who received the same treatment over 3 hours later. After analysing the first 300 patients, the Safety Monitoring Committee recommended that recruitment be halted because of an increase in mortality caused by intracerebral hemorrhage.

Recombinant tissue plasminogen activator (rt-PA)

A promising but risky option: most efforts, hopes and controversies have recently addressed the use of rt-PA for acute stroke management.

Intravenous rt-PA

Following a series of pilot studies aimed toward evaluating the safety of rt-PA in acute ischemic stroke, a two-part, four-armed study of rt-PA with entry before 90 minutes or between 91 and 180 minutes from the onset of symptoms, was completed by the National Institute of Neurological Disorders and Stroke (NINDS).[17] Patients eligible for the study were diagnosed as those suffering from ischemic stroke with a baseline CT scan of the brain to exclude hemorrhage and a defined time of symptom onset. Angiographic demonstration of the arterial occlusion was not required for inclusion in the study. Both parts of the NINDS trial employed an intravenous dose of 0.9 mg/kg of rt-PA. Part 1 assessed changes in neurologic deficits 24 hours after the onset of stroke as a measure of the activity of t-PA and 291 patients were randomized to rt-PA or placebo. At 24 hours, no difference in neurologic status was observed between the two groups. Part 2 of the NINDS study evaluated results at 3 months among 333 patients randomized to receive t-PA or placebo. A favorable outcome was demonstrated when patients were given rt-PA: complete neurologic recovery increased from 20% for the placebo group to 31% for the rt-PA group, while the rate of complete recovery to full independence in performing daily activities increased from 38% to 50%. The benefit was reported for all subtypes of ischemic stroke. In the combined experiences of both parts, symptomatic hemorrhage was more frequent among rt-PA-treated patients and it contributed significantly to mortality at 3 months for this group of patients. Nevertheless, overall mortality was not higher with rt-PA than with placebo (17 versus 21%).

The optimistic conclusions of the NINDS study eventually convinced the Federal Drugs Administration (FDA) to approve the use of t-PA for the treatment of acute stroke. The Committee of the American Heart Association[18] and the American Academy of Neurology[19] issued guidelines favoring thrombolysis treatment with t-PA for acute ischemic stroke, given within 3 hours of the onset of symptoms, and after exclusion of any recent major brain infarction per CT.

A recent update of the NINDS study reported a sustained long term advantage for t-PA treated patients, with a favorable clinical outcome at 12 months.[20]

Soon after the NINDS report, a large randomized, blinded study failed to confirm the benefit of high-dose rt-PA in acute ischemic stroke. In the European Cooperative Acute Stroke Study (ECASS),[21] 620 acute ischemic stroke patients with moderate to severe neurologic deficit were randomized to 1.1 mg/kg rt-PA or placebo within 6 hours of the onset of symptoms. The inclusion of 109 patients with large regions of hemispheric injury on admission, unappreciated by the investigators on initial CT scan, was a major flaw of the study. Even though these patients were excluded from the target population analysis, the occurrence of large parenchymal hemorrhages was more frequent among rt-PA-treated patients.

Following the conflicting results of the NINDS and ECASS I rt-PA trials, the ECASS II study results were anticipated with great interest.[22] The ECASS II tested whether a lower dose of 0.9 mg/kg rt-PA, given within 6 hours of onset of stroke, could improve neurologic outcome at 3 months in comparison with placebo. A total of 800 patients, of whom 341 had no record of infarction on baseline CT brain scan, were recruited in both arms. No significant difference was evident between the rt-PA and the placebo group. The hemorrhagic price paid by t PA patients was high. Parenchymal hemorrhage was four times more common in the rt-PA group than in the placebo group, and large, confluent space occupying intracranial hemorrhages occurred 10 times more often.

Intra-arterial thrombolysis

Studies of intra-arterial rt-PA delivery have shown the effectiveness of this therapy in cerebral arterial recanalization shortly after acute ischemic stroke. Recanalization has been observed in about half of acutely treated patients in mostly uncontrolled studies.[23] The reported incidence of hemorrhagic transformation (hemorrhagic infarction and parenchymal hematoma) after intra-arterial thrombolysis with u-PA, streptokinase or rt-PA is around 25%, 60% of which was symptomatic.[24] In order to assess the benefit and safety of intra-arterial thrombolysis, a prospective trial of recombinant prourokinase (rpro-UK) versus placebo was undertaken.

The Prolyse in Acute Cerebral Thromboembolism (PROACT)[25] trial tested the rate of recanalization, safety and efficacy of 6 mg intra-arterial rpro-UK given within 6 hours after stroke due to occlusion of the middle cerebral artery, together with low or high doses of heparin.

Recanalization of the middle cerebral artery occurred in 58% in the rpro-UK group and in only 14% in the placebo group. Transluminal angioplasty is often necessary to keep arteries open after intra-arterial thrombolysis.

Thrombolysis in stroke: conclusions

Controversial but investigational, thrombolysis is feasible in the setting of acute stroke and may be helpful in a limited subset of patients. However the systematic use of fibrinolysis cannot be justified until its exact indications and contraindications are better defined by more efficacy trials. Selection of patients should be improved using better diagnostic tools. Clinical evaluation and CT scanning are unreliable for the diagnosis of conditions that could mimic stroke, such as migraines or seizures.[26] The causes of stroke are heterogeneous and only patients with lysable clots should be eligible for thrombolytic therapy. Pinpointing the exact location of the occlusion is essential to the decision of choosing between intravenous and intra-arterial thrombolysis. This is based on the fact that occlusions of the main stem, divisional middle cerebral and basilar artery respond better to intra-arterial thrombolysis, while intravenous therapy seems to be better for occlusions of middle cerebral artery branches than it is for main stem occlusions.[27] Obvious limitations are the time and expertise required to perform an angiography: 'time is brain.'[28] Finally, patients should give their consent to a possible benefit in long-term independence and neurologic improvement after being informed of the higher risk of early hemorrhagic death.

For all these reasons, thrombolytic therapy for stroke should still be reserved for clinical trials performed in specialized centers.

Aspirin in acute stroke

Aspirin is a logical therapy choice in the acute phase of the stroke, during which there is a massive activation of platelets in the peri-infarct zone with sludging in the microcirculation, and production of thromboxane, which is a highly thrombogenic and neurotoxic eicosenoid.[3]

Three large trials were designed to determine the possible effectiveness of early aspirin in acute ischemic stroke. The early and small, Multicenter Acute Stroke Trial — Italy (MAST-I),[15] was conducted in order to determine whether, prescribed separately or together, streptokinase and aspirin have clinical benefits in acute ischemic stroke.

In this trial, 300 mg aspirin daily, was initiated within 6 hours of onset of the neurologic deficit for a duration of 10 days in 309 patients (aspirin alone or with streptokinase). Aspirin reduced the short- and long-term fatality rates, but statistical significance was not reached. Patients treated with aspirin suffered a slightly higher risk of intracerebral hemorrhage than those given placebo (2 versus 0.6%).

The International Stroke Trial (IST)[29] randomized some 20 000 patients to receive aspirin (300 mg daily), heparin, both or neither, within 48 hours of onset of acute stroke for a duration of 14 days. The primary outcomes were death within 14 days and death or dependency at 6 months. Aspirin did not improve the early death rate as compared with the control group (9.0 versus 9.4%). The aspirin group exhibited a mild, but significant, reduction in recurrent ischemic stroke within 14 days with no excess of hemorrhagic strokes.

The Chinese Acute Stroke Trial (CAST)[30] was prospectively planned to be analysed together with its contemporary IST. In the Chinese trial, 20 000 patients were randomized to receive 160 mg aspirin daily, starting within 48 hours of the onset of acute stroke, for a duration of 4 weeks. Primary endpoints were similar to those defined in the IST.

Pooled results for both CAST and IST show that aspirin, given within 48 hours of acute stroke, produces a marginal but significant reduction of about 10 deaths or recurrent strokes per 1000 in the first few weeks.

Heparins

A survey conducted 10 years ago among 247 American neurologists revealed broad use of early heparin therapy in acute ischemic stroke, as a method of preventing stroke progression and recurrent cerebral embolism. This policy is still controversial after several large trials failed to prove any advantage of intravenous unfractionated heparin or subcutaneous low molecular weight heparin over placebo in ischemic stroke. In the IST,[29] 9717 patients were allocated to receive unfractionated heparin (5000 or 12 500 units intravenously twice daily) early after stroke. The percentage dead within 14 days and the percentage dead or dependent at 6 months was identical in both groups and similar to the control group. Heparin-treated patients had fewer recurrent

strokes at day 14 but suffered an increased risk of hemorrhagic stroke. Heparin was also associated with an excess of fatal extracranial bleeds.

Checking the hypothesis that low molecular weight heparin could be as efficacious but safer than unfractionated heparin, Kay et al[31] randomly assigned 312 patients to receive, shortly after the onset of the symptoms, one of two regimens of subcutaneous nadroparin (4100 antifactor X units once or twice daily) for 10 days or placebo. No significant difference was found between the three groups in terms of deaths or complications at 10 days and 3 months. At 6 months, nadroparin was superior to placebo in terms of survival and dependency. The discordance between the 3-month and the 6-month outcomes raises questions about whether a true therapeutic effect was indeed observed.

Danaparoid sodium (ORG 10172) is a mixture of glycosaminoglycans with an antifactor X activity due to its heparin sulfate component with a high affinity for antithrombin.

The Trial of ORG 10172 in Acute Stroke Treatment (TOAST)[32] was designed to test whether danaparoid is an effective therapy to improve outcome at 3 months. Of the 641 patients assigned to receive ORG 10172, 482 (75.2%) had favorable outcomes at 3 months as compared to 467 of 634 (73.7%) of placebo-treated patients.

Conclusions

Studies of unfractionated heparin and low molecular weight heparin treatment for acute stroke management can hardly be compared since their protocols are heterogeneous: dosages, routes of administration and follow-up methods differ from one trial to another. Nevertheless, the lack of benefit found in the IST and TOAST trials does not support the clinical use of heparin derivatives in acute stroke. Their use can still be justified for the prevention of venous thromboembolism in stroke patients.

Secondary prevention of ischemic stroke

While therapies to reduce brain injury caused by acute stroke are being developed, leading to contradictory results and controversial guidelines, prevention — control of hypertension, cessation of cigarette smoking and increased physical activity — is still the most effective strategy for high-risk patients.

Antiplatelet agents seem to be effective adjuvants in reducing vascular events in secondary prevention of stroke. In 1994, the Antiplatelet Trialists' Collaboration[33] published an overview of 145 trials of prolonged antiplatelet therapy in the prevention of death, MI and stroke in various categories of patients.

Early aspirin trials in the 1970s reported an impressive reduction in stroke incidence among men only.[34] The European Stroke Prevention Study (ESPS)[35] compared the clinical outcome at 24 months of 2500 patients with transient ischemic attack (TIA) or stroke, treated with either aspirin 975 mg daily and dipyridamole, or placebo only. Stroke and death rates decreased by 36.5% with the aspirin–dipyridamole combination in men and women alike.

In the Swedish Aspirin Low-dose Trial (SALT),[36] a daily intake of 75 mg aspirin resulted in an 18% decrease in stroke recurrence and death compared to placebo. The Dutch TIA Trial Study Group[37] compared two doses of aspirin (30 mg and 283 mg daily) in patients after TIA or minor ischemic stroke and found that both doses of aspirin are equally effective in reducing vascular death, stroke or MI.

There is still no evidence that low to intermediate doses of aspirin (30–325 mg daily) are as effective for secondary prevention of stroke as 975 mg daily or more. Ticlopidine, or its newer derivative, clopidogrel, have been tested in several recent studies for patients at risk who do not tolerate high-dose aspirin. The Canadian American Ticlopidine Study (CATS),[38] enrolled 1072 patients after a recent stroke, to receive either ticlopidine 500 mg daily or placebo. Therapy was initiated within 1 week to 4 months after stroke. Ticlopidine reduced the incidence of stroke, MI or vascular death by 30%.

Aspirin or ticlopidine?

Contemporary with CATS, a trial comparing ticlopidine with aspirin for the prevention of stroke in high-risk patients[39] favored ticlopidine, with a mild benefit at 3 years: 10% stroke recurrence versus 13% for aspirin. However, side-effects were more frequent with ticlopidine.

Comparable results have been obtained with clopidogrel, a thienopyridine derivative, similar to ticlopidine. In the CAPRIE trial,[40] more than 19 000 patients with recent MI, ischemic stroke or peripheral arterial disease were randomized to clopidogrel (75 mg daily) or 35 mg aspirin daily. Long-term clopidogrel therapy reduced the risk of ischemic stroke, MI or vascular death by 8.7% compared to aspirin. The overall annual risk for vascular complications was 5.32% for the clopidogrel group and 5.83% for aspirin.

Since the two antiplatelet agents act on different pathways and both are effective in the prevention of vascular events, a combination of aspirin and clopidogrel could eventually improve the outcome over their separate use, without excessive toxicity. Such an hypothesis deserves testing in further clinical trials.

Primary stroke prevention

While secondary stroke prevention with long-term antiplatelet therapy in high-risk patients has been demonstrated beyond doubt, clinical trials of aspirin in the low-risk population (primary prevention) have led to controversial and paradoxical results. The Antiplatelet Trialists' Collaboration report[33] showed a statistically insignificant 21% increase of nonfatal stroke among low-risk patients treated with aspirin. A recent report by the Cardiovascular Health Study has confirmed the increased risk of stroke in a cohort of 5000 elderly patients.[41] Frequent aspirin use was associated with an increased number of ischemic strokes in women and hemorrhagic strokes in both genders.

The actual accountability of aspirin for the higher risk of ischemic stroke has still to be confirmed. The Women's Health Study randomized 40 000 female health professionals aged 45 years and older in order to evaluate the affect of aspirin among low-risk patients.[42] Results of this large trial are not available to date.

The possible benefit of primary stroke prevention with antiplatelet therapy may be difficult to show because of the low incidence of vascular events in this population. Present data do not support the systematic use of aspirin in the primary prevention of cardiovascular disease and stroke.

Atrial fibrillation

Atrial fibrillation (AF), even in the absence of valvulopathy, is associated with an impressive risk of thromboembolic events, especially stroke, which may be as high as 8% a year.[43] The risk increases up to 17 times in valvular AF with mitral stenosis. Stroke secondary to AF has a high recurrence rate and is more likely to be associated with severe neurological deficits. In addition to AF, age, prior stroke or TIA, hypertension and diabetes are major risk factors for stroke. Several placebo-controlled trials have tested the effect of warfarin and aspirin in stroke prevention in AF.[44] In all of these trials, which included thousands of randomized patients, warfarin resulted in a reduction of 70% in the incidence of ischemic stroke, provided that an international normalized ratio (INR) in the range of 1.5–4.0 was respected.

Reduction of stroke was not observed in patients younger than 65 years with no concomitant risk factors. In this subgroup, the incidence of stroke was 1.0% per year with or without antithrombotic therapy. Despite these compelling data, most AF patients at high risk of stroke do not receive adequate anticoagulation agents because of the fear of bleeding complications and the need for regular laboratory testing.[45]

The preventive effect of aspirin has been investigated in several trials comparing aspirin to warfarin and placebo. The ASAFAK I and II,[46] and the SPAF (1–3)[47] showed divergent results and have not completely clarified the effect of aspirin on stroke prevention in AF. Presently available data support the use of adjusted-dose warfarin for most patients with AF (target INR: 2.0–3.0). Fixed-dose low-intensity warfarin is ineffective and is not recommended. The addition of aspirin to low-dose warfarin is unjustified. Patients younger than 65 with no other risk factor can receive aspirin 325 mg daily.

Carotid endarterectomy

Several large trials have considered carotid endarterectomy in patients with recent TIA or nondisabling ischemic stroke.

The North American Symptomatic Carotid Endarterectomy Trial (NASCET)[48] and the European Carotid Surgery Trial (ECST)[49] have shown the advantage of surgery over medical therapy for prevention of stroke in patients with high grade carotid stenosis ($\geq$70%). This advantage is less pronounced among patients with symptomatic but moderate carotid stenosis (50–69%): in order to prevent one single stroke in this subgroup, 15 patients should undergo endarterectomy. Patients with mild stenosis (less than 50%) do not benefit from surgery.[50] The low complication rates observed in these large studies (5–7%) are due to selection of highly specialized centers by the trial organizing committee. Unfortunately, most candidates for surgery are not selectively referred to hospitals with high volumes of procedures and low mortality rates. It is therefore doubtful whether the recommendations issued after these clinical trials can be safely extended to the general population of patients in the community setting.

The value of carotid endarterectomy in asymptomatic stenosis (primary prevention) has recently been assessed in a meta-analysis of six randomized trials.[51] Although endarterectomy reduces the incidence of ipsilateral stroke by some 30%, the absolute benefit of the procedure is marginal because the overall risk of stroke in asymptomatic stenosis is low. Patients should be aware of the earlier risks of surgery compared to latter occurrence of stroke in unoperated patients. It seems that the logical recommendation for asymptomatic carotid stenosis is still to 'spare the knife' until high-risk subgroups will be reliably identified as appropriate candidates for endarterectomy.

References

1. American Heart Association. *1993 Heart and Stroke Facts Statistics*. Dallas: American Heart Association, 1993.

2. Marcus HS, Hambley H. Neurology and the blood: haematological abnormalities in ischaemic stroke. *J Neurol Neurosurg Psychiatry* 1998; **64**: 150–159.

3. Van Kooten F, Ciabattoni G, Patrono C et al. Evidence for episodic platelet activation in stroke. *Stroke* 1994; **25**: 278–281.

4. Lugassy G, Filin I. Study of fibrinolytic parameters in different types of polycythemia. *Am J Hematol* 1999; **60**: 196–199.

5. Ridker PM, Hennekens CH, Stampfer MJ et al. Prospective study of endogenous tissue plasminogen activator and risk of stroke. *Lancet* 1994, **343**: 940–943.

6. Catto AJ, Carter AM, Stickland MH et al. Elevated levels of plasminogen activator inhibitor-I (PAI-I) 4G/5G promoter polymorphism and the development of atherothrombotic and hemorrhagic stroke (abstr). *Thromb Haemost* 1995; **74**: 1399.

7. Clarke R, Kaly I, Robinson K et al. Hyperhomocysteinemia: an independent risk factor for vascular disease. *N Engl J Med* 1991; **324**: 1149–1155.

8. The Antiphospholipid Antibodies in Stroke Study (APASS) Group. Anticardiolipin antibodies are an independent risk factor for first ischemic stroke. *Neurology* 1993; **43**: 2069–2073.

9. Ridker PM, Hennekens CH, Lindpainter K et al. Mutation in the gene coding for coagulation factor V and the risk of myocardial infarction, stroke, and venous thrombosis in apparently healthy men. *N Engl J Med* 1995; **332**: 912–917.

10. Consensus Statement of the Royal College of Physicians of Edinburgh Consensus Conference on Medical Management of Stroke, 26–27 May 1998. *Br J Haematol* 1998; **102**: 1107–1113.

11. Stroke Unit Trialists' Collaboration. Collaborative systematic review of the randomized trials of organized inpatient (stroke unit) care after stroke. *BMJ* 1997; **314**: 1151–1159.

12. The GUSTO Investigators. An international trial comparing four thrombolytic strategies for acute myocardial infarction. *N Engl J Med* 1993; **329**: 673–682.

13. Zivin JA, Grotta JC. Animal stroke models:

they are relevant to human disease. *Stroke* 1990; **21**: 982–983.

14. Multicentre Acute Stroke Trial — Europe Group. Thrombolytic therapy with streptokinase in acute ischemic stroke. *N Engl J Med* 1996; **335**: 145–150.

15. Multicentre Acute Stroke Trial — Italy Group. Randomized controlled trial of streptokinase, aspirin, and combination of both in treatment of acute ischemic stroke. *Lancet* 1995; **346**: 509–514.

16. Donnan GA, Davis SM, Chambers BR et al. Streptokinase for acute ischemic stroke with relationship to time of administration. *JAMA* 1996; **276**: 961–966.

17. NINDS rtPA Stroke Study Group. Tissue plasminogen activator for acute ischemic stroke. *N Engl J Med* 1995; **333**: 1581–1587.

18. Adams HP Jr, Brott TG, Furlan AJ et al. Guidelines for thrombolytic therapy for acute stroke: a supplement to the guidelines for the management of patients with acute ischemic stroke. *Circulation* 1996; **94**: 1167–1174.

19. Quality Standards Subcommittee of the American Academy of Neurology. Practice advisory: thrombolytic therapy for acute ischemic stroke — summary statement. *Neurology* 1996; **47**: 835–839.

20. Kwiatkovski TG, Libman RB, Frankel M et al. Effects of tissue plasminogen activator for acute ischemic stroke at one year. *N Engl J Med* 1999; **340**: 1781–1787.

21. Hacke W, Kaste M, Fieschi C et al. Intravenous thrombolysis with recombinant tissue plasminogen activator for acute hemispheric stroke: the European Cooperative Acute Stroke Study (ECASS). *JAMA* 1995; **274**: 1017–1025.

22. Hacke W, Kaste M, Fieschi C et al. Randomised double-blind placebo-controlled trial of thrombolytic therapy with intravenous alteplase in acute ischemic stroke (ECASS II). *Lancet* 1998; **352**: 245–251.

23. Pessin MS, del Zoppo GJ, Furlan AJ. Thrombolytic treatment in acute stroke: review and update of selective topics. In: Moskowitz MA, Caplan LR (eds). *Cerebrovascular Diseases: Nineteenth Princeton Stroke Conference.* Boston: Butterworth-Heinemann, 1995: 409–418.

24. Del Zoppo GJ. Antithrombotic therapy of acute stroke: thrombolytic agents. *Thromb Haemost* 1997; **78**: 183–190.

25. Del Zoppo GJ, Higashida RT, Furlan AJ et al and the PROACT Investigators. PROACT: A phase II randomized trial of recombinant pro-urokinase by direct arterial delivery in acute middle cerebral artery stroke. *Stroke* 1998; **29**: 4–10.

26. Van Gijn J, Dennis MS. Issues and answers in stroke care. *Lancet* 1998; **352**(Suppl II): 23–27.

27. Caplan LR, Mohr JP, Kistler JP, Koroshetz W. Should thrombolytic therapy be the first-line treatment for acute ischemic stroke? *N Engl J Med* 1998; **337**: 1309–1310.

28. Hill MD, Hachinski V. Stroke treatment: time is brain. *Lancet* 1998; **352** (Suppl III): 10–14.

29. International Stroke Trial Collaborative Group. The International Stroke Trial (IST): a randomized trial of aspirin, subcutaneous heparin, both or neither among 19 435 patients with acute ischaemic stroke. *Lancet* 1997; **349**: 1569–1581.

30. CAST (Chinese Acute Stroke Trial) Collaborative Group. CAST: randomised placebo-controlled trial of early aspirin use in

20 000 patients with acute ischaemic stroke. *Lancet* 1997; **349**: 1641–1649.

31. Kay R, Wong K, Yu YL et al. Low-molecular-weight heparin for the treatment of acute ischemic stroke. *N Engl J Med* 1995; **333**: 1588–1593.

32. The Trial of ORG 10172 in Acute Stroke treatment (TOAST) Investigators. Low molecular weight heparinoid, ORG 10172 (Danaparoid), and outcome after acute ischemic stroke. *JAMA* 1998; **279**: 1265–1272.

33. Antiplatelet Trialists' Collaboration. Collaborative overview of randomised trials of antiplatelet therapy — I: Prevention of death, myocardial infarction, and stroke by prolonged antiplatelet therapy in various categories of patients. *BMJ* 1994; **308**: 81–106.

34. Canadian Cooperative Study Group. A randomized trial of aspirin and sulfinpyrazone in treated stroke. *N Engl J Med* 1970, **299**: 53–59.

35. The ESPS Group. The European Stroke Prevention Study (ESPS): principal end-points. *Lancet* 1987; **ii**: 1351–1354.

36. The SALT Collaborative Group. Swedish Aspirin Low dose Trial (SALT) of 75 mg aspirin as secondary prophylaxis after cerebrovascular ischaemic events. *Lancet* 1991; **338**: 1345–1349.

37. The Dutch TIA Trial Study Group. A comparison of two doses of aspirin (30 mg vs. 283 mg a day) in patients after a transient ischemic attack or minor ischemic stroke. *N Engl J Med* 1991; **325**: 1261–1266.

38. Gent M, Blakely JA, Easton DJ et al. The Canadian American Ticlopidine Study (CATS) in Thromboembolic Stroke. *Lancet* 1989; **ii**: 1215–1220.

39. Hass WK, Easton DJ, Adams HP et al. A randomized trial comparing ticlopidine hydrochloride with aspirin for the prevention of stroke in high-risk patients. *N Engl J Med* 1989; **321**: 501–507.

40. CAPRIE Steering Committee. Clopidogrel reduced stroke, MI, and vascular death compared with aspirin. *Lancet* 1996; **348**: 1329–1339.

41. Manolio TA, Kronmal RA, Burke GL et al for the CHS Collaborative Research Group. Short-term predictors of incident stroke in older adults: the Cardiovascular Health Study. *Stroke* 1996; **27**: 1479–1486.

42. Tell GS, Fried LP, Hermanson BH et al. Recruitment of adults 65 years and older as participants in the Cardiovascular Health Study. *Ann Epidemiol* 1991; **3**: 358–366.

43. The Stroke Prevention in Atrial Fibrillation Investigators. Predictors of thromboembolism in atrial fibrillation: I. Clinical features of patients at risk. *Ann Intern Med* 1992; **116**: 1–5.

44. Koefoed BG, Gulløv AL, Petersen P. Prevention of thromboembolic events in atrial fibrillation. *Thromb Haemost* 1997; **78**: 377–381.

45. Kutner M, Nixon G, Silverstone F. Physicians' attitudes toward oral anticoagulants and antiplatelet agents for stroke prevention in elderly patients with atrial fibrillation. *Arch Intern Med* 1991; **151**: 1950–1953.

46. Gulløv AL, Koefoed BG, Petersen P et al. Fixed minidose warfarin and aspirin alone in and in combination vs. adjusted-dose warfarin for stroke prevention in atrial fibrillation: Second Copenhagen Atrial Fibrillation, Aspirin and Anticoagulation Study. *Arch Intern Med* 1998; **158**: 1513–1521.

47. The SPAF III Writing Committee for the Stroke Prevention in Atrial Fibrillation Investigators. Patients with nonvalvular atrial fibrillation at low risk of stroke during treatment with aspirin: Stroke Prevention in Atrial Fibrillation III Study. *JAMA* 1998; **279**: 1273–1277.

48. North American Symptomatic Carotid Endarterectomy Trial Collaborators. Beneficial effect of carotid endarterectomy in symptomatic patients with high-grade carotid stenosis. *N Engl J Med* 1991; **325**: 445–453.

49. European Carotid Surgery Trialists' Collaborative Group. Endarterectomy for moderate symptomatic carotid stenosis: interim results from the MRC European Carotid Surgery Trial. *Lancet* 1996; **347**: 1591–1593.

50. Barnett HJM, Taylor W, Eliasziw M et al. Benefit of carotid endarterectomy in patients with symptomatic moderate or severe stenosis. *N Engl J Med* 1998; **339**: 1415–1425.

51. Benavente O, Moher D, Pham B. Carotid endarterectomy for asymptomatic carotid stenosis: a meta-analysis. *BMJ* 1998; **317**: 1477–1480.

Peripheral arterial thrombosis

Gilles Lugassy

13

Peripheral arterial thrombosis is the clinical result of a longstanding process of atheromatous accumulation, complicated by plaque rupture, excessive platelet aggregation and a reduced fibrinolytic system, unable to lyse the thrombus.[1] Known atherothrombotic risk factors include hypertension, elevated serum cholesterol and triglyceride levels, diabetes mellitus and increased plasma viscosity. Above all, peripheral arterial disease correlates strongly with cigarette smoking.[2]

Other newly defined risk factors include markers of inflammation such as fibrinogen, serum amyloid A and C reactive protein, which have predictive value in determining risk for future atherothrombotic disease, independently of other cardiovascular risk factors.[3] Hyperhomocysteinemia is a common finding among patients with atherosclerosis, particularly among those who suffer clinical events at a young age.[4]

Arterial thrombosis mostly involves the lower limbs, but may also affect other vascular territories such as the coronary and cerebral arteries. This associated pathology accounts for the high morbidity and mortality encountered in this population of patients during the perioperative period.

The natural history of peripheral arterial disease is characterized by progressive narrowing of the vessels up to total occlusion. Patients may present with intermittent claudication or pain at rest, with or without cutaneous lesions.

In the presence of clinical manifestations of acute arterial occlusion or chronic symptoms of ischemia at rest (longer than 2 weeks), revascularizaton should be attempted.

Invasive procedures

Invasive strategies include the following.[5]

- Disobliteration by removal of an occlusive thrombus, embolus or atherosclerotic plaque: thromboembolectomy or endarterectomy.
- Transluminal dilatation of atherosclerotic plaque with a percutaneously introduced balloon catheter.
- Bypass graft using autologous vessel, mostly the saphenous vein, or prosthetic grafts. Knitted Dacron or polytetrafluoroethylene (PTFE) are preferred.

Thrombolytic therapy

Fibrinolytic therapy is an alternative and an adjuvant method to invasive treatment of arterial occlusive disease.

Fibrinolytic agents ideally activate fibrin-bound plasminogen, which in turn generates a high concentration of plasmin within the thrombus. Fibrinolytic therapy can be administered either systematically or locally. Systemic infusion appears to be poorly effective since the plasminogen activator given intravenously has a minimal surface contact with the thrombus. In a meta-analysis of 11 studies involving 2265 patients who received systemic fibrinolytic therapy for occlusive arterial disease, only 20% of all patients benefited from substantial lysis, while 80% had either incomplete or no lysis.[6] Regional intra-arterial delivery directed to the thrombus reaches the plasminogen activator where it is protected from circulating inhibitors with minimal systemic activation of plasminogen. Although theoretical considerations favor local delivery (intra-arterial) of fibrinolytic agents, a comparative efficacy trial of regional versus systemic administration has not been performed yet.

The most important step for a successful intra-arterial delivery is the correct lodging of the infusion catheter into the occluded vessel and penetration into the thrombus with the guidewire.

Thrombolytic agents include streptokinase, urokinase, tissue plasminogen activator (t-PA) and the recent pro-urokinase (single chain urokinase plasminogen activator or scu-PA).

Streptokinase was the first effective thrombolytic agent approved for clinical use. However, severe antigenicity and excessive systemic fibrinolysis resulting in high bleeding complication rates, have led most investigators to bar its use in favor of urokinase or recombinant-PA (rt-PA).

The initial dose of urokinase usually consists of a bolus of 250–500 000 units, followed by 4000 IU/min for 4 hours, then 2000 units/min for up to 36–44 hours. When using rt-PA, a dose of 0.05 mg/kg per hour is given for up to 12 hours. Heparin is sometimes added to the thrombolytic agents to reduce pericatheter thrombosis, usually with a higher hemorrhagic complication risk.

Complications of thrombolytic therapy

Bleeding is common during thrombolytic therapy. Incidence of major bleeding is higher with streptokinase (up to 26%) than with other agents (4–7%).[7] Hemorrhages tend to occur at the site of the invasive procedure. Intracerebral bleeding may also complicate thrombolytic therapy in hypertensive, diabetic and elderly patients. Laboratory values of prothrombin time, partial prothrombin time, fibrinogen and D-dimer do not correlate with the risk and the severity of bleeding complications.

Other complications may occur during intra-arterial fibrinolysis:

- Extravasation of contrast material or blood in knitted Dacron grafts.
- Distal emboli during revascularization of thrombosed PTFE grafts, due to thrombus fragments carried distally.

Clinical experience with intra-arterial thrombolytic therapy for vascular occlusion

Intra-arterial catheter-directed fibrinolysis for arterial obstruction was performed for the first time in 1974 by Dotter.[8] Since then, many investigators have adopted the regional approach, either alone, or in association with percutaneous angioplasty, and/or surgery. However, only few of the clinical trials in this field are prospective, randomized and controlled studies. Moreover, variation in patient selection, methods and endpoint analysis, make it difficult to determine the appropriate applications to individual clinical decision-making.

Parent et al[9] administered 40 courses of intra-arterial UK to 33 patients with acute ischemia due to thromboembolism of a native artery or bypass graft. Heparin was also given to prevent pericatheter thrombosis during urokinase infusion. The majority of patients presented with rest pain of 2 weeks' duration. Short-term outcome of intra-arterial urokinase was better in patients with prosthetic grafts (94% successful revascularization) than with autologous grafts or native arteries (55 and

54%, respectively). Successful thrombolysis was dependent on the physician's ability to insert the catheter in the thrombus. On long-term follow-up, prognosis was poor for autologous grafts, with none patent at 10 months, while 47% of the synthetic grafts and 100% of the native arteries in which complete lysis was obtained, were patent at 1 year.

In a prospective randomized placebo-controlled study that included 134 patients undergoing operative lower extremity revascularization, Comerota et al[10] evaluated the safety and the effect of three different doses of intra-arterial urokinase on fibrinolytic laboratory parameters. A dose-related effect was noted on plasminogen levels, plasma fibrinogen degradation products and D-dimer, in both regional and systemic circulations, with no excessive operative blood loss.

The issue of the best approach for ischemia of the lower extremity has been addressed by several multicenter trials that compared surgery with thrombolysis. The first large trial was the Surgery versus Thrombolysis for Ischemia of the Lower Extremity (STILE).[11] The purpose of the study was to compare thrombolysis and surgery for the occurrence of a composite clinical outcome, in patients suffering from nonembolic arterial and graft occlusion.

The composite clinical outcome included ongoing or recurrent ischemia, death, major amputation, and life threatening hemorrhage and severe perioperative complications (cerebrovascular accident, pulmonary oedema, and pulmonary embolism). Patients were randomized to either catheter-directed thrombolysis with rt-PA (0.05 mg/kg per hour for 12 hours) or urokinase infusion (250 000 units bolus followed by 4000 units/min for 4 hours, then 2000 units/min for up to 36 hours) or operative revascularization. Patient recruitment was terminated early with only 393 patients randomized, after surgical therapy was proven to be significantly better than thrombolysis in reducing ischemic events at 30 days: 23.6% versus 45.4%. The rate of failure of catheter placement (in 28% of patients randomized to lysis) was an important factor in the relatively poor results obtained with thrombolytic therapy. However, stratification by duration of ischemia showed that patients with acute (less than 14 days) ischemic deterioration had lower amputation rates and shorter hospital stays when treated with thrombolysis. Efficacy was similar between patients treated with urokinase or rt-PA. Bleeding was more frequent in the thrombolysis treated group (urokinase and rt-PA alike) than in the surgical group: 6.2% versus 0.8%.

A subgroup of patients recruited in the STILE study, who suffered from occluded lower extremity bypass grafts, was evaluated separately.[12] Methods of treatment and endpoints were those of the STILE study. In this cohort of 124 patients, catheter positioning failed in 39% of the 78 lysis intention-to-treat patients. Successful catheter placement was not dependent upon the age or the type of the graft, or the duration of the occlusion. Patency of the occluded graft was restored in 84% after successful positioning in the catheter, in the thrombolytic group. Once successful regional lytic therapy re-established patency of the occluded graft, long-term outcomes were similar to surgery. Acutely ischemic patients treated with thrombolysis had lower major amputation rates at 30 days and 1 year compared with surgical patients. The STILE study and its subtype analysis for bypass grafts illustrates the difficulty of interpreting results of trials designed to compare thrombolytic with surgical therapy in patients with peripheral arterial thromboembolic occlusion. For instance, the primary endpoint of the bypass graft study indicated that surgery was the best primary treatment for lower extremity bypass graft thrombosis. However, the study attributed the same importance for major limb loss and for correctable ongoing ischemia. Conclusions were different when one considered, not the composite clinical outcome, but the clinical outcome classification. Improvement in the clinical outcome classification considered improvement by at least one clinical category at 30 days. When taking into account the clinical outcome classification, thrombolysis-treated patients fared better than surgically treated patients. This discordance was due to the fact that the clinical outcome

classifications of thrombolysis patients reflected the results of combined lytic and surgical revascularization (when performed after primary failure of lysis), while clinical outcome classification of surgical patients was the result of surgery alone.

Ouriel et al performed two important large studies to compare the efficacy of thrombolytic with surgical therapy. The first trial[13] randomized 114 patients with limb-threatening ischemia of less than 7 days' duration to either intra-arterial catheter directed urokinase, or surgery. Primary endpoints included limb salvage and survival. While limb salvage was similar for both groups (82% at 12 months), survival was better in the thrombolysis group: 84 versus 58% at 12 months.

Preliminary results of the Thrombolysis or Peripheral Arterial Surgery (TOPAS) trial[14] suggested that an initial dose of urokinase of 4000 units/min for 4 hours, followed by 2000 units/min to a maximum of 48 hours, is safe and associated with limb salvage and survival rates similar to those achieved with surgery. The final report of the TOPAS study was published recently.[15] In total 548 patients with arterial obstruction of the legs for 14 days or less, due to embolism, or thrombosis of a native artery, prosthetic or vein graft, were recruited from 113 centers. Patients were randomized to either intra-arterial urokinase or surgery. The primary end point was amputation-free survival at 6 months.

In the urokinase group, amputation-free survival was 71.8% at 6 months and 65% at 12 months, compared with 74.8% and 69.9% in the surgery group, respectively. At 6 months the surgery group had undergone more operative procedures, excluding amputations, as compared with the thrombolysis group. Major bleedings were more frequent in the lysis group. The TOPAS investigators concluded that urokinase may reduce the need for surgical procedures with no increased risk of amputation or death in patients with acute arterial occlusion of the legs. These conclusions were soon criticized on the grounds of a possible selection bias and inappropriate choice of primary endpoints.[16]

Thrombolysis for artery occlusion: a temporary conclusion

Thrombolytic therapy is most effective when given regionally, after successful insertion of the catheter into the thrombus, for patients with acute ischemia (up to 14 days) due to thrombosed lower extremity bypass graft. Since advantage of lytic therapy over surgery as first line treatment, is not proven, most authors still recommend the use of lytic agents in combination with surgery. Since complete removal of the thrombus is often not obtained by surgery, residual distal thrombotic material can be lysed with intraoperative intra-arterial infusions.

Heparins for arterial occlusion

Intravenous unfractionated heparin is usually given immediately after diagnosis of acute arterial occlusion due to thrombosis or system emboli is undertaken, but little has been done in evaluating heparins in patients undergoing arterial revascularization.

Unfractionated heparin was held responsible for the high rates of intracranial hemorrhage when given concurrently to intra-arterial urokinase in several trials, including in the TOPAS trial.[15]

Samama et al[17] studied the role of heparin in the prevention of early graft thrombosis in 201 patients undergoing femorodistal reconstructive surgery. Patients received either enoxaparin or unfractionated heparin before clamping and for another 10 days after surgery. Two-thirds of the patients had autologous venous grafts and 25% had PTFE grafts. At day 10, angiography-proven thrombosed grafts occurred in only 8% of the enoxaparin group compared with 22% in the unfractionated heparin group. Major hemorrhages were similar in both groups. The higher efficacy of enoxaparin in preventing early graft thrombosis was attributed by the investigators to its greater bioavailability and consistent anticoagulant effect.

Efficacy of dalteparin on long-term femoropopliteal graft patency was evaluated by Edmonson et al[18] in 200 patients scheduled to undergo bypass surgery. All patients received dalteparin 2000 units daily during the first week after surgery and were then randomized to either dalteparin 2500 units daily or aspirin 300 mg plus dipyridamole 100 mg every 8 hours for 3 months. The authors concluded that dalteparin was better than the aspirin–dipyridamole combination in maintaining graft patency in patients with critical limb ischemia undergoing surgery. These conclusions were criticized because dalteparin was given to all patients after surgery and before randomization.

Antiplatelet therapy

The Antiplatelet Trialists' Collaboration has reviewed 39 randomized trials of antiplatelet therapy versus control among some 3000 patients with peripheral arterial disease or procedures.[19] Considering only the 14 trials in which vascular occlusion was monitored, antiplatelet therapy was associated with a reduction of 43% in vascular occlusion.

Antiplatelet therapy, when given for an average period of 19 months, produced an absolute reduction of 92 per 1000 patients in the risk of peripheral arterial occlusion: 15.7% in the antiplatelet treated group versus 24.9% in the control group.

Which antiplatelet agent for arterial occlusion?

Although aspirin is an accepted and widely used option for secondary prophylaxis,[20] its

efficiency is still to be proven, and several trials have failed to show significant benefits of aspirin, alone or in association with dipyridamole, as compared with placebo. Kohler et al[21] reported a 2-year patency rate of 58% among patients with infrainguinal saphenous vein grafts assigned to receive aspirin and dipyridamole, a result worse than the 73% rate of patency for the placebo group. McCollum et al[22] confirmed the lack of efficiency of aspirin with dipyridamole, while in contrast, Sheehan et al[23] did find a benefit for the combination in patients with infrainguinal prosthetic grafts. Other newer antiplatelet agents have been developed, among them ticlopidine, clopidogrel and satigrel.[24]

Ticlopidine has been shown to be effective in patients at high risk of arterial thromboembolic events, including transient ischemic attack, stroke, ischemic heart disease and peripheral arterial disease.[25,26]

In a study of patients suffering from intermittent claudication, Bergqvist et al[27] found that ticlopidine is effective in reducing the need for vascular surgery by almost 50%.

In a recently published prospective, double-blind randomized study that included 243 patients, Becquemin[28] assessed the efficacy of ticlopidine on the long-term patency of saphenous vein bypass graft in peripheral vascular disease. At 2 years, ticlopidine significantly improved the patency of the grafts: 66.4% compared with 51.2% in the placebo group. There were also fewer major amputations in the ticlopidine group.

No randomized study has yet compared the effect of combined ticlopidine and aspirin therapy with each drug alone in reducing poststenting thrombotic complications. Bossavy et al[29] used an ex vivo model to study the effect of combined aspirin, 325 mg daily and ticlopidine, 500 mg daily, versus aspirin and ticlopidine alone on arterial thrombogenesis. Platelet thrombus formation was more effectively blocked by the aspirin–ticlopidine combination than by aspirin or ticlopidine alone: 90% reduction of thrombus formation, versus 29 and 15% respectively.

Another 2-thienopyridine derivative, clopidogrel, is 40 times as active as ticlopidine in inhibiting ADP-induced platelet aggregation in animal models. The Clopidogrel versus Aspirin in Patients at Risk of Ischemic Events (CAPRIE) trial,[30] included patients with ischemic cerebrovsacular, cardiac and peripheral arterial disease, to receive clopidogrel 75 mg once daily, or aspirin 325 mg once daily for a minimum of 1 year and a maximum of 3 years. Patients treated with clopidogrel had an annual 5.3% risk of composite outcome of ischemic stroke, myocardial infarction or vascular death compared with 5.8% in the aspirin group, with a similar overall safety profile. In fact those with peripheral arterial disease constituted the only subgroup that had a statistically significant benefit from clopidogrel.

Satigrel is a new antiplatelet agent that strongly inhibits cyclo-oxygenase and phosphodiesterase in vitro and in vivo, platelet adhesion, aggregation and release reaction. A recent small study of nine patients with arteriosclerosis obliterans has shown that satigrel can inhibit platelet accumulation in vascular grafts, and can be useful for preventing postoperative graft occlusion.[31]

When should antiplatelet therapy be started, and for how long?

The Antiplatelet Trialists recommend that antiplatelet therapy be started just before or as early as possible after vascular procedure.[19] The average duration of antiplatelet therapy in most clinical trials is 1 year. Since no comparison of different durations of treatment has been performed so far, it seems logical and safe to continue therapy with platelet antiaggregants for as long as the patient remains at high risk for occlusive vascular complications.

Iloprost

Iloprost is a chemically stable analogue of prostacyclin (epoprostenol) and an effective inhibitor of platelet aggregation.[32] Other biological properties of clinical importance include inhibition of the release reaction of dense granule contents, enhancement of fibrinolytic activity and arterial vasodilation.

Tissue protective properties have also been described. Iloprost has greater metabolic stability than prostacyclin and is given as an intravenous infusion of up to 2 ng/kg per minute for 2–4 weeks. Iloprost has proven beneficial clinical effect in patients with peripheral atherosclerotic obliterative disease, diabetic angiopathy, intermittent claudication, thromboangitis obliterans and Raynaud's phenomenon.

Prostaglandin E₁ (PGE₁)

The efficacy of PGE_1 in severe intermittent claudication has been recently reported in a multicenter double-blind trial[33] in which a 4-week course of PGE_1 improved the walking distance by an average 100%.

PGE_1 improves the perfusion to occluded vessels, possesses important vasodilating and antithrombotic properties, and induces endothelial stabilizing effects.[33]

Direct thrombin inhibitors

Direct thrombin inhibitors have been extensively investigated in acute coronary syndromes.[34–36] Direct thrombin inhibitors, of which recombinant hirudin is the prototype, also include bivalirudin, hirulog, hirugen and argatroban. The potential benefit of these new antithrombotic agents for peripheral arterial disease, deserves to be evaluated in well-designed large-scale multicenter trials.

Oral anticoagulants

Kretschmer and Holzenbein[37] have recently shown the favorable outcome of long-term anticoagulant therapy concerning bypass function, limb salvage and patient survival among 130 patients who received a femoropopliteal bypass.

References

1. Fowkes FGR. Epidemiology of peripheral arterial disease. In: Tooke J, Lowe G, (eds). *A Textbook of Vascular Medicine*. London. Arnold, 1996: 149–161.

2. Murabito JM, D'Agostino RB, Silbershatz H et al. Intermittent claudication: a risk profile from the Framingham study. *Circulation* 1997; **96:** 44–49.

3. Ridker PM. Fibrinolytic and inflammatory markers of arterial occlusion: the evolving epidemiology of thrombosis and hemostasis. *Thromb Haemost* 1997; **78:** 53–59.

4. Clarke R, Daly L, Robinson K et al. Hyperhomocysteinemia: an independent risk factor for vascular disease. *N Engl J Med* 1991; **324:** 1149–1155.

5. Blaisdell FW, Steele M, Allen RE. Management of acute lower extremity arterial ischemia due to embolism and thrombosis. *Surgery* 1978; **84:** 822–834.

6. Frandness DE Jr, Salzman EW, Shortell CK, Marder VJ. Management of peripheral arterial disease. In: Colman RW (ed). *Hemostasis and Thrombosis: Basic Principles and Clinical Practice*. Philadelphia: JB Lippincott, 1994.

7. Marder VJ. Thrombolytic therapy: overview

of results in major vascular occlusions. *Thromb Haemost* 1995; **74**: 101–105.

8. Dotter CT, Rosch J, Seamen AJ. Selective clot lysis with low dose streptokinase. *Radiology* 1974; **111**: 31–37.

9. Parent F III, Plotrowski JJ, Bernhard VM et al. Outcome of intraarterial urokinase for acute vascular occlusion. *J Cardiovasc Surg* 1991; **32**: 680–690.

10. Comerota AJ, Rao AK, Throm RC et al. A prospective, randomized, blinded and placebo-controlled trial of intraoperative intra-arterial urokinase infusion during lower extremity revascularization. *Ann Surg* 1993; **218**: 534–543.

11. Results of a prospective randomized trial evaluating surgery versus thrombolysis for ischemia of the lower extremity: the STILE trial. *Ann Surg* 1994; **220**: 251–268.

12. Comerota AJ, Weaver FA, Hosking JD et al. Results of a prospective randomized trial of surgery versus thrombolysis for occluded lower extremity bypass grafts. *Am J Surg* 1996; **172**: 105–112.

13. Ouriel K, Shortell CK, De Weese JA et al. A comparison of thrombolytic therapy with operative revascularization in the initial treatment of acute peripheral arterial ischemia. *J Vasc Surg* 1985; **2**: 65–78.

14. Ouriel K, Veith FJ, Sasahara AA. Thrombolysis or peripheral arterial surgery: phase I results. *J Vasc Surg* 1996; **23**: 64–73.

15. Ouriel K, Veith FJ, Sasahara AA. A comparison of recombinant urokinase with vascular surgery as initial treatment for acute arterial occlusion of the legs. *N Engl J Med* 1998; **338**: 1105–1111.

16. Porter JM. Thrombolysis for acute arterial occlusion of the legs (editorial). *N Engl J Med* 1998; **338**: 1148–1149.

17. Samama C, Batre E, Combe S. A pilot study on the use of low molecular weight heparin (enoxaparin) in arterial reconstructive surgery. *Thromb Haemost* 1991; **17**: 367–370.

18. Edmondson RA, Cohen AT, Das SK et al. Low-molecular weight heparin versus aspirin and dipyridamole after femoropopliteal bypass grafting. *Lancet* 1994; **344**: 914–918.

19. Antiplatelet Trialists' Collaboration. Collaborative overview of randomised trials of antiplatelet therapy. II: Maintenance of vascular graft or arterial patency by antiplatelet therapy. *BMJ* 1994; **308**: 159–168.

20. Guidelines on oral anticoagulation: third edition. *Br J Haematol* 1998; **101**: 374–387.

21. Kohler TR, Kaufman HJI, Kacoyanis G et al. Effect of aspirin and dipyridamole on the patency of lower extremity bypass grafts. *Surgery* 1984; **96**: 462–466.

22. McCollum C, Alexander C, Kenchington G et al. Antiplatelet drugs in femoropopliteal vein bypasses: a multicenter trial. *J Vasc Surg* 1991; **13**: 150–161.

23. Sheehan SJ, Salter MCP, Donaldson DR et al. Five year follow up of long-term aspirin/dipyridamole in femoropopliteal Dacron bypass grafts (abstract). *Br J Surg* 1987; **74**: 330.

24. Verstraete M, Zoldhelic P. Novel antithrombotic drugs in development. *Drugs* 1995; **49**: 856–884.

25. Gent M, Blakely JA, Easton JD et al. The Canadian American Ticlopidine Study (CATS) in thromboembolic stroke. *Lancet* 1989; **i**: 1215–1220.

26. Hass WK, Easton JD, Adams HP et al. A

randomized trial comparing ticlopidine hydrochloride with aspirin for the prevention of stroke in high-risk patients. *N Engl J Med* 1989; **321**: 501–502.

27. Bergqvist D, Almgren B, Dickinson JP. Reduction of requirement for leg vascular surgery during long term treatment of claudicant patients with ticlopidine: results from the Swedish Ticlopidine Multicentre study (STMS). *Eur J Vasc Endovasc Surg* 1995; **10**: 69–76.

28. Becquemin JP. Effect of ticlopidine on the long-term patency of saphenous-vein-by-pass grafts in the legs. *N Engl J Med* 1997; **337**: 1726–1731.

29. Bossavy JP, Thalarnas C, Sagnard L et al. A double-blind randomized comparison of combined aspirin and ticlopidine therapy versus aspirin or ticlopidine alone on experimental arterial thrombogenesis in humans. *Blood* 1998; **92**: 1518–1525.

30. CAPRIE Steering Committee. A randomised, blinded, trial of clopidogrel versus aspirin in patients at risk of ischaemic events (CAPRIE). *Lancet* 1996; **348**: 1329–1339.

31. Esato K, Kubo Y, Yauda K et al. Satigrel, a new antiplatelet agent, inhibits platelet accumulation in prosthetic arterial grafts. *Am J Surg* 1998; **175**: 56–60.

32. Grant SM, Goa KL. Iloprost. A review of its pharmacodynamic and pharmacokinetic properties, and therapeutic potential in peripheral vascular disease, myocardial ischaemia and extracorporeal circulation procedures. *Drugs* 1992; **43**: 889–924.

33. Belcaro G, Laurora G, Nicolaides AN et al. Treatment of severe intermittent claudication with PGE$_1$. A short-term versus a long-term infusion plan. *Angiology* 1998; **49**: 885–895.

34. The Global Use of Strategies to Open Occluded Coronary Arteries (GUSTO) IIb Investigators. A comparison of recombinant hirudin with heparin for the treatment of acute coronary syndromes. *N Engl J Med* 1996; **335**: 775–782.

35. Antman EM. Hirudin in acute myocardial infarction. Thrombolysis and Thrombin Inhibition in Myocardial Infarction (TIMI) 9B trial. *Circulation* 1996; **94**: 911–921.

36. Serruys PW, Herman JP, Simon P et al. for the HELVETICA Investigators. A comparison of hirudin with heparin in the prevention of restenosis after coronary angioplasty. *N Engl J Med* 1995; **333**: 757–763.

37. Kretschmer G, Holzenbein T. Oral anticoagulation in peripheral vascular surgery: how intense, for how long, or at all? *J Int Med* 1999; **245**: 389–397.

Prevention and treatment of venous thrombosis and pulmonary embolism

14

Sam Schulman

In the prevention of venous thromboembolism, the risk of haemorrhagic complications of the chosen method has always to be weighed against the potential benefit achieved. The haemorrhagic risk is negligible with physical methods of prevention, but these techniques are not sufficiently effective on their own. Pharmacological methods of prevention carry a risk of bleeding that is usually proportional to the intensity of the preventive effect. The benefit that can be expected, depends not only on the effectiveness of the technique but also on the magnitude of the risk of thromboembolism. Thus, in situations with a pronounced risk of thromboembolism, highly effective prophylactic agents are required, and a slightly increased risk of bleeding may be justified. However, in some situations haemorrhagic complications will have detrimental results, for example in neurosurgery, and a moderate risk of thromboembolism has to be accepted. The acquired risk factors for thrombosis are reviewed in Chapter 4 whereas inherited risks are discussed in Chapter 3.

Thromboprophylactic methods

General

Simple and sometimes obvious ways of reducing the risk of thromboembolism include discontinuation of combined oral contraceptives a month before elective surgery, appropriate perioperative fluid substitution, the use of local or regional rather than general anaesthesia, atraumatic surgical technique, prompt treatment of infections and early mobilization after surgery, trauma, stroke or myocardial infarction. The difference between the modes of anaesthesia can be explained by the fact that an epidural block postpones the increase of factor VIII and von Willebrand factor, induced by trauma,[1] and this is associated with the blocking of nociceptive afferents.

Physical methods

The effects of physiotherapy and early mobilization after surgery have not been assessed objectively. The prophylactic effect of compression stockings, which should be graduated, has been quite variable in different studies. In a meta-analysis of 12 trials the risk reduction was 68% (95% confidence interval 53–73%).[2] The studies included concerned mainly abdominal, gynaecological and neurosurgery. The addition of low molecular weight heparin to compression stockings in neurosurgery decreased the incidence of

thrombosis further from 32 to 17%.[3] In another meta-analysis, intermittent pneumatic compression of the legs resulted in a 62% reduction of deep-vein thrombosis, compared to placebo. Furthermore, the effect was 42% better than with compression stockings (*Figure 14.1*).[4] Still, intermittent pneumatic compression is regarded as a cumbersome technique and has not been widely adopted.

Pharmacological methods

The agents most commonly used are unfractionated heparin alone or in combination with dihydroergotamine, low molecular weight heparins, heparinoids, dextran and vitamin K antagonists. Recent trials have demonstrated that direct thrombin inhibitors, such as desirudin and napsagatran also may become valuable alternatives (see Chapter 9).

Unfractionated heparin is either given in a fixed dose, which is usually 5000 U, starting from 2 hours before surgery and repeated every 8–12 hours, or in a dose, which is adjusted postoperatively to maintain a slight prolongation of the activated partial thromboplastin time. In an overview of more than 70 randomized trials with 16 000 patients in general orthopaedic and urological surgery low-dose heparin resulted in a risk reduction of deep-vein thrombosis of 67%, 68% and 75%, respectively.[5] There was also a 64% reduction of fatal pulmonary embolism

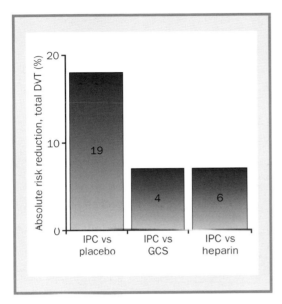

Figure 14.1
Pooled analysis of effectiveness of intermittent pneumatic compression (IPC) devices versus placebo, graduated compression stockings (GCS) or minidose heparin, measured as absolute risk reduction of total deep-vein thrombosis. Numbers inside bars are number of studies included. Data adapted from Vanek.[4]

from 0.9 to 0.3%. The risk of bleeding, but not of fatal haemorrhage, increased, especially in patients with urological surgery.[5]

The regimen with dihydroergotamine in combination with low-dose heparin has largely been abandoned due to the risk of vasospasm.[6]

Low molecular weight heparins (see also Chapters 7 and 8) have mainly been compared with unfractionated heparin rather than placebo for ethical reasons. It has not been possible to demonstrate a further reduction of pulmonary embolism, whether fatal or not, by low molecular weight heparin in comparison with unfractionated heparin. The efficacy in

general surgery has been comparable, whereas low molecular weight heparin is more effective than fixed-dose unfractionated heparin and than warfarin in total hip replacement and more effective than warfarin in total knee replacement.[7] In hip fracture surgery low molecular weight heparins are equally effective to adjusted-dose vitamin K antagonists.[7] The benefits of low molecular weight heparins are that they can be given once daily, that there is no need for monitoring and adjustment of the dose and that there is a lower risk of heparin-induced thrombocytopenia than with unfractionated heparin.[7]

Dextran is a branched polysaccharide and

it is usually the 70 000 Da variant (dextran 70) that has been used in thromboprophylaxis, mainly in Scandinavia. Dextran lowers the risk of fatal pulmonary embolism[8] but it is inferior to unfractionated and low molecular weight heparin in the prevention of deep-vein thrombosis. Dextran is expensive, causes anaphylactic reactions — albeit preventable with a haptene — and sometimes volume overload. The latter feature can be turned into an advantage, by using dextran as a simultaneous plasma expander.

Vitamin K antagonists, mostly warfarin, are used in different dose ranges. Minidose warfarin, which is approximately 1 mg daily, does not require monitoring, prevents thrombus formation on indwelling catheters[9] and prevents venous thromboembolism in gynaecological surgery[10] and in patients with metastatic breast cancer treated with chemotherapy.[11] For other situations, when a higher intensity of anticoagulation is needed, for example orthopaedic surgery, minidose is not sufficient and the dose has to be adjusted to maintain an international normalized ratio (INR) of about 2–3. This requires daily monitoring during the perioperative period, or else the risk of haemorrhage becomes high, and therefore this method is chosen infrequently. In the secondary prophylaxis after venous thromboembolism adjusted dose of a vitamin K antagonist is, however, standard, since the risk of haemorrhage is much lower than perioperatively and monitoring during long-term prophylaxis can be less frequent (see below).

Strategies for prevention of venous thromboembolism

Low-risk surgery

When minor surgery or procedures lasting less than 30 minutes are performed or the patients are under 40 years of age the risk of thromboembolic complications is low and prophylactic methods are only required in case additional risk factors are present, such as inherited thrombophilia (Chapter 3) or cancer. It may be sufficient to use elastic stockings for some of those patients with additional risks, but intermittent pneumatic compression, unfractionated or low molecular weight heparin are more effective.

Intermediate-risk surgery

In case of general surgery lasting longer than 30 minutes in patients older than 40 years without additional risk factors the risk is considered as 'intermediate.' The same is valid for women less than 40 years of age, in whom combined oral contraceptives were not discontinued 1 month before surgery. The prophylactic methods that provide efficacy and safety are intermittent pneumatic compression, unfractionated heparin 5000 U every 12 hours or low molecular weight heparin once daily. The latter includes dalteparin 2500 U, enoxaparin 20 mg or 2000 U, nadroparin 3100 U and tinzaparin 3500 U.[7] The first dose of all these agents is usually injected 1–2 hours before surgery.

High-risk surgery

The risk is high when the operated patient has had previous venous thromboembolism, when major surgery is performed for malignant disease or in case of major orthopaedic surgery of the lower limbs or pelvis. For gynaecological surgery, including cancer surgery, minidose warfarin is also effective and safe.[10] In other kinds of high-risk surgery, unfractionated heparin 5000 U every 8 hours, low molecular weight heparin once or twice daily, dextran or intermittent pneumatic compression are appropriate alternatives. The regimens evaluated with low molecular weight heparins are: ardeparin 50 U/kg twice daily, dalteparin 5000 U once daily, enoxaparin 4000 U (40 mg) once daily or 3000 U (30 mg) twice daily, nadroparin 40 U/kg once daily for 3 days followed by 60 U/kg once daily, tinzaparin 75 U/kg once daily or 50 U/kg twice daily.[7] The first dose has for some of these agents been given before surgery (2, 8 or 12 hours) and for others 12–24 hours after surgery. The former probably reduces the risk of thromboembolism further and the latter the risk of haemorrhage.

Multiple trauma

In the prevention of venous thromboembolism after major trauma, enoxaparin at a dose of 30 mg once daily was more effective than low-dose unfractionated heparin.[12] Although there were five and one major haemorrhages, respectively, this difference was not statistically significant. In subacute myelopathy, whether traumatic or due to a medical disease, the risk of venous thromboembolism is high and also here enoxaparin seems to be more effective than unfractionated heparin.[13]

Nonhaemorrhagic stroke

The hemiparesis and immobilization result in an incidence of deep-vein thrombosis of 63% in pooled analysis,[7] and subsequent pulmonary embolism is responsible for 5% of early deaths. In trials with low-dose heparin, an average relative risk reduction of 63% was achieved, and with low molecular weight heparin the corresponding figure was 75%.[7]

Myocardial Infarction

The incidence of deep-vein thrombosis of 24% in patients with myocardial infarction is reduced by 71% with low-dose heparin and by 86% with high-dose heparin in pooled analysis.[7]

Other medical conditions

The reason for pulmonary embolism remaining a major cause of death, as evidenced by a general autopsy material,[14] is not only insufficient postoperative prophylaxis but to a large extent a neglect of the risk in medical patients. With the relatively lower risk of haemorrhage these patients are excellent candidates for prophylaxis with low-dose heparin, low molecular weight heparin or for long-term prophylaxis with vitamin K antagonists.

In a large multicentre trial (MEDENOX) 866 evaluable patients had received 20 or 40 mg enoxaparin or placebo once daily.[15] There was a significant reduction of venographically detected deep-vein thrombosis in the 40 mg group, and a non-significant reduction of mortality at 110 days. Since only six of the cases with deep-vein thrombosis were symptomatic (3, 1 and 2, respectively, in the groups) and there was no fatal pulmonary embolism, the cost–benefit of this approach requires clarification.

In patients with cancer, prophylaxis with adjusted-dose warfarin may be difficult to stabilize if the patient has frequent courses of chemotherapy with concomitant drug interactions. Furthermore, it is not unusual that patients with adenocarcinoma suffer from a pronounced tendency to develop deep-vein thrombosis with recurrence while on therapeutic anticoagulation with vitamin K antagonists. In these cases long-term prophylaxis with low molecular weight heparin is a promising alternative.

Pregnancy

In patients with inherited thrombophilia and/or with previous thromboembolic episodes the risk of new events during pregnancy and especially during the puerperium is high (see also Chapter 3). In a series of 34 pregnant patients with a moderate–high risk of recurrence, dalteparin, adjusted to achieve a peak antifactor Xa level of 0.4–0.6 IU/ml and a nadir of 0.15–0.20 IU/ml, proved effective and safe.[16]

Treatment of venous thromboembolism

Acute phase

The concept that it is crucial to anticoagulate in case of established venous thromboembolism derives partly from a controlled study in patients with pulmonary embolism, in which none of 16 patients treated with heparin but 10 of 19 control patients had a recurrence during 14 days of follow-up.[17] That this is also true for proximal deep-vein thrombosis was demonstrated in a trial where initial treatment with heparin in combination with secondary prophylaxis with a vitamin K antagonist was compared with the latter alone.[18] The rate of recurrence during 6 months of follow-up was 6.7 and 20%, respectively. The same kind of evidence does not exist for calf-vein thrombosis. Nevertheless, this is not a harmless condition, since in a comparison of initial heparin therapy combined with maintenance prophylaxis with warfarin versus warfarin alone, 4.3% versus 32.1%, respectively, suffered from a recurrent episode during the following year.[19]

Treatment with unfractionated heparin requires monitoring to verify adequate prolongation of the activated partial thromboplastin time (APTT) to 2–3 times the control value. By the use of a weight-based nomogram for dosing of heparin a higher proportion of the APTTs is within the therapeutic range and the risk of recurrence during 3 months can be reduced from 25% with the standard dosing of heparin to 5%.[20] Unfractionated heparin had been administered intravenously for decades until it was shown that subcutaneous injections twice daily are feasible and permit faster mobilization of the patients. In a meta-analysis of six trials subcutaneously injected unfractionated heparin was more effective than intravenous infusion, with an incidence of recurrent venous thromboembolism of 6.4 versus 10.5%, respectively.[21]

Low molecular weight heparin

During the past decade a substantial number of trials and also several meta-analyses have demonstrated that low molecular weight heparins are effective and safe in the treatment of deep-vein thrombosis. The comparison was invariably with unfractionated heparin intravenously, which is unfortunate, since that mode of administration appears to be disadvantageous. The odds ratios in favour of low molecular weight heparin were in one of these meta-analyses 0.53 for recurrent episodes, 0.68 for clinically important bleeding and 0.47 for death[22] (*Figure 14.2*). The difference in the rate of major haemorrhage relies heavily on one large trial, in which 75% of the patients allocated to unfractionated heparin received initially a rather high dose of 40 000 IU/24h, which may have been a disadvantage to that group.[23]

Patients with symptomatic pulmonary embolism were excluded in all these trials, although it is widely accepted that deep-vein thrombosis and pulmonary embolism are one and the same disease. During recent years it has, however, been shown that subcutaneous low molecular weight heparin is equally effective and safe in symptomatic, submassive pulmonary embolism, both for fraxiparine,[24] dalteparin,[25] reviparin[26] and tinzaparin.[27]

Owing to the almost complete bioavailability of low molecular weight heparins after subcutaneous injections, there is a predictable dose–response relationship and with a weight-adjusted dose there is no need for monitoring antifactor Xa-levels, at least during short-term therapy but probably during prophylaxis in connection with pregnancy. Another advantageous feature of

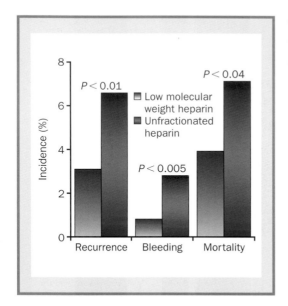

Figure 14.2
Comparison of outcome and adverse events of low molecular weight heparin and unfractionated heparin in the treatment of deep-vein thrombosis. (Data adapted from Lensing et al.[22])

the low molecular weight heparins is the longer half-life compared to unfractionated heparin, allowing for once daily injections in most situations. In a randomized comparison nadroparin once daily was at least as effective and safe as the same dose divided into two daily injections in the treatment of deep-vein thrombosis.[28] Owing to these features low molecular weight heparins are suitable for outpatient treatment. Two multicentre randomized trials have convincingly demonstrated the safety and efficacy of an outpatient regimen for the initial treatment of deep-vein thrombosis (*Figure 14.3*).[29,30]

Thrombolysis

The rationale for thrombolytic therapy in deep-vein thrombosis is to rapidly resolve the thrombus before permanent damage has occurred to the venous valves, in order to avoid the postthrombotic syndrome in the future. Although many studies have demonstrated a higher number of cases with completely resolved thrombus within the first 1–2 weeks, few have included a long-term follow-up in the design. In a pooled analysis of four randomized studies, comparing unfractionated heparin with streptokinase and with follow-up for 7–134 months, 67 and 28%, respectively, of the patients had

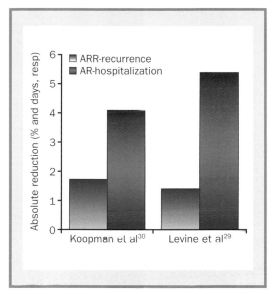

Figure 14.3
Absolute reduction of risk of recurrent venous thromboembolism (%) and of days of hospitalization with low molecular weight heparin subcutaneously versus unfractionated heparin intravenously. (Data adapted from Levine et al[29] and Koopman et al.[30])

symptoms compatible with the postthrombotic syndrome.[31–34] There was, however, only a total of 120 patients in these studies, with a follow up of less than 2 years in two of those.

Recombinant human tissue-type plasminogen activator (rt-PA), whether given alone at a dose of 0.05 mg/kg per hour or together with heparin for 24 h resulted in a greater than 50% lysis in 28–29% of the patients versus 0% with heparin alone in another trial with relatively few patients.[35] One of the 53 patients treated with rt-PA had a nonfatal intracranial haemorrhage. This dreaded complication is taking its toll in patients treated with streptokinase. In a review

of 28 studies of deep-vein thrombosis with 1127 and 2305 patients treated with streptokinase and heparin, respectively, the incidence of fatal complications was 1.8 and 0.6%, respectively.[36] In a pooled analysis of three randomized trials major haemorrhage was 2.9 times more prevalent in patients treated with streptokinase than with heparin.[37]

Based on these data it is prudent to refrain from thrombolytic therapy in the vast majority of patients with deep-vein thrombosis. Only for young patients with a very low risk of haemorrhage and iliofemoral thrombosis or phlegmasia coerulea dolens should this alternative be considered.

In pulmonary embolism, treatment with urokinase or streptokinase provides, in comparison with heparin, a more rapid resolution of the emboli on repeated lung scanning and faster haemodynamic normalization, but no study has demonstrated any benefit regarding mortality.[38,39] The thrombolytic effect of rt-PA is even faster than with urokinase, resulting in clot lysis after 2 h in 82 and 48%, respectively, but after 24 h the scintigraphic result is equal.[40] Although rt-PA improves right ventricular wall motion after 24 h to a much higher extent than does heparin,[41] again a possible benefit on mortality or long-term outcome has never been demonstrated. The choice of thrombolytic therapy should therefore be reserved for patients with a haemodynamically unstable condition due to massive pulmonary embolism or due to submassive embolism in combination with pre-existing cardiopulmonary disease with limited function. Established regimens are shown in *Table 14.1*.

Interruption of inferior vena cava

The major indication for insertion of a filter in inferior vena cava is recurrent pulmonary embolism in spite of adequate anticoagulant therapy. There is rarely a situation when the procedure is required due to contraindication for anticoagulation, since the latter is hardly ever absolute. Although the filter reduces the risk of short-term pulmonary embolism compared to heparin, there is no difference in mortality after 2 years and almost twice as many patients treated with the filter have a recurrent deep-vein thrombosis within 2 years.[43]

Secondary prophylaxis

When the initial treatment for venous thromboembolism is not accompanied by secondary prophylaxis the risk of an early recurrence is high, even for patients with calf-vein thrombosis — recurrence rate 32% during the first year.[44] Maintenance

Table 14.1
Recommended regimens for the treatment of venous thromboembolism.[20,42] For the low molecular weight heparins the doses are different for each product.

Agent	Bolus dose	Maintenance dose	Duration
Unfractionated heparin	80 U/kg	500 U/kg per 24 h	≥ 5 days
Streptokinase	250 000 IU	100 000 IU/h	DVT: 72 h; PE: 24 h
Urokinase	4400 IU/kg	2200 IU/kg	DVT: 48 h; PE: 12 h
rt-PA	10 mg/1–2 min	45 mg/h	PE: 2 h

prophylaxis is usually provided with vitamin K antagonists, aiming at an INR of 2.0–3.0.[45] The prophylaxis may be discontinued after 6 weeks in patients with calf-vein thrombosis and an identified temporary risk factor, such as surgery.[46] In all other subgroups the risk of recurrence during 2 years is reduced to half if the prophylaxis is prolonged from 6 weeks to 6 months, and there is no appreciable increase in the risk of haemorrhage.[46] For the patients who discontinue the anticoagulation after 6 weeks there is a rapid accumulation of recurrent events up to 6 months (*Figure 14.4*). The same is true if the prophylaxis is discontinued after 3 months in patients with idiopathic venous thromboembolism.[47] The

impact of a proximal extension of the deep-vein thrombus or presence of symptomatic pulmonary embolism is equal to the importance of absence of known risk factors.[48] For patients with a second episode of venous thromboembolism extended anticoagulation is far more effective than 6 months but there is a trend to more major haemorrhages after 4 years with the former alternative.[49] This suggests two possible solutions, either a period of full anticoagulation, limited to 1–2 years, or a switch after 6 or 12 months to a lower intensity of anticoagulation to avoid haemorrhages. The latter is currently being evaluated in multicentre randomized trials. For patients with antiphospholipid

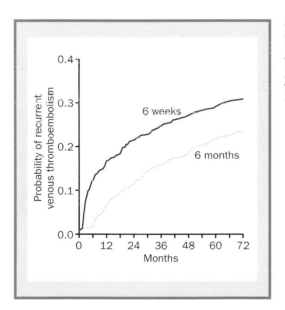

Figure 14.4
*Probability of recurrent venous thromboembolism during 6 years in patients treated with vitamin K antagonists for 6 weeks or 6 months after the first event. (From Schulman et al.[49] Wien med Wschr 1999; **149**: 67 with permission from Blackwell Wissenschafts-Verlag GmbH.)*

antibodies,[50] hyperhomocysteinemia[51] or active cancer there is a need for long-term anticoagulation due to the high risk of recurrence (see also Chapter 4).

As an alternative to vitamin K antagonists low molecular weight heparin may be used, as demonstrated in three randomized trials.[52–54] It seems, however, as if the dose of dalteparin 5000 IU or of enoxaparin 4000 IU (40 mg) once daily is slightly too low and that efficacy would improve with a dose that is 50–100% higher. For patients with a short duration of secondary prophylaxis, unstable prothrombin times, increased risk of haemorrhage, difficulties in arranging for proper monitoring or pregnancy, low molecular weight heparin is definitely an attractive alternative.

Conclusion

The current knowledge and recommendations for prophylaxis and treatment of venous thromboembolism are based on a large number of randomized, controlled trials of sufficient size. Each trial, which results in a valid conclusion will naturally evoke new questions. One example is the study demonstrating that 6 months of secondary prophylaxis with vitamin K antagonists is superior to 6 weeks in most cases. This leads to questions whether even further extension of the prophylaxis would be optimal, what subgroups benefit more than others and if the

intensity should be lowered at any certain time point. However, some of those may not require new trials in case novel, simple oral anticoagulants, such as direct thrombin inhibitors will prove to be safer, easier to use and effective. The ideal drug should be administered orally, have a rapid onset of its effect, have a wide therapeutic margin and no interactions with other drugs or food.

References

1. Bredbacka S, Blombäck M, Hägnevik K et al. Per- and postoperative changes in coagulation and fibrinolytic variables during abdominal hysterectomy under epidural or general anaesthesia. *Acta Anaesthesiol Scand* 1986; **30**: 204–210.

2. Wells PS, Lensing AW, Hirsh J. Graduated compression stockings in the prevention of postoperative venous thromboembolism. A meta-analysis. *Arch Intern Med* 1994; **154**: 67–72.

3. Agnelli G, Piovella F, Buoncristiani P et al. Enoxaparin plus compression stockings compared with compression stockings alone in the prevention of venous thromboembolism after elective neurosurgery. *N Engl J Med* 1998; **339**: 80–85.

4. Vanek VW. Meta-analysis of effectiveness of intermittent pneumatic compression devices with a comparison of thigh-high to knee-high sleeves. *Am Surg* 1998; **64**: 1050–1058.

5. Collins R, Scrimgeour A, Yusuf S, Peto R. Reduction in fatal pulmonary embolism and venous thrombosis by perioperative administration of subcutaneous heparin. *N Engl J Med* 1988; **318**: 1162–1173.

6. European Consensus Statement. Prevention of venous thromboembolism. *Int Angiol* 1992; **11**: 151–159.

7. Clagett GP, Anderson FA, Geerts WH et al. Prevention of venous thromboembolism. *Chest* 1998; **114** (Suppl): 531S–560S.

8. Kline A, Hughes LE, Campbell H et al. Dextran 70 in prophylaxis of thromboembolic disease after surgery: a clinically oriented randomized double-blind trial. *BMJ* 1975; **ii:** 109–112.

9. Bern MM, Lokich JJ, Wallach SR et al. Very low doses of warfarin can prevent thrombosis in central venous catheters. A randomized prospective trial. *Ann Intern Med* 1990; **112:** 423–428.

10. Poller L, McKernan A, Thomson JM et al. Fixed minidose warfarin: a new approach to prophylaxis against venous thrombosis after major surgery. *Br Med J Clin Res Ed* 1987; **295:** 1309–1312.

11. Levine M, Hirsh J, Gent M et al. Double-blind randomised trial of a very-low-dose warfarin for prevention of thromboembolism in stage IV breast cancer. *Lancet* 1994; **343:** 886–889.

12. Geerts WH, Jay RM, Code KI et al. A comparison of low-dose heparin with low-molecular-weight heparin as prophylaxis against venous thromboembolism after major trauma. *N Engl J Med* 1996; **335:** 701–707.

13. Spivack SB, Aisen ML. A comparison of low molecular weight heparin and low dose unfractionated heparin prophylaxis in subacute myelopathy. *J Spinal Cord Med* 1997; **20:** 402–405.

14. Karwinsky B. The significance of autopsy in modern medicine. A study from western Norway. Thesis, University of Bergen, Norway, 1995.

15. Samama MM, Cohen AT, Darmon J-Y et al. A comparison of enoxaparin with placebo for the prevention of venous thromboembolism in acutely ill medical patients. *N Engl J Med* 1999; **341:** 793–800.

16. Hunt BJ, Doughty H-A, Majumdar G et al. Thromboprophylaxis with low molecular weight heparin (Fragmin) in high risk pregnancies. *Thromb Haemost* 1997; **77:** 39–43.

17. Barritt DW, Jordan SC. Anticoagulant drugs in the treatment of pulmonary embolism. *Lancet* 1960; **i:** 1309–1312.

18. Brandjes DPM, Heijboer H, Büller HM et al. Acenocoumarol and heparin compared with acenocoumarol alone in the initial treatment of proximal-vein thrombosis. *N Engl J Med* 1992; **327:** 1485–1489.

19. Lagerstedt CL, Olsson CG, Fagher BO et al. Need for long-term anticoagulant treatment in symptomatic calf deep-vein thrombosis. *Lancet* 1985; **ii:** 515–518.

20. Raschke RA, Reilly BM, Guidry JR et al. The weight-based heparin dosing nomogram compared with a 'standard care nomogram'. *Ann Intern Med* 1993; **119:** 874–881.

21. Hommes DW, Bura A, Mazzolai L et al. Subcutaneous heparin compared with continuous intravenous heparin administration in the initial treatment of deep vein thrombosis. *Ann Intern Med* 1992; **116:** 279–284.

22. Lensing AWA, Prins MH, Davidson BL, Hirsh J. Treatment of deep venous thrombosis with low-molecular-weight heparins. *Arch Intern Med* 1995; **155:** 601–607.

23. Hull RD, Raskob GE, Pineo GF et al. Subcutaneous low-molecular-weight heparin compared with continuous intravenous

heparin in the treatment of proximal-vein thrombosis. *N Engl J Med* 1992; **326:** 975–982.

24. Théry C, Simonneau G, Meyer G et al. Randomized trial of subcutaneous low-molecular-weight heparin CY 216 (fraxiparine) compared with intravenous unfractionated heparin in the curative treatment of submassive pulmonary embolism. A dose-ranging study. *Circulation* 1992; **85:** 1380–1389.

25. Meyer G, Brenot F, Pacouret G et al. Subcutaneous low-molecular-weight heparin Fragmin versus intravenous unfractionated heparin in the treatment of acute non massive pulmonary embolism: an open randomized pilot study. *Thromb Haemost* 1995; **74:** 1432–1435.

26. The Columbus Investigators. Low-molecular-weight heparin in the treatment of patients with venous thromboembolism. *N Engl J Med* 1997; **337:** 657–662.

27. Simmoneau G, Sors H, Charbonnier B et al. A comparison of low-molecular-weight heparin with unfractionated heparin for acute pulmonary embolism. *N Engl J Med* 1997; **337:** 663–669.

28. Charbonnier BA, Fiessinger J-N, Banga JD et al. Comparison of a once daily with a twice daily subcutaneous low molecular weight heparin in the treatment of deep vein thrombosis. *Thromb Haemost* 1998; **79:** 897–901.

29. Levine M, Gent M, Hirsh J et al. A comparison of low-molecular-weight heparin administered primarily at home with unfractionated heparin administered in the hospital for proximal deep-vein thrombosis. *N Engl J Med* 1996; **334:** 677–681.

30. Koopman MM, Prandoni P, Piovella F et al.

Treatment of venous thrombosis with intravenous unfractionated heparin administered in the hospital as compared with subcutaneous low-molecular-weight heparin administered at home. *N Engl J Med* 1996; **334:** 682–687.

31. Common HH, Seaman AJ, Rösch J et al. Deep vein thrombosis treated with streptokinase or heparin. Follow-up of a randomized study. *Angiology* 1976; **27:** 645–654.

32. Elliot MS, Immelman EJ, Jeffery P et al. A comparative randomized trial of heparin versus streptokinase in the treatment of acute proximal venous thrombosis: an interim report of a prospective trial. *Br J Surg* 1979; **66:** 838–843.

33. Johansson L, Nylander G, Hedner U, Nilsson IM. Comparison of streptokinase with heparin: late results in the treatment of deep venous thrombosis. *Acta Med Scand* 1979; **206:** 93–98.

34. Arnesen H, Høiseth A, Ly B. Streptokinase or heparin in the treatment of deep vein thrombosis. Follow-up results of a prospective study. *Acta Med Scand* 1982; **211:** 65–68.

35. Goldhaber SZ, Meyerovitz MF, Green D et al. Randomized controlled trial of tissue plasminogen activator in proximal deep venous thrombosis. *Am J Med* 1990; **88:** 235–240.

36. Schulman S. Studies on the medical treatment of deep vein thrombosis. *Acta Med Scand* 1985; Suppl 704: 1–68.

37. Goldhaber SZ, Buring JE, Lipnick RJ, Hennekens CH. Pooled analysis of randomized trials of streptokinase and heparin in phlebographically documented acute deep venous thrombosis. *Am J Med* 1984; **76:** 393–397.

38. Urokinase Pulmonary Embolism Trial. Phase I results. *JAMA* 1970; **214**: 2163–2172.

39. Urokinase Streptokinase Pulmonary Embolism Trial. Phase II results. *JAMA* 1974; **229**: 1606–1613.

40. Goldhaber SZ, Kessler CM, Heit J et al. Randomised controlled trial of recombinant tissue plasminogen activator versus urokinase in the treatment of acute pulmonary embolism. *Lancet* 1988; **ii**: 293–298.

41. Goldhaber SZ, Haire WD, Feldstein ML et al. Alteplase versus heparin in acute pulmonary embolism: randomised trial assessing right-ventricular function and pulmonary perfusion. *Lancet* 1993; **341**: 507–511.

42. Hyers TM, Agnelli G, Hull RD et al. Antithrombotic therapy for venous thromboembolic disease. *Chest* 1998; **114** (Suppl): 561S–578S.

43. Decousus H, Leizorovicz A, Parent F et al. A clinical trial of vena caval filters in the prevention of pulmonary embolism in patients with proximal deep-vein thrombosis. *N Engl J Med* 1998; **338**: 409–415.

44. Lagerstedt CL, Olsson CG, Fagher BO et al. Need for long-term anticoagulant treatment in symptomatic calf deep-vein thrombosis. *Lancet* 1985; **ii**: 515–518.

45. Hull R, Hirsh J, Jay R et al. Different intensities of oral anticoagulant therapy in the treatment of proximal-vein thrombosis. *N Engl J Med* 1982; **307**: 1676–1681.

46. Schulman S, Rhedin A-S, Lindmarker P et al. A comparison of six weeks with six months of oral anticoagulant therapy after a first therapy of venous thromboembolism. *N Engl J Med* 1995; **332**: 1661–1665.

47. Kearon C, Gent M, Hirsh J et al. A comparison of three months of anticoagulation with extended anticoagulation for a first episode of idiopathic venous thromboembolism. *N Engl J Med* 1999; **340**: 901–907.

48. Schulman S and the Duration of Anticoagulation Study Group. The effect of the duration of anticoagulation and other risk factors on the recurrence of venous thromboembolism. *Wien Med Wochenschr* 1999; **149**: 66–69.

49. Schulman S, Granqvist S, Holmström M et al. The duration of oral anticoagulant therapy after a second episode of venous thromboembolism. *N Engl J Med* 1997; **336**: 393–398.

50. Schulman S, Svenungsson E, Granqvist S and the Duration of Anticoagulation Trial Study Group. The predictive value of anticardiolipin antibodies in patients with venous thromboembolism. *Am J Med* 1998; **104**: 332–338.

51. Eichinger S, Stümpflen A, Hirschl M et al. Hyperhomocysteinemia is a risk factor of recurrent venous thromboembolism. *Thromb Haemost* 1998; **80**: 566–569.

52. Monreal M, Lafoz E, Olive A et al. Comparison of subcutaneous unfractionated heparin with a low molecular weight heparin (Fragmin) in patients with venous thromboembolism and contraindications to coumarin. *Thromb Haemost* 1994; **71**: 7–11.

53. Pini M, Aiello S, Manotti C et al. Low molecular weight heparin versus warfarin in the prevention of recurrences after deep vein thrombosis. *Thromb Haemost* 1994; **72**: 191–197.

54. Das SK, Cohen AT, Edmondson RA et al. Low molecular weight heparin versus warfarin for prevention of recurrent venous thromboembolism: a randomized trial. *World J Surg* 1996; **20**: 521–527.

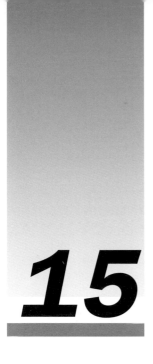

Gestational thrombosis and pregnancy loss: role of antithrombotic therapy

Benjamin Brenner

15

Epidemiology of gestational venous thrombosis

The risk of venous thromboembolism increases two- to four-fold during pregnancy, and increases significantly in the postpartum period. The risk is higher in patients with heritable or acquired thrombophilia, and in fact, most gestational venous thrombotic events can be related to thrombophilia, in particular to factor V Leiden, factor II G20210A mutation, hyperhomocysteinemia and antiphospholipid syndrome.[1,2] Women with other less common inherited thrombophilias such as protein C or protein S deficiency may also manifest thrombosis during pregnancy or the postpartum period.[3,4] In particular, up to 50% of women with antithrombin deficiency may manifest thrombosis during pregnancy (Chapter 3).[5]

Retrospective studies have reported the incidence of recurrent venous thromboembolism to be as high as 15% in women with a previous episode of deep-vein thrombosis.[6] Venous thrombosis during gestation mostly involves the leg veins, more often on the left side due to an increased abdominal pressure on the veins at that side. Other contributing factors include immobilization, cesarean section and gestational vascular complications such as pre-eclampsia, placental abruption and disseminated intravascular coagulation (DIC). Pulmonary embolism occurs in pregnant women usually as a complication of venous thrombosis of the legs or the pelvic veins. Occasionally, pulmonary embolism manifests itself as a sole thrombotic phenomenon without apparent origin.

Amniotic fluid embolism

Amniotic fluid embolism is a dreadful complication of late pregnancy with mortality in over 80% of women. The clinical manifestations include sudden onset of dyspnea, tachycardia, diaphoresis, hypoxemia and shock, which usually appear during labor or shortly after delivery.[7] The placenta is an organ rich in procoagulants including tissue factor, cancer procoagulant, and some other less well-defined procoagulants.[8] During labor, these procoagulants may generate extreme thrombotic activity in the placenta and amniotic fluid. A physiological placental barrier prevents this procoagulant activity from pouring into the systemic maternal circulation. However, occasionally amniotic fluid and debris may infiltrate into the maternal circulation, thereby resulting in this catastrophic thrombotic manifestation. Serological assays and immunohistochemical staining designed to detect sialyl Tn antigen have been employed successfully in the diagnosis of amniotic fluid embolism.[9]

Diagnosis of venous thromboembolism in pregnancy

Women who present with clinical manifestations suggestive of venous thrombosis during gestation should undergo evaluation to document thrombosis. Doppler ultrasound studies of the venous system are simple and safe and have a high accuracy rate reaching 96%.[10]

Venography should, at best, be avoided during pregnancy particularly during the first trimester. Isotope studies utilizing fibrinogen ^{131}I should also not be performed in pregnant women. Recently, assays of crosslinked fibrin degradation products have been reported to increase the diagnostic accuracy of noninvasive tests such as Doppler ultrasound. These D-dimer tests, which have a high sensitivity but low specificity resulting in a high (95–98%) negative predictive value, are used to rule out venous thrombosis and pulmonary embolism.[11]

Following diagnosis of deep vein thrombosis or pulmonary embolism, a battery of tests for thrombophilia workup should be sent to the coagulation laboratory (see Chapter 5).

Treatment and prevention of venous thrombosis (Table 15.1)

Warfarin

Warfarin is contraindicated during the first trimester as the drug crosses the placental barrier and may result in teratogenicity and carries a risk of fetal hemorrhage throughout pregnancy. Fetal embryopathy syndrome is characterized by certain skeletal deformities such as nasal hypoplasia and epiphysis stippling.[12]

A recent report demonstrated that a knockout model of murine γ-glutamyl carboxylase results in a phenotype similar to the warfarin embryopathy syndrome in human fetuses.[13]

Unfractionated and low molecular weight heparin

Unfractionated heparin and low molecular weight heparin are the drugs of choice for prevention and treatment of venous thromboembolism in pregnancy. Several case-control studies have reported the efficacy and safety of these drugs in pregnant women. The rate of major bleeding in pregnant women treated with heparin is about 2%[14] and the

Table 15.1
Antithrombotic therapy in pregnancy

Indication	Drug	Therapeutic benefit
Prevention of venous thromboembolism	Unfractionated heparin	+++
	Low molecular weight heparin	+++
Treatment of venous thromboembolism	Unfractionated heparin	+++
	Low molecular weight heparin	+++
Mechanical heart valves	Unfractionated heparin	++
	Low molecular weight heparin	ND
	Warfarin	++
Arterial thrombosis	Unfractionated heparin	+++
	Low molecular weight heparin	++ +
	Aspirin	++

++, Substantial; +++, high; ND, not determined.

anticoagulant effect of heparin may increase postpartum bleeding. Long-term heparin therapy may cause osteoporosis. Although symptomatic fractures occur in less than 2%, a subclinical effect of bone density reduction may occur in up to 30% of women receiving heparin over 1 month.[15] It has been suggested that low molecular weight heparin may induce less osteoporosis than unfractionated heparin. Unfractionated heparin, low molecular weight heparin and warfarin are not secreted in breast milk and therefore can be administered safely to nursing mothers. Heparin-induced thrombocytopenia may occur during heparin therapy. In pregnant women, the diagnosis of heparin-induced thrombocytopenia may pose a diagnostic problem with other causes of thrombocytopenia. These include mild thrombocytopenia associated with pregnancy, autoimmune thrombocytopenia associated with antiphospholipid syndrome and thrombocytopenia resulting from increased platelet consumption in patients with pre-eclampsia and HELLP syndrome. A search for antiplatelet antibodies, antiphospholipid antibodies and signs of hemolysis and elevation of liver enzymes should be performed in addition to tests directed to diagnose heparin-induced thrombocytopenia. In case of heparin-induced thrombocytopenia, heparin should be stopped and therapy with the heparinoid danaparoid should be instituted.

Efficacy data of anticoagulants in the prevention of venous thromboembolism during pregnancy are largely uncontrolled and consist of small case series. Recommendations for treatment are based upon extrapolation from data in nonpregnant patients with venous thromboembolism. Following an episode of deep-vein thrombosis in pregnancy, the immediate therapy is either unfractionated heparin or low molecular weight heparin. Unfractionated heparin is usually given intravenously for 1 week followed by subcutaneous injection twice daily aiming to increase the activated partial thromboplastin time (APTT) by two- to three-fold. If low molecular weight heparin is given, the regimen is every 12 hours aiming to achieve an anti-Xa of 0.5–1.2 U/ml. Based on the current state of knowledge, there are two general approaches to pregnant patients with previous venous thromboembolism: (1) active prophylaxis with heparin or low molecular weight heparin; and (2) clinical surveillance. There is a concern that a dose of heparin 5000 U subcutaneously every 12 hours, may be insufficient in high-risk situations because it does not reliably produce detectable heparin levels. More intense heparin therapy, in doses that produce plasma heparin levels (measured as anti-factor Xa activity) of 0.1–0.2 IU/ml, is associated with low recurrence rates in pregnant women with previous venous thromboembolism.[16] In addition, low recurrence rates have been reported with the use of low molecular weight heparin once daily.

Mechanical heart valves

Management of women at the reproductive age with valvular heart disease is problematic because of the lack of reliable data on the efficacy and safety of antithrombotic therapy during pregnancy.[17] In a recent retrospective survey describing outcomes in pregnant women with mechanical heart valves, it was concluded that warfarin was safe and not associated with embryopathy and that heparin was associated with more thromboembolic and bleeding complications than warfarin.[18]

It is reasonable to use subcutaneous heparin during 6–12 weeks of gestation and during the last month of pregnancy. Warfarin, targeted at an international normalized ratio (INR) of 2.5–3.5 can be used for the rest of time during pregnancy. The other possibility is to use heparin throughout pregnancy. In addition, European experts have recommended warfarin therapy throughout pregnancy in view of the reports of unfavorable outcomes with heparin, and the impression that the risk of embryopathy with warfarin derivatives has been overstated.[19] Subcutaneous heparin should be initiated in doses of 17 500 units every 12 hours and adjusted to prolong a 6-hour postinjection APTT into the therapeutic range. It should be emphasized that inadequate doses of heparin are ineffective in prevention of thrombosis in women with mechanical heart valves.

Theoretically, low molecular weight heparins or heparinoids are probably reasonable substitutes for unfractionated heparin because they appear to reduce the risk of bleeding and osteoporosis and do not cross the placenta, but clinical information is required before these agents can be recommended for use in women with mechanical heart valves. In addition, for some high-risk patients, addition of low-dose aspirin 80 mg daily may reduce the risk of thrombosis, although it may increase the risk of bleeding.[20]

Safety of aspirin during pregnancy

Potential complications of aspirin during pregnancy include birth defects and bleeding in the neonate and in the mother. The results of large randomized studies (over 10 000 patients)[21,22] demonstrated that low-dose aspirin (60–150 mg/day) therapy administered during the second and third trimesters of pregnancy was safe for the mother and fetus. However, the safety of higher doses of aspirin and/or aspirin ingestion during the first trimester remains a subject of debate.

Thrombophilia and pregnancy

Pregnancy loss

Recurrent pregnancy loss is a common health problem with three or more losses affecting 1–2% and two or more losses affecting up to 5% of women at the reproductive age.[23,24] Several etiologies have been implicated to play a role in recurrent pregnancy loss. These include chromosomal translocations and inversions, anatomic alterations of the uterus, endocrinologic abnormalities and autoimmune disorders.[25,26] However, until recently, the majority of recurrent pregnancy losses remained unexplained.

Recurrrent pregnancy loss is a well-established finding in certain acquired thrombophilic disorders like antiphospholipid syndrome[27] and essential thrombocythemia.[28] Several earlier reports demonstrated an increased thrombotic risk during gestation and puerperium in women with the inherited thrombophilic states antithrombin, protein C and protein S deficiencies.[29,30] More recently a case control study in 60 women with these inherited thrombophilias documented an increased risk for recurrent pregnancy loss as well.[31] A total of 42 of 188 pregnancies (22%) in women with thrombophilia resulted in pregnancy loss compared to 23 of 202 (11%) in controls (OR = 2.0; 95% CI 1.2–3.3).[31] In addition, a high incidence of gestational abnormalities was reported in 15 women with dysfibrinogenemia associated with thrombosis. Of 64 pregnancies, 39% ended by miscarriage and 9% by intrauterine fetal death.[32]

Certain women with recurrent pregnancy loss exhibit hypofibrinolysis related to abnormal plasma levels of activators and inhibitors of fibrinolysis. It appears that these patients may have functional abnormalities of the vascular endothelium characterized by high plasma levels of von Willebrand factor, tissue plasminogen activator, and plasminogen activator inhibitor-1, which may be associated with increased thrombin formation.[33,34]

Factor V Leiden mutation, factor II G20210A mutation and hyperhomocysteinemia account for the majority of venous thromboembolic events particularly during gestation or in association with usage of oral contraceptives. Factor V Leiden mutation can be found in over 50% of women with gestational thrombosis.[35] Factor II G20210A mutation is associated with a 20–50% increase in prothrombin plasma levels and a three-fold increased risk for venous thrombosis.[36]

Transient activated protein C (APC) resistance can be documented during normal gestations in women with normal factor V genotype. APC-sensitivity ratio shows a progressive fall through normal pregnancy in correlation with changes in factor VIII, factor V and protein S.[37] APC-sensitivity ratios may decrease further during gestation in women with factor V Leiden mutation.

Likewise, APC-sensitivity ratios were reported to be decreased in patients with recurrent pregnancy loss.[38–41] While APC-resistance is more common in women with second trimester losses,[38] it can also be found in women with first trimester recurrent pregnancy loss.[39] Indeed, APC-resistance was documented in 20 of 41 (49%) of women experiencing second trimester recurrent pregnancy loss compared to 10 of 37 (27%) of women with only first trimester abortions ($P < 0.05$).[39] Several case studies have suggested a potential association between factor V Leiden and recurrent pregnancy loss[40,41] while others have not found such a correlation.[42] These discrepancies may be explained in part by differences in study populations regarding ethnic origin and selection criteria of study groups. For example, the European Prospective Cohort on Thrombophilia (EPCOT) study analysed the risk for fetal loss in a cohort of 571 women with known inherited thrombophilia of various types and found that the odds ratio for stillbirth was 3.6 (1.4–9.4), and for miscarriages 1.27 (0.94–1.71).[43] For factor V Leiden, the odds ratio was 2.0 (0.5–1.77) for stillbirth and 0.9 (0.5–1.5) for miscarriages.

Three recent case control studies have evaluated the prevalence of factor V Leiden mutation in women with recurrent pregnancy loss (*Table 15.2*). Despite differences in ethnic Caucasian subpopulations and selection criteria for recurrent pregnancy loss, all three studies documented significantly increased prevalence of factor V Leiden mutation in women with recurrent pregnancy loss. A potential interpretation of these four studies[43–46] is that factor V Leiden, which is a mild risk factor for thrombosis, is also a mild risk factor for recurrent pregnancy loss and that in the majority of women who are carriers of the mutation it will not result in recurrent pregnancy loss. However, some women with factor V Leiden mutation will present with recurrent pregnancy loss and the prevalence of the mutation in the general population will determine in part, its prevalence in women with recurrent pregnancy loss from the same population.

Plasma homocysteine levels decrease during normal pregnancy compared to levels in nonpregnant women. Several recent studies have shown that homozygosity for the MTHFR C677T mutation is not predictive for recurrent pregnancy loss,[46,47] while other studies reported a potential association between recurrent pregnancy loss, hyperhomocysteinemia and homozygosity for MTHFR C677T.[48,49] Moreover, plasma homocysteine levels can increase in pregnant women with folic acid or vitamin B12 deficiency particularly in the presence of homozygosity for MTHFR C677T, and this may result in recurrent pregnancy loss.[49] It is well established that combinations of inherited or acquired thrombophilic states increase the risk for thrombosis.[50,51] Likewise,

Table 15.2
Factor V Leiden mutation in women with recurrent pregnancy loss

Study (reference)	Selection	Patients	Controls	OR	95% CI	P
Ridker et al[44]	No	9/113(8%)	16/437(3.7%)	2.3	1.0–5.2	0.05
Grandone et al[45]	Yes	7/43(16%)	5/118(4%)	4.4	1.3–14.7	0.01
Brenner et al[46]	Yes	24/76(32%)	11/106(10%)	4.0	1.8–8.8	0.001

combinations of thrombophilic states may further increase the risk for recurrent pregnancy loss. For example, coexistence of factor V Leiden and homozygous hyperhomocysteinemia[52] and combination of factor V Leiden with familial antiphospholipid syndrome[53] was reported to result in thrombosis and recurrent fetal loss. It is therefore not surprising that the EPCOT study documented the highest odds ratio for stillbirth in women with combined thrombophilia.[43] In our recent study on 76 women with recurrent pregnancy loss 6 (7.9%) had combined thrombophilia compared to 1 of 106 (0.9%) controls ($P < 0.02$).[46]

In view of the high prevalence of the three common thrombophilic mutations in the general population, we have evaluated their prevalence in women with recurrent pregnancy loss. At least one of the three common mutations, factor V Leiden, factor II G20210A and MTHFR C677T was found in 49% of women with recurrent pregnancy loss of unknown cause compared to 23% in controls (OR = 3.2; 95% CI: 1.7–6.1, $P = 0.0002$).[46]

Gestational vascular complications (Table 15.3)

Pre-eclampsia characterized by gestational hypertension, edema and proteinuria has long been associated with an abnormal placental vasculature. Activation of blood coagulation and endothelial cell stimulation are fundamental findings in pre-eclampsia.[54,55] Activation of the coagulation and fibrinolytic systems is more marked in the uteroplacental circulation than in the systemic circulation,[56] and an abnormal pattern of hemostasis has been reported to operate in the uteroplacental circulation in women with pre-eclampsia.[56]

Several recent reports suggest an association between APC-resistance, factor V Leiden mutation and early onset of severe pre-

Table 15.3
Placental vascular complications associated with thrombophilia

	Miscarriages	IUFD	Pre-eclampsia	HELLP	Placental abruption
Antithrombin deficiency	++	++	+		
Protein C deficiency	+	++	+		
Protein S deficiency	+	++	+	+	
Dysfibrinogenemia	+	+			
Activated protein C resistance	++	++	++	+	
Factor V Leiden	++	++	++	+	++
MTHFR C677T	+	+	+		+
Hyperhomocysteinemia	+	+	++	++	++
Factor II G20210A	+	+	+	++	++
Antiphospholipid syndrome	++	++	++	+	
Combined defects	++	++		+	

IUFD, intrauterine fetal death; HELLP, hemolysis, elevated liver enzymes, low platelet counts.
Degree of association: +, possible association; ++, established association.

eclampsia. In one study, 14 of 158 women with severe pre-eclampsia (8.9%) were found to be heterozygous for the factor V Leiden mutation compared with 17 of 403 normotensive gravida controls (4.2%; $P = 0.03$).[57] Likewise, in another study, factor V Leiden mutation was documented in 19% of women with pre-eclampsia compared to 7% of control.[58]

The HELLP syndrome is a severe presentation of pre-eclampsia manifested by Hemolysis, Elevated levels of Liver enzymes and Low Platelet count. A potential association between factor V Leiden mutation and HELLP syndrome in two women has been reported.[59] Therapy with low molecular weight heparin throughout pregnancy in three successive pregnancies resulted in normal delivery. Another study has documented APC-resistance in a third of 21 women with HELLP syndrome.[60] Dekker et al[61] have found in 85 women with a history of severe early-onset pre-eclampsia a variety of thrombophilic defects including protein S deficiency (25%) anticardiolipin antibodies (29%), APC-resistance (16%) and hyperhomocysteinemia (18%). Thirteen patients had combinations of thrombophilic defects emphasizing the role of combined thrombophilia in the observed placental vascular pathology.[61] Interestingly, 53% of women with severe early-onset pre-eclampsia in Dekker's report had HELLP syndrome.[61] Recently, Grandone et al[62] have shown a predisposition for pre-eclampsia in women with either factor V Leiden or MTHFR C677T mutations.

A recent study has evaluated the association of the genetic thrombophilias with gestational vascular complications in 110 women with pre-eclampsia, intrauterine growth restriction, placental abruption or stillbirth who were compared to 110 women with normal gestations.[63] One of the three common thrombophilic mutations, factor V Leiden, factor II G20210A or MTHFR C677T was found in 57/110 (52%) of women with gestational vascular complications compared to only 19/110 (17%) of controls (OR = 5.2; 95% CI: 2.8–9.6). Additional patients had other thrombophilias accounting for a total of 71/110 (65%) compared to only 20/110 (18%) in controls ($P < 0.001$). Patient and control groups differ in parity with 92/110 of patients being in their first pregnancy compared to only 62/110 of controls ($P < 0.001$).[63]

The three inherited thrombophilias were more common in women with severe pre-eclampsia (OR = 5.4; 95% CI; 2.3–12.4), placental abruption (OR = 7.2; 95% CI: 2.3–20), intrauterine growth restriction (OR = 4.8; 95% CI: 2.2–10.3) and stillbirth (OR = 3.4; 95% CI: 1.0–11.9). These resulted in earlier delivery, 32 weeks versus 39 weeks, and decreased birth weight, 1375 g versus 3400 g, in patients with gestational vascular complications compared to controls.[63]

As up to 65% of vascular gestational abnormalities can be accounted for by genetic thrombophilias,[46,63] the implication is to screen for these mutations in all women with vascular gestational abnormalities. Furthermore, this high prevalence of genetic thrombophilias, which is similar to the findings in women with pregnancy-related venous thromboembolism,[64] suggests that usage of antithrombotic drugs may also have potential therapeutic benefit in women with gestational vascular complications.

Therapeutic regimens (Table 15.4)

Recently, two prospective randomized studies have shown that heparin plus low-dose aspirin results in significantly better gestational outcome than low-dose aspirin alone in women with antiphospholipid syndrome who had experienced recurrent pregnancy loss. In the study by Kutteh[65] viable infants were delivered in only 11 of 25 (44%) women receiving aspirin compared to 20 of 25 (80%) women receiving aspirin and subcutaneous heparin ($P < 0.05$). In the study by Rai et

Table 15.4
Therapeutic modalities for prevention of pregnancy loss in thrombophilic patients

	Steroids	Aspirin	Heparin	Low molecular weight heparin	Factor concentrates
Antithrombin deficiency			+++	+++	+
Protein C deficiency			+++	+++	
Protein S deficiency			+++	+++	
Factor V Leiden		+		+++	
Antiphospholipid syndrome	+	++	+++	+++	
Combined defects		+	+++	+++	

Therapeutic benefit: +, equivocal; ++, substantial; +++, high.

al,[66] the rate of live births for patients treated with low-dose aspirin and heparin was 71% (32/45 pregnancies) compared to only 42% (19/45 pregnancies) for women treated with aspirin alone ($P < 0.01$).

Emerging data on therapy of women with inherited thrombophilia and pregnancy loss are mostly uncontrolled and include small series of patients. A recent collaborative study has demonstrated the safety of using low molecular weight heparin during 486 gestations.[67] Successful outcome was reported in 83 of 93 (89%) gestations in women with recurrent pregnancy loss and in all 28 gestations in women with pre-eclampsia in a previous pregnancy.[57] Administration of the low molecular weight heparin, enoxaparin 20 mg/day to women with primary early recurrent pregnancy loss and impaired fibrinolytic capacity resulted in normalization of impaired fibrinolysis, conception in 16 of 20 (80%) and successful live births in 13 of 16 (81%).[68]

During the past 4 years we have treated 63 pregnancies in 42 women with thrombophilia who presented with thromboembolism and/or recurrent pregnancy loss with enoxaparin throughout gestation (B Brenner unpublished data). Enoxaparin dosage was 40 mg/day, except for patients with combined thrombophilia or in the case of abnormal Doppler velocimetry suggesting decreased placental perfusion, where the dosage was increased to 40 mg twice daily aimed toward an anti-Xa level of 0.3–0.4. Plasma anti-Xa levels may decrease in late pregnancy implying a potential need for increase in low molecular weight heparin dosage at that stage.

In the case of previous thrombosis low molecular weight heparin therapy was continued for 6 weeks after delivery. Forty-five of the 63 pregnancies (71%) resulted in live births. In women with inherited thrombophilia and recurrent pregnancy loss, the percentage of live births increased from 20% without therapy to 75% following enoxaparin treatment.

A beneficial effect for aspirin in secondary prevention of pre-eclampsia has been suggested.[69] However, these observations have not been confirmed by more recent studies.[70] Recent preliminary reports suggest that low molecular weight heparin with or without aspirin has a beneficial role in women with thrombophilia and vascular gestational abnormalities including recurrent pregnancy loss, pre-eclampsia and fetal growth retardation.[71,72] The role of aspirin in the setting of thrombophilia and vascular gestational abnormalities remains to be confirmed. In patients with antiphospholipid syndrome or in those with combined thrombophilia, aspirin is given along with low molecular weight heparin. However, whether aspirin has an added benefit to heparin or low molecular weight heparin alone has not been evaluated. Prospective randomized, dose-finding studies, are warranted to assess the potential advantage of low molecular weight heparin in women with thrombophilia and vascular gestational abnormalities.

Future perspectives

Currently 30–50% of vascular gestational pathologies cannot be accounted for by thrombophilia. Whether novel genetic or acquired thrombophilia will be found to play a role remains to be determined. Recent observations suggest that presence of antiendothelial cell antibodies[73] and complement-fixing antibodies to trophoblasts[74] may be associated with recurrent pregnancy loss. These studies as well as those suggesting the presence of antibodies directed toward specific phospholipids, or inhibiting protective molecules such as annexin V[75] imply a broader spectrum for recurrent pregnancy loss related to autoantibodies.

The pathogenetic mechanisms responsible for placental vascular pathologies in women with thrombophilia have not been elucidated. Furthermore, it is still unknown why only some women with thrombophilia express vascular gestational pathologies while others do not. It is possible that this may relate to local factors affecting coagulation, fibrinolysis and vascular tone at the placental vessels level.

Finally, the role of antithrombotic therapeutic modalities deserves prospective clinical trials in order to improve outcome for

a large population of women who currently experience poor gestational outcome.

References

1. Long AA, Ginsberg JS, Brill-Edwards P et al. The relationship of antiphospholipid antibodies to thromboembolic disease in systemic lupus erythematosus: a cross-sectional study. *Thromb Haemost* 1991; **66**: 520–524.

2. Bonnar J, Green R, Norris L. Inherited thrombophilia and pregnancy. The obstetric perspective. *Semin Thromb Hemost* 1998; **24**: 49–54

3. Brenner B, Fishman A, Goldsher O et al. Cerebral thrombosis in a newborn with congenital deficiency of antithrombin III. *Am J Hematol* 1988; **27**: 209–212.

4. Brenner B, Shapira A, Bahari C et al. Hereditary protein C deficiency during pregnancy. *Am J Obstet Gynecol* 1987; **157**: 160–61.

5. Conard J, Horellou MI, Van Dreden P et al. Thrombosis and pregnancy in congenital deficiencies in ATIII, protein C or protein S: study of 78 women. *Thromb Haemost* 1990; **63**: 319–320.

6. Ginsberg JS, Hirsh J, Turner DC et al. Risks to the fetus of anticoagulant therapy during pregnancy. *Thromb Haemost* 1989; **61**: 197–203.

7. Clark SL. Amniotic fluid embolism: analysis of the national registry. *Am J Obstet Gynecol* 1995; **172**: 1158–1169.

8. Gordon SG, Hasiba U, Cross BA et al. Cysteine proteinase procoagulant from amnion-chorion. *Blood* 1985; **66**: 1261–1265.

9. Oi H, Kolayashi H, Hiroshima Y et al. Serological and immunohistochemical diagnosis of amniotic fluid embolism. *Semin Thromb Hemost* 1998; **24:** 479–484.

10. Strothman G, Blebea J, Fowl RJ, Rosenthal G. Contralateral duplex scanning for deep venous thrombosis is unnecessary in patients with symptoms. *J Vasc Surg* 1995; **22:** 543–547.

11. Brenner B, Pery M, Lanir N et al. Application of a bedside whole blood D-dimer assay in the diagnosis of deep vein thrombosis. *Blood Coag Fibrinol* 1995; **6:** 219–222.

12. Hall JAG, Paul RM, Wilson KM. Maternal and fetal sequelae of anticoagulation during pregnancy. *Am J Med* 1980; **68:** 122–140.

13. Zhu A, Raymond R, Zheng X et al. Abnormalities of development and hemostasis in γ-carboxylase deficient mice (abstract). *Blood* 1998; **92:** 611.

14. Ginbsberg JS, Kowalchuk G, Hirsh J et al. Heparin therapy during pregnancy: risks to the fetus and mother. *Arch Intern Med* 1989; **149:** 2233–2236.

15. Douketis JD, Ginsberg JS, Burrows RD et al. The effects of long-term heparin therapy on bone density. A prospective matched cohort study. *Thromb Haemost* 1996; **75:** 254–257.

16. Dahlman TC. Osteoporotic fractures and the recurrence of thromboembolism during pregnancy and the puerperium in 184 women undergoing thromboprophylaxis with heparin. *Am J Obstet Gynecol* 1993; **168:** 1265–1278.

17. Caruso A, De Carolis S, Ferrazzani S. Pregnancy outcome in women with cardiac valve prosthesis. *Eur J Obstet Gynecol Reprod Biol* 1994; **54:** 77–81.

18. Iturbe-Alessio I, Fonseca MC, Mutchnik O et al. Risks of anticoagulant therapy in pregnant women with artificial heart valves. *N Engl J Med* 1986; **315:** 1390–1393.

19. Sbarouni E, Oakley CM. Outcome of pregnancy in women with valve prosthesis. *Br Heart J* 1994; **71:** 196–201.

20. Turpie AGG, Gent M, Laupacis A et al. A comparison of aspirin with placebo in patients treated with warfarin after heart-valve replacement. *N Engl J Med* 1993; **329:** 524–529.

21. Sibai BM, Caritis SN, Thom E et al. Prevention of preeclampsia with low dose aspirin in healthy nulliparous pregnant women. *N Engl J Med* 1993; **339:** 1213–1218.

22. CLAPS Collaborative Group. A randomized trial of low dose aspirin for the prevention and treatment of pre-eclampsia among 9364 pregnant women. *Lancet* 1994; **343:** 619–629.

23. Cook CL, Pridham DD. Recurrent pregnancy loss. *Curr Opin Obstet Gynecol*, 1995; **7:** 357–366.

24. Clifford K, Rai R, Watson H, Regan L. An informative protocol for the investigation of recurrent miscarriage: preliminary experience of 500 consecutive cases. *Human Reprod* 1994; **9:** 1328–1332.

25. Hatasaka HH. Recurrent miscarriage: epidemiologic factors, definitions, and incidence. *Clin Obstet Gynecol* 1994; **37:** 625–634.

26. Raziel A, Arieli S, Bukovsky I et al. Investigation of the uterine cavity in recurrent aborters. *Fertil Steril* 1994; **62:** 1080–1082.

27. Triplett DA, Harris EN. Antiphospholipid antibodies and reproduction. *Am J Reprod Immunol* 1989; **21:** 123–131.

28. Beressi AH, Tefferi A, Silverstein MN et al.

Outcome analysis of 34 pregnancies in women with essential thrombocythemia. *Arch Intern Med* 1995; **155**: 1217–1222.

29. Hellgren M, Tengborn L, Abildgaard U. Pregnancy in women with congenital antithrombin III deficiency: experience of treatment with heparin and antithrombin. *Gynecol Obstet Invest* 1982; **14**: 127–141.

30. Conard J, Horellou MH, Van Dreden P et al. Thrombosis and pregnancy in congenital deficiencies in ATIII, protein C or protein S. *Thromb Haemost* 1990; **63**: 319–320.

31. Sanson BJ, Friederich PW, Simioni P et al. The risk of abortion and stillbirth in antithrombin, protein C, and protein S-deficient women. *Thromb Haemost* 1996; **75**: 387–388.

32. Haverkate F, Samama M. Familial dysfibrinogenemia and thrombophilia. Report on a study of the SSC Subcommittee on Fibrinogen. *Thromb Haemost* 1995; **73**: 151–161.

33. Gris JC, Schved JF, Neveu S et al. Impaired fibrinolytic capacity and early recurrent spontaneous abortions. *BMJ* 1990; **300**: 1500

34. Gris JC, Neveu S, Mares P et al. Plasma fibrinolytic activators and their inhibitors in women suffering from early recurrent abortions of unknown etiology. *J Lab Clin Med* 1993; **122**: 606–615.

35. Hellgren M, Svensson PJ, Dahlbäck B. Resistance to activated protein C as a basis for venous thromboembolism associated with pregnancy and oral contraceptives. *Am J Obstet Gynecol* 1995; **173**: 210–213.

36. Poort SR, Rosendaal FR, Reitsma PH, Bertina RM. A common genetic variation in the 3'-untranslated region of the prothrombin gene is associated with elevated plasma prothrombin levels and an increase in venous thrombosis. *Blood* 1996; **88**: 3698–3703.

37. Clark P, Brennand J, Conkie JA et al. Activated protein C sensitivity ratio, protein C, protein S and coagulation in normal pregnancy. *Thromb Haemost* 1998; **79**: 1166–1170.

38. Rai R, Regan L, Hadley E et al. Second trimester pregnancy loss is associated with activated protein C resistance. *Br J Haematol* 1996; **92**: 489–490.

39. Younis JS, Brenner B, Ohel G et al. Factor V Leiden mutation is associated with first as well as second trimester recurrent fetal loss. *Fertil Steril* 1998; **70** (Suppl 3): S55.

40. Brenner B, Mandel H, Lanir N et al. Activated protein C resistance can be associated with recurrent fetal loss. *Br J Haematol* 1997; **97**: 551–554.

41. Rotmensch S, Liberati M, Mittlemann M, Ben-Rafael Z. Activated protein C resistance and adverse pregnancy outcome. *Am J Obstet Gynecol* 1997; **177**: 170–173.

42. Dizon-Townson DS, Kinney S, Branch DW, Ward K. The factor V Leiden mutation is not a common cause of recurrent miscarriage. *J Reprod Immunol* 1997; **34**: 217–223.

43. Preston FE, Rosendaal FR, Walker ID et al. Increased fetal loss in women with heritable thrombophilia. *Lancet* 1996; **348**: 913–916.

44. Rikder PM, Miletich JP, Buring JE et al. Factor V Leiden mutation as a risk factor for recurrent pregnancy loss. *Ann Intern Med* 1998; **128**: 1000-1003.

45. Grandone E, Margaglione M, Colaizzo D et al. Factor V Leiden is associated with repeated and recurrent unexplained fetal osses. *Thromb Haemost* 1997; **77**: 822–824.

46. Brenner B, Sarig G, Weiner Z et al.

Thrombophilic polymorphisms are common in women with fetal loss without apparent cause. *Thromb Haemost* 1999; **82**: 6–9.

47. Deitcher SR, Park VM, Kutteh WH. Methylene tetrahydrofolate reductase 667C→T mutation analysis in Caucasian women with early first trimester recurrent pregnancy loss. *Blood* 1998; **92** (Suppl 1): 117B.

48. Kornberg A, Raziel A, Rahimini-Levene N et al. Hypercoagulability and recurrent abortions. *Blood* 1998; **92** (Suppl 1): 121B.

49. Nelen WL, Blom HJ, Thomas CM et al. Methylenetetrahydrofolate reductase polymorphism affects the change in homocysteine and folate concentrations resulting from low dose folic acid supplementation in women with unexplained recurrent miscarriages. *J Nutr* 1998; **128**: 1336–1341.

50. Zöller B, Berntsdotter A, Garcia de Frutos P, Dahlbäck B. Resistance to activated protein C as an additional genetic risk factor in hereditary deficiency of protein S. *Blood* 1995; **85**: 3518–3523.

51. Brenner B, Zivelin A, Lanir N et al. Venous thromboembolism associated with double heterozygosity for R506Q mutation of factor V and for T298M mutation of protein C in a large family of a previously described homozygous protein C deficient newborn with massive thrombosis. *Blood* 1996; **88**: 877–880.

52. Mandel H, Brenner B, Berant M et al. Coexistence of hereditary homocysteinuria and factor V Leiden: effect on thrombosis. *N Engl J Med* 1996; **334**: 763–768.

53. Brenner B, Vulfsons SL, Lanir N, Nahir M. Coexistence of familial antiphospholipid syndrome and factor V Leiden: impact on thrombotic diathesis. *Br J Haematol* 1996; **94**: 166–167.

54. Brenner B. Zwang E, Bronshtein M, Seligsohn U. von Willebrand factor multimer patterns in pregnancy-induced hypertension. *Thromb Haemost* 1989; **62**: 715–717.

55. Cadroy Y, Grandjean H, Pichon J et al. Evaluation of six markers of haemostatic system in normal pregnancy and pregnancy complicated by hypertension or preeclampsia. *Br J Obstet Gynecol* 1993; **100**: 416–420.

56. Higgins JR, Walshe JJ, Darling MR et al. Hemostasis in the uteroplacental and peripheral circulations in normotensive and pre-eclamptic pregnancies. *Am J Obstet Gynecol* 1998; **179**: 520–526.

57. Dizon-Townson DS, Nelson LM, Easton K, Ward K. The factor V Leiden mutation may predispose women to severe preeclampsia. *Am J Obstet Gynecol* 1996; **175**: 902–905.

58. Nagy B, Toth T, Rigo J Jr et al. Detection of Factor V Leiden mutation in severe pre-eclamptic Hungarian Women. *Clin Genet* 1998; **53**: 478–481.

59. Brenner B, Lanir N, Thaler I. HELLP syndrome associated with factor V R506Q mutation. *Br J Haematol* 1996; **92**: 999–1001.

60. Krauss T, Augustin HG, Osmers R et al. Activated protein C resistance and factor V Leiden in patients with hemolysis, elevated liver enzymes, low platelet syndrome. *Obstet Gynecol* 1998; **92**: 457–460.

61. Dekker GA, de Vries JI, Doelitzsch PM et al. Underlying disorders associated with severe early onset preeclampsia. *Am J Obstet Gynecol* 1995; **173**: 1042–1048.

62. Grandone E, Margaglione M, Colaizzo D et al. Factor V Leiden, C→T MTHFR

polymorphism and genetic susceptibility to preeclampsia. *Thromb Haemost* 1997; **77:** 1052–1054.

63. Kupferminc MJ, Eldor A, Steinman N et al. Increased frequency of genetic thrombophilias in women with complications of pregnancy. *N Engl J Med* 1999; **340:** 9–13.

64. Grandone E, Margaglione M, Colaizzo D et al. Genetic susceptibility to pregnancy-related venous thromboembolism: roles of factor V Leiden, prothrombin G20210A, and methylenetetrahydrofolate reductase C677T mutations. *Am J Obstet Gynecol* 1998; **179:** 1324–1328.

65. Kutteh WH. Antiphospholipid antibody-associated recurrent pregnancy loss: treatment with heparin and low-dose aspirin is superior to low-dose aspirin alone. *Am J Obstet Gynecol* 1996; **174:** 1584–1589.

66. Rai R, Cohen H, Dave M, Regan L. Randomised controlled trial of aspirin and aspirin plus heparin in pregnant women with recurrent miscarriage associated with antiphospholipid antibodies. *BMJ* 1997; **314:** 253–257.

67. Sanson BJ, Lensing AWA, Prins MH et al. The use of low molecular weight heparin in pregnancy. *Blood* 1998; **92** (Suppl 1): 360A.

68. Gris JC, Neveu S, Tailland ML et al. Use of low-molecular weight heparin (enoxaparin) or of a phenformin-like substance (moroxydine chloride) in primary early recurrent aborters with an impaired fibrinolytic capacity. *Thromb Haemost* 1995; **73:** 362–367.

69. Benigni A, Gregorini G, Frusca T et al. Effect of low dose aspirin on fetal and maternal generation of thromboxane by platelets in

women at risk for pregnancy induced hypertension. *N Engl J Med* 1989; **321:** 357–362.

70. Caritis S, Sibai B, Hauth J et al. Low-dose aspirin to prevent preeclampsia in women at high risk. National Institute of Child Health and Human Development Network of Maternal-Fetal Medicine Units. *N Engl J Med* 1998; **38:** 701–705.

71. Riyazi N, Leeda M, de Vries JI et al. Low-molecular-weight heparin combined with aspirin in pregnant women with thrombophilia and a history of preeclampsia or fetal growth restriction: a preliminary study. *Eur J Obstet Reprod Biol* 1998; **80:** 49–54.

72. Eldor A, Kupferminc MJ, Steinman N et al. High incidence of thrombophilia in women with obstetric complications and the beneficial effects of LMW heparin and aspirin in subsequent pregnancies. *Blood* 1998; **92** (Suppl 1): 556A.

73. Roussev RG, Stern JJ, Kaider BD, Thaler CJ. Anti-endothelial cell antibodies: another cause for pregnancy loss? *Am J Reprod Immunol* 1998; **39:** 89–95.

74. Tedesco F, Pausa M, Nardon E et al. Prevalence and biological effects of anti-trophoblast and anti-endothelial cell antibodies in patients with recurrent spontaneous abortions. *Am J Reprod Immunol* 1997; **38:** 205–211.

75. Rand JH, Wu X-X, Andree HAM et al. Pregnancy loss in the antiphospholipid-antibody syndrome: a possible thrombogenic mechanism. *N Engl J Med* 1997; **337:** 154–160.

Thrombosis and cancer

16

Gilles Lugassy

1865 was a busy year: Wagner produced *Tristan and Isolde,*
Manet painted Olympia, Lewis Carroll published *Alice in
Wonderland,* Lincoln was assassinated, Mendel discovered
heredity and Armand Trousseau lectured on phlegmasia alba
dolens. In his lecture, Trousseau described the occurrence of
unexplained episodes of migratory thrombophlebitis in
patients with visceral cancer.[1] He concluded that spontaneous
coagulation is common in cancer patients because of a 'special
crasis' in their blood.

It is now common knowledge that thromboembolic
disease is often the earliest manifestation and also the most
frequent complication of cancer. It is the second cause of
death in patients with an overt malignancy.[2] Evidence of
thromboembolism is seen in up to half of all cancer patients
studied at autopsy, particularly with tumors of the pancreas,
lung and gastrointestinal tract.[2] Recent studies have
investigated the mechanisms by which cancer causes
thrombosis and emphasized the importance of the coagulation
system in angiogenesis and tumor metastasis.[3]

Pathogenesis of thrombosis in cancer

The activation of the clotting process in the genesis of cancer-associated thrombosis is multifactorial. It includes the following.

- Tumor interaction with the vascular endothelium
- Platelet activation
- Abnormal activation of the coagulation pathway
- Failure of natural anticoagulant mechanisms

Tumor interaction with endothelium

The normal endothelium maintains blood fluidity by producing inhibitors of blood coagulation and platelet aggregation, and by providing a protective envelope separating hemostatic blood components from reactive subendothelial structure. Recent observations have shown the ability of blood-circulating malignant cells to adhere to the endothelial lining and cause injury to endothelial cells.[4] A vascular permeability factor (VPF), secreted by tumor cells of human and animal origin, causes a separation of endothelial cells in postcapillary venules without damaging these cells or provoking inflammation.[5]

Such injuries may damage the endothelium, prevent the natural release of anticoagulants, platelet antiaggregants and vasodilators by the endothelial cells, and lead to vasospasm and thrombosis.

Platelet activation

Platelets are an integral part of the microthrombus involved in the arrest and lodgement of circulating malignant cells. The role of platelets in tumor cell adhesion and metastasis via platelet integrin, glycoprotein (GP) IIb/IIIa, fibronectin and von Willebrand factor, has been recently reviewed.[6]

Quantitative platelet abnormalities have been described in solid tumors and in myeloproliferative disorders.[7] Modest thrombocytosis, up to 800 000/mm^3 may occur in patients with untreated lung and liver carcinomas. More severe thrombocytosis, over 10×10^6/mm^3, is a landmark of myeloproliferative disorders and is associated with the development of thromboembolic complications.[8]

Qualitative platelet abnormalities in malignancy include thrombotic as well as antithrombotic properties: aggregation may increase, be impaired or occur spontaneously. Tumor cells can cause platelet aggregation in vitro.[9] Intravenous tumor cell injection causes thrombocytopenia in mice.[9] The platelet aggregative activity of the tumor cells is due to sialic acid and complementary components released from plasma membrane vesicles shed by the malignant cells.[10]

Tumor cells are also able to activate platelets directly and generate thrombin and ADP release, contributing to the process of coagulation pathway activation.

Coagulation pathway activation

Tumor procoagulant activity (PCA) can be detected in various tumor cell lines and it seems to exist in the shed membrane vesicles.[11] Two main categories of procoagulants are known: tissue factor and cancer procoagulant.

Tissue factor (TF)

TF, a potent natural activator of factor VII found in most normal tissues (pancreas excluded), is expressed in pancreatic, gastric, ovary and kidney tumors.[3] TF is also generated indirectly by mononuclear cells (monocytes, macrophages) when activated by the tumor cells.[12]

Measurements of elevated plasma levels of TF and activated factor VII in patients with solid tumors demonstrated that the extrinsic pathway is an important determinant of activated coagulation in cancer patients.[13]

Cancer procoagulant

Tumor cells produce a single chain cystein protease with factor VII-independent procoagulant activity. This cancer procoagulant (CP) activates factor X directly, to set off coagulation.[14] CP is expressed by a broad spectrum of malignant cells and tissues but not by normal tissues. CP represents the main procoagulant activity of cells from human acute promyelocytic leukemia (APL), the prototype of malignant cells inducing blood clotting activation.[15] Donati et al[16] have shown that CP levels in bone marrow and peripheral blasts of APL patients closely correlate with the disease activity: CP was not found in cells of leukemic remission but reappeared when relapse occurred.

CP is a possible marker of cell differentiation: it is expressed by amnio chorionic undifferentiated tissue from human placenta and by dedifferentiated malignant tissue.[17] Once normal differentiation occurs, expression of CP is repressed.

Failure of natural anticoagulant mechanisms

There are several reasons for suggesting that hypercoagulation of malignancy may also be due to consumption and/or failure of the natural anticoagulant systems, in addition to the procoagulant activity of tumor cells and tumor-associated monocytes.[18] Antithrombin and protein C are major natural anticoagulants produced by the liver. Several studies have suggested that hepatic synthesis of these anticoagulants is decreased in metastatic cancer.[19] Low antithrombin levels have been found in patients with metastatic carcinomas of colon, ovary and prostate, but do not predict the development of thromboembolic complications in cancer patients.

Venous thromboembolism can be the first clinical manifestation of an occult cancer (Trousseau dixit)

Thrombosis is often the first and earliest clinical manifestation of cancer. The prognostic importance of discovering cancer at its earliest stage in patients with thromboembolic disease has prompted clinical investigators to determine the most efficient (and cost effective) workup study for the detection of cancer at an early stage and estimation of the incidence and type of cancer among patients with 'idiopathic' deep-vein thrombosis.

Only recently have large clinical studies been performed to determine whether symptomatic deep-vein thrombosis is associated with the presence of malignancy at diagnosis or during follow-up. In a retrospective cohort study of 136 patients with deep-vein thrombosis, cancer was diagnosed in 16 patients at the initial evaluation.[20] All 16 patients had at least one abnormal finding in their medical history, physical examination, and basic laboratory testing or chest radiography. Cancer was diagnosed in none of the patients with a normal initial evaluation. Prandoni et al[21] evaluated the occurrence of cancer after a first episode of idiopathic thrombosis, among 250 patients with venographically proven deep-vein thrombosis, and no evidence of cancer on routine examination at time of referral. The incidence of subsequently detected, overt, symptomatic malignancy in the 145 patients with idiopathic thrombosis was compared with the incidence of cancer developing in the 105 patients with secondary venous thrombosis. During the 2-year follow-up, cancer was diagnosed in two patients (1.9%) with secondary thrombosis and 11 patients (7.6%) with idiopathic thrombosis. Cancers were mainly adenocarcinomas of the brain, breasts, and gastrointestinal, respiratory and urogenital tracts. The incidence of cancer was even higher in the group of patients with recurrent idiopathic venous thrombosis: 17.1%. Sorensen et al[22] confirmed the excess cancer in a cohort of over 15 000 patients with deep-vein thrombosis and 11 000 patients with pulmonary emboli. The risk of developing cancer was only elevated during the first 6 months of follow-up, meaning that most of these cancers were probably present at the time of thrombosis diagnosis.

Which workup for deep-vein thrombosis patients?

The appropriate workup study for searching for a hidden cancer at time of deep-vein thrombosis, or during follow-up, should not include invasive procedures.[23] According to Monreal et al[24] such a workup should include routine laboratory tests, such as erythrocyte sedimentation rate (ESR), lactate dehydrogenase (LDH) and carcino embryonic antigen (CEA) levels, chest radiography and abdominal ultrasound or computed tomography (CT) scan. Additional testing should be guided by abnormalities detected in the initial workups. More extensive screening is not cost effective and may cause physical discomfort and psychological stress. A prospective study, the SOMIT (Screening for Occult Malignancy in patients with Thromboembolism) is being conducted to establish the best screening policies for patients with idiopathic deep-vein thrombosis.[25]

Thrombotic complications of cancer

The overall incidence of thromboembolic manifestations in malignancy is about 5% (range: 1–11%). Thromboembolism is more common in patients with adenocarcinomas of the pancreas, stomach, colon, lung and metastatic disease.[26]

Venous thrombosis is often migratory, and may involve superficial veins, and unusual sites such as the upper extremities and the chest wall.[27] Arterial thrombosis is less common than venous thrombosis and occurs in tumors of the pancreas, lung and colon.[27]

Microvascular arterial thrombosis is observed in patients with myeloproliferative disorders.[8] Paraneoplastic digital gangrene with Raynaud's phenomenon has been described.[27]

Venous thromboembolism in cancer surgery

Patients suffering from a malignant disease are at high risk for postoperative venous thromboembolic complications, compared to patients undergoing major orthopedic surgery. The incidence of postsurgery deep-vein thrombosis and pulmonary embolism (PE) in cancer patients is 3–5 times more frequent than in nonneoplastic patients undergoing the same type of surgery.[25] The excess risk of deep-vein thrombosis following cancer surgery is the consequence of the malignancy itself as well as other factors frequently encountered in this population of patients: older age, prolonged immobilization, difficult surgery and infectious complications.[28] Two studies evaluated the frequency of deep-vein thrombosis in cancer patients in the preoperative period.[29,30] Venography confirmed that deep-vein thrombosis was found in 20% of cancer patients and in 13% of patients with benign disorders before surgery.

A subpopulation of cancer patients with higher risk of postoperative deep-vein thrombosis can be identified by their elevated preoperative plasma levels of thrombin–anti-thrombin (TAT) complex and prothrombin fragment 1 + 2 (F1 + 2).[31]

Regardless of the importance of each risk factor, the presence of cancer as the reason for major surgery indicates a high risk of deep-vein thrombosis and justifies prophylaxis.

Thromboembolism and chemotherapy

An increased risk for venous thromboembolism has been observed with cytotoxic and hormonal therapies in cancer patients. The thrombogenic effect of anticancer therapy has been elegantly proven by Levine et al.[32] In a randomized trial comparing a 12-week to a 36-week course of chemohormonal therapy in 205 women with stage II breast cancer, thrombosis occurred more often among patients treated for 36 weeks. The addition of tamoxifen to chemotherapy increases the thrombotic risk over chemotherapy alone.[33] Cytoxic therapy with L asparaginase, mitomycin and cisplatinum has been associated with a high incidence of thromboembolism, as well as the intensive chemotherapy regimen used before bone marrow transplantation.[34] Several mechanisms have been advanced to explain the thrombotic effect of chemotherapy:[35–37]

- Release of procoagulants and cytokines from tumor cells
- Reduced fibrinolytic activity
- Reduced levels of antithrombin (estrogenic effects of tamoxifen)
- Fall of protein C, protein S and antithrombin levels due to hepatotoxicity
- Direct damage to vascular endothelium
- Interaction between the cytotoxic drugs and increased number of large multimers of von Willebrand factor

Thrombosis and venous access devices

Thrombosis of central venous access devices has been described in up to 40% of patients and may be as frequent as infectious complications among cancer patients.[38] Conlan et al have reported a 41% rate of central venous catheter thrombosis in patients with relapsed lymphoma undergoing autologous stem cell transplantation.[39]

The true incidence of thrombosis due to the catheter alone is difficult to estimate in a population of patients with other risk factors for thrombosis such as the cancer itself, and cytotoxic therapy. Since central catheters are located deep in the mediastinum, thrombosis may be clinically occult for a long period. It has been advanced that patients with elevated platelet counts may be at a higher risk of developing subclavian deep-vein thrombosis.

Prevention and treatment of cancer-associated thrombosis

Primary prevention

Thrombosis prevention in cancer surgery

For cancer patients, who are at a high risk for perioperative thromboembolic complications, effective prophylactic anticoagulation is indicated.

Available modalities include unfractionated heparin, low molecular weight heparin and physical methods. Early randomized clinical trials[40] have shown the effectiveness of prophylactic low-dose unfractionated heparin (5000 units, twice daily) in general surgery. The benefit of unfractionated heparin was greater in benign than in malignant disease: thromboembolic risk was reduced from 53 to 30% in the malignant population, and from 28 to 7% in the nonmalignant population. These results indicate that cancer patients may need a stronger anticoagulation agent in order to achieve maximum benefit. Increasing the 12-hourly unfractionated heparin dose from 5000 to 7000 units had no detectable impact.

Low molecular weight heparins are effective and safe for thromboprophylaxis after major general and orthopedic surgeries.[41] They have been compared with unfractionated heparin in cancer patients undergoing major abdominal surgery. In a double-blind randomized multicenter study,[42] danaparoid (Orgaran, The Netherlands) reduced the frequency of deep-vein thrombosis after cancer surgery to 10.4% (25 out of 241 patients) compared to 14.9% (37 out of 249 patients) with unfractionated heparin, a statistically insignificant advantage for danaparoid. In another large clinical study, 1115 patients undergoing elective curative abdominal or pelvic surgery for cancer were randomized to receive prophylactic enoxaparin (40 mg subcutaneously once daily) or unfractionated heparin (5000 units subcutaneously three times daily).[43] The primary endpoint was the frequency of deep-vein thrombosis (per phlebography) after 10 days of therapy. The frequency of thromboembolic complications was similar in both groups: 18.2% for the unfractionated heparin group and 14.7% for enoxaparin. There were no differences in bleeding events or in mortality at 30 days and 3 months between the two populations of patients.

Prophylactic low molecular weight heparins in cancer surgery — which dose?

Bergqvist et al[44] confirmed the hypothesis that a higher dose of low molecular weight heparins may be more effective in reducing thrombosis in the perioperative period in cancer patients. The authors compared two doses of dalteparin, 2500 and 5000 units once daily, in 2070 patients undergoing major abdominal surgery, 63% of whom had cancer. The higher dose of low molecular weight heparins reduced the incidence of perioperative thrombosis from 12.6 to 6.7%.

Prophylactic low molecular weight heparins in cancer surgery — how long?

Deep-vein thrombosis may occur late in the postoperative course in high-risk patients. Isotopically detectable deep-vein thrombosis develops in some 25% of patients during the first month after discharge from hospital. The persistent occurrence of venous thromboembolism observed after 7–10 days of anticoagulant prophylaxis with unfractionated heparin or low molecular weight heparins supports the need for continuation of preventive therapy in the high-risk population, long after hospital discharge.

Thrombosis prevention during chemotherapy

Long-term prophylactic anticoagulation may be justified in metastatic cancer patients treated with chemotherapy, balancing the bleeding risk against a possible benefit of thrombosis prevention.

There is only one trial that tested prophylactic anticoagulation in ambulatory cancer patients treated with chemotherapy. Levine et al[45] randomized 311 metastatic

breast cancer patients undergoing chemotherapy, to receive either minidose warfarin or placebo. The warfarin dose was 1 mg daily for 6 weeks and then adjusted to obtain an international normalized ratio (INR) between 1.3 and 1.9. Prophylaxis was continued until 1 week after the end of chemotherapy. An 85% risk reduction in thrombotic events (deep-vein thrombosis, pulmonary embolism) was observed in the warfarin group compared to the placebo group. Major bleeding was rare and similar in both groups. A cost effectiveness analysis on the results showed that very low-dose warfarin can be given to patients receiving chemotherapy for metastatic breast carcinoma without an increase in healthcare costs. It is still not known whether this strategy can be safely and effectively applied to other forms of cancer.

A logical approach could be to reserve warfarin prophylaxis for high-risk situations such as large abdominal or pelvic mass, previous thromboses, etc. in patients receiving chemotherapy.

Thrombosis prevention in cancer patients with central venous access devices

Several randomized controlled studies have documented the efficiency of warfarin, 1 mg daily, in prophylaxis of thrombosis related to an indwelling central venous catheter.

Bern et al[46] found that patients receiving low-dose warfarin had a 9.5% risk of upper extremity deep-vein thrombosis compared to 37.5% in the placebo group. Monreal et al[47] conducted an open prospective study to determine the efficacy and safety of long-term administration of a low molecular weight heparin (Fragmin) to reduce the incidence of deep-vein thrombosis in cancer patients with a subclavian venous catheter. Patients received either 2500 units Fragmin subcutaneously, once daily, for 90 days, or placebo. Patients underwent upper extremity venography at 90 days or earlier, if deep-vein thrombosis symptoms had appeared. Patient recruitment was terminated early after eight of 13 control patients developed deep-vein thrombosis compared to one patient receiving low molecular weight heparins. No bleeding complications were reported in the low molecular weight heparins group.

Treatment and secondary prevention of deep-vein thrombosis in the cancer population

An effective and safe policy for the therapy of acute deep-vein thrombosis in cancer patients is yet to be determined. It should consider the fact that the presence of active cancer is a risk factor for recurrence of venous thrombosis, even under warfarin therapy. Cancer patients who develop acute venous thrombosis should receive heparin (unfractionated heparin or low molecular weight heparins) for 5–7 days, overlapped and followed by warfarin. Oral anticoagulation medication (target INR: 2.0–3.0) should be prescribed as long as the cancer is active, or at least during the period of chemotherapy. Persistent or recurrent thrombosis while on anticoagulation is a difficult challenge. Full-dose unfractionated heparin or low molecular weight heparins, followed by warfarin, with a target INR of 3.0–4.5 is an option. Vena caval filters as a prevention of pulmonary embolism in high risk patients, given together with unfractionated heparin or low molecular weight heparins, is effective in the short term, with no difference in mortality and at a higher price of late deep-vein thrombosis.[48]

Is the hemorrhagic risk increased in cancer patients receiving anticoagulant therapy?

Classic risk factors for excessive bleeding during oral anticoagulation once included cancer, together with age, previous gastrointestinal tract bleeding and previous stroke. A study from the Mayo Clinic[49] apparently confirmed that cancer patients are at an increased risk of hemorrhage while on warfarin. In this population-based study, major hemorrhages occurred mainly when the INR was greater than 4.0. Two other prospective studies[50,51] did not confirm the extra hemorrhagic risk of cancer patients during anticoagulation. In a cohort study of 355 patients (58 cancer and 297 noncancer patients), treated with heparin followed by 3 months of warfarin, the risk of bleeding was not different in patients with or without cancer: 8.6 versus 9.8% respectively, including for major bleeding: 3.4 versus 3.0%, respectively.[50]

Bona et al[51] also concluded that major hemorrhagic risk in cancer patients is similar to those without cancer. It seems that as long as the INR is kept between 2.0 and 4.0, major hemorrhagic risk is not excessive in cancer patients receiving long-term oral anticoagulation.

Antimalignant properties of antithrombotic agents

Intravascular coagulation activation and tumor fibrin deposition play an important part in oncogenesis and in metastatic spread.[3] It can therefore be expected that anticoagulant therapy may have antimalignant properties. Indeed, the antitumor effect of antithrombotic agents has been proven in experimental animals and has led to clinical trials in human cancer.

Antiplatelet agents, such as aspirin, dipyridamole and ticlopidine, have proven to be effective in preventing metastasis in experimental systems.

In several clinical trials of human cancers, warfarin lowered the recurrence rate of malignant melanoma after surgical resection and prolonged survival in recurrent colon cancer and small cell lung cancer.[52,53] A study by Carpi et al[54] suggested that oral anticoagulants may reduce both cancer incidence and mortality.

As early as 1930, Goerner demonstrated that heparin inhibits tumor growth in animals. The anticancer effect of heparin is multifactorial. Heparin affects cells directly via interaction with growth factors, enzymes and structural proteins within the extracellular matrix. Heparin can also influence tumor cells by modulating cellular immunity and angiogenesis.[55]

In two recent studies that compared the effectiveness of unfractionated heparin with that of low molecular weight heparins in the treatment of deep-vein thrombosis, mortality was lower in patients randomized to low molecular weight heparins. The advantage of low molecular weight heparins over unfractionated heparin was not attributed to thrombotic or bleeding events.[56–58] These results suggest that low molecular weight heparin exerts an inhibitory effect on tumor growth that is not obtained with unfractionated heparin.

References

1. Trousseau A. *Phlegamasia alba dolens. Lectures on clinical medicine, delivered at the Hôtel Dieu Paris.* London: New Sydenham Society 1872; 281–295.

2. Donati MB. Cancer and thrombosis: from phlegmasia alba dolens to transgenic mice. *Thromb Haemost* 1995; **74**: 278–281.

3. Francis JL, Biggerstaff J, Amirkhosravi A. Hemostasis and malignancy. *Semin Thromb Haemost* 1998; **24**: 93–109.

4. Nand S, Messmore H. Hemostasis in malignancy. *Am J Hematol* 1990; **35**: 45–55.

5. Senger DR, Galli SJ, Dvorak AM et al. Tumor cells secrete a vascular permeability factor that promotes accumulation of ascitic fluid. *Science* 1983; **21**: 983–985.

6. Nierodzik ML, Klepfish A, Karpatkin S. Role of platelets, thrombin, integrin IIb–IIIa, fibronectin and von Willebrand factor on tumor adhesion in vitro and metastasis in vivo. *Thromb Haemost* 1995; **74**: 282–290.

7. Sun NC, McAfee Wm, Hum GJ et al. Hemostatic abnormality in malignancy. A prospective study of 108 patients. *Am J Clin Pathol* 1979; **71**: 10–16.

8. Lugassy G. Essential thrombocythemia — update on pathogenesis and therapy. *Cancer J* 1998; **11**: 57–59.

9. Gasic GJ, Gasic TB, Galanti N et al. Platelet–tumor cell interactions in mice. The role of platelets in the spread of malignant disease. *Int J Cancer* 1973; **11**: 704–718.

10. Grignani G, Pacchiarini I, Ricetti MM et al. Mechanisms of platelet activation by cultured human cancer cells and cells freshly isolated from tumor tissues. *Invasion Metastasis* 1989; **9**: 298–309.

11. Dvorak HF, Van De Water L, Blither LAM et al. Procoagulant activity associated with plasma membrane vesicles shed by cultured tumor cells. *Cancer Res* 1983; **43**: 4434–4442.

12. Edwards RL, Rickles FR, Cronlund M. Abnormalities of blood coagulation in patients with cancer. Mononuclear cell tissue factor generation. *J Lab Clin Invest* 1981; **98**: 917–928.

13. Kakkar AK, DeRuvo N, Chinswangwatanakul V et al. Extrinsic-pathway activation in cancer with high factor VIIa and tissue factor. *Lancet* 1995; **346**: 1004–1005.

14. Falanga A, Bolognese D'Alessandro AP et al. Several murine metastasizing tumors possess a cysteine proteinase with cancer procoagulant characteristics. *Int J Cancer* 1987; **39**: 774–777.

15. Falanga A, Alessio MG, Donati MB, Barbui T. A new procoagulant in acute leukemia. *Blood* 1988; **71**: 870–875.

16. Donati MB, Falanga A, Consonni R et al. Cancer procoagulant in acute non lymphoid leukemia: relationship of enzyme detection to disease activity. *Thromb Haemost* 1990; **64**: 11–16.

17. Gordon SG, Hashiba V, Poole MA et al. A cysteine proteinase procoagulant for amniochorion. *Blood* 1985; **66**: 1261–1266.

18. Nand S, Fisher SG, Salgia R, Fisher RI. Hemostatic abnormalities in untreated cancer. Incidence and correlation with thrombotic and hemorrhagic complications. *J Clin Oncol* 1987; **5**: 1998–2003.

19. Rubin RN, Kies MS, Posch JJ. Measurement of antithrombin III in solid tumor patients with and without hepatic metastases. *Thromb Res* 1980; **18**: 353–360.

20. Cornuz J, Pearson SD, Creager M et al. Importance of findings on the initial evaluation for cancer in patients with symptomatic idiopathic deep venous thrombosis. *Ann Intern Med* 1996; **125**: 785–793.

21. Prandoni P, Lensing AWA, Bollen HR et al.

Deep vein thrombosis and the incidence of subsequent symptomatic cancer. *N Engl J Med* 1992; **327**: 1128–1133.

22. Sorensen HT, Mellemkjaer L, Steffensen FH et al. The risk of a diagnosis of cancer after primary deep venous thrombosis or pulmonary embolism. *N Engl J Med* 1998; **338**: 1169–1173.

23. Prins H, Hettiarachchi JK, Lensing WA, Hirsh J. Newly diagnosed malignancy in patients with venous thromboembolism. Search or wait and see? *Thromb Haemost* 1997; **78**: 121–125.

24. Monreal M, Lafoz E, Casals A et al. Occult cancer in patients with deep venous thrombosis: a systematic approach. *Cancer* 1991; **67**: 541–545.

25. Agnelli G. Venous thromboembolism and cancer: a two-way clinical association. *Thromb Haemost* 1997; **78**: 117–120.

26. Bona RD, Dhami MS. Thrombosis in patients with cancer. *Postgrad Med* 1993; **93**: 131–140.

27. Naschitz JE, Yeshurun D, Eldar S, Lev L. Diagnosis of cancer-associated vascular disorders. *Cancer* 1996; 77: 1759–1767.

28. Gallus AS. Prevention of post-operative deep leg vein thrombosis in patients with cancer. *Thromb Haemost* 1997; **78**: 126–132.

29. Heatley RV, Hughes LE, Morgan A, Okwonga W. Preoperative or postoperative deep-vein thrombosis? *Lancet* 1976; **i**: 437–439.

30. Rodzynek JJ, Damien J, Huberty M et al. Incidence of pre-operative deep venous thrombosis in abdominal surgery. *Br J Surg* 1984; **71**: 731–732.

31. Falanga A, Ofosu PA, Cortelazzo S et al. Preliminary study to identify cancer patients

at high risk of venous thrombosis following major surgery. *Br J Haematol* 1993; **85**: 745–750.

32. Levine MN, Gent M, Hirsh J et al. The thrombogenic effect of anticancer drug therapy in women with stage II breast cancer. *N Engl J Med* 1988; **318**: 404–407.

33. Pritchard KI, Paterson AHG, Paul NA et al. Increased thromboembolic complications with concurrent tamoxifen and chemotherapy in a randomized trial of adjuvant therapy for women with breast cancer. *J Clin Oncol* 1996; **14**: 2731–2737.

34. Goodnough LT, Saito H, Manni A et al. Increased incidence of thromboembolism in stage IV breast cancer patients treated with a five-drug chemotherapy regimen: a study of 159 patients. *Cancer* 1984; **54**: 1264–1268.

35. Aranda A, Patamo JA, Cuesta B et al. Fibrinolytic activity in malignancy (abstract). *Thromb Haemost* 1987; **58**: 110.

36. Jordan VC, Fritz NF, Tormey DC. Long-term adjuvant therapy with tamoxifen: effects on sex hormone binding globulin and antithrombin III. *Cancer Res* 1987; **47**: 4517–4519.

37. Nicolson GL, Custead SE. Effects of chemotherapeutic drugs on platelet and metastatic tumor cell–endothelial cells interactions as a model for assessing vascular endothelial integrity. *Cancer Res* 1985; **45**: 331–336.

38. Lokich JJ, Becker B. Subclavian vein thrombosis in patients treated with infusion chemotherapy for advanced malignancy. *Cancer* 1983; **52**: 1586–1589.

39. Conlan MG, Haire WD, Liberman RP et al. Catheter-related thrombosis in patients with refractory lymphoma undergoing autologous

stem cell transplantation. *Bone Marrow Transplant* 1991; **7**: 235–240.

40. Gallus A, Hirsh J, O'Brien SE et al. Prevention of venous thrombosis with small subcutaneous doses of heparin. *JAMA* 1976; **235**: 1980–1982.

41. Samama M, Bernard P, Bonnardot JP et al. Low molecular weight heparin compared with unfractionated heparin in prevention of postoperative thrombosis. *Br J Surg* 1988; **75**: 128–131.

42. Gallus A, Cade J, Ockelford et al. Orgaran (Org 10172) or heparin for preventing venous thrombosis after elective surgery for malignant disease? A double-blind randomised multicentre comparison. *Thromb Haemost* 1993; **70**: 562–567.

43. ENOXACAN Study Group. Efficacy and safety of enoxaparin versus unfractionated heparin for prevention of deep vein thrombosis in elective cancer surgery: a double-blind randomized multicentre trial with venographic assessment. *Br J Surg* 1997; **84**: 1099–1103.

44. Bergqvist D, Burmark US, Flordal PA et al. Low molecular weight heparin started before surgery as prophylaxis against deep vein thrombosis: 2500 versus 5000 Xal units in 2070 patients. *Br J Surg* 1995; **82**: 496–501.

45. Levine M, Hirsh J, Gent M et al. Double-blind randomised trial of very-low-dose warfarin for prevention of thromboembolism in stage IV breast cancer. *Lancet* 1994; **343**: 886–889.

46. Bern MM, Lokich JJ, Wallach SR et al. Very low doses of warfarin can prevent thrombosis in central venous catheters: a randomized prospective trial. *Ann Intern Med* 1990; **112**: 423–428.

47. Monreal M, Alastrue A, Rull M et al. Upper extremity deep venous thrombosis in cancer patients with venous access devices. Prophylaxis with a low molecular weight heparin (Fragmin). *Thromb Haemost* 1996; **75**: 251–253.

48. Decousus H, Leizorovicz A, Parent F et al. A clinical trial of vena caval filters in the prevention of pulmonary embolism in patients with proximal deep vein thrombosis. *New Engl J Med* 1998; **338**: 409–415.

49. Gitter MJ, Jaeger TM, Petterson TM et al. Bleeding and thromboembolism during anticoagulant therapy: a population-based study in Rochester, Minnesota. *Mayo Clin Proc* 1995; **70**: 725–733.

50. Prandoni P, Lensing AWA, Cogo A et al. The long term clinical course of acute deep venous thrombosis. *Ann Intern Med* 1996; **125**: 1–70.

51. Bona RD, Sivjec KY, Hickey AD et al. The efficacy and safety of oral anticoagulation in patients with cancer. *Thromb Haemost* 1995; **74**: 1055–1058.

52. Zacharski LR, Henderson WG, Rickles FR et al. Effect of warfarin anticoagulation on survival in carcinoma of the lung, colon head and neck, and prostate. Final report of VA cooperative study 475. *Cancer* 1984; **53**: 2046–2052.

53. Chlebowski RT, Gota CH, Chan KK et al. Clinical and pharmacokinetic effects of combined warfarin and 5-fluorouracil in advanced colon cancer. *Cancer Res* 1982; **42**: 4827–4830.

54. Carpi A, Sagripanti A, Poddigle R et al. Cancer incidence and mortality in patients with heart disease. Effect of oral anticoagulant therapy. *Am J Clin Oncol* 1995; **18**: 15–18.

55. Engelberg H. Actions of heparin that may affect the malignant process. *Cancer* 1999; **85**: 257–272.

56. Prandoni P, Lesing AWA, Buller HR et al. Comparison of subcutaneous low-molecular-weight heparin with intravenous standard heparin in proximal deep-vein thrombosis. *Lancet* 1992; **339**: 441–445.

57. Hull RD, Raskob GL, Pineo GF et al. Subcutaneous low-molecular weight heparin compared with intravenous heparin in the treatment of proximal-vein thrombosis. *New Engl J Med* 1992; **326**: 975–982.

58. Green D, Hull RD, Brant R, Pineo GF. Lower mortality in cancer patients treated with low-molecular weight versus standard heparin. *Lancet* 1992; **339**: 1476.

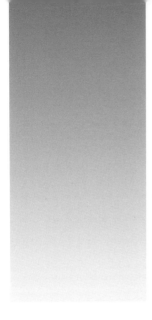

Index